GROWING UP WITH AUTISM

Growing Up with Autism

Working with School-Age Children and Adolescents

Edited by

Robin L. Gabriels
Dina E. Hill

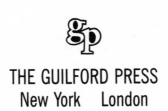

THE GUILFORD PRESS
New York   London

© 2007 The Guilford Press
A Division of Guilford Publications, Inc.
72 Spring Street, New York, NY 10012
www.guilford.com

Printed in the United States of America

This book is printed on acid-free paper.

Last digit is print number: 9   8   7   6   5   4   3   2   1

Library of Congress Cataloging-in-Publication Data

Growing up with autism : working with school-age children and adolescents / edited by
Robin L. Gabriels, Dina E. Hill.
    p. cm.
Includes bibliographical references and index.
ISBN-13: 978-1-59385-459-1 (hardcover : alk. paper)
ISBN-10: 1-59385-459-5 (hardcover : alk. paper)
    1. Autism in children. 2. Autism in adolescence. I. Gabriels, Robin L., 1962– II.
Hill, Dina E., 1965–
    RJ506.A9G76 2007
    618.92'85882—dc22
                                                                            2007008807

*To the memory of Shirley Riley, MFCC, ATR,
one of my very best teachers and mentors, whose
amazingly creative talents with family systems therapy
continue to guide my work with many systems*

*And to my nearest and dearest—Mark Gabriels—
spouse extraordinaire*

—R. L. G.

*To my mentors, Richard Campbell and Ronald Yeo,
for their ongoing encouragement and support*

*And to my husband, Robert Thoma, and daughter,
Elizabeth, with much love and gratitude*

—D. E. H.

About the Editors

Robin L. Gabriels, PsyD, is a licensed clinical psychologist and on the faculty in the Departments of Psychiatry and Pediatrics, University of Colorado at Denver and Health Sciences Center. She is also the Clinical Director and founder of the Neuropsychiatric Special Care Program at The Children's Hospital, Denver, Colorado, an intensive day treatment and inpatient program for children and adolescents with comorbid developmental, psychiatric, and/or medical diagnoses. Dr. Gabriels is the coeditor (with Dina E. Hill) of *Autism: From Research to Individualized Practice* and has published in the fields of art therapy, asthma, and autism. She has lectured nationally and internationally and conducts research related to improving autism interventions.

Dina E. Hill, PhD, is a licensed clinical psychologist and Assistant Professor in the Department of Psychiatry, University of New Mexico (UNM) School of Medicine. She works as a pediatric neuropsychologist at the UNM Center for Neuropsychological Services. Dr. Hill is the coeditor of *Autism: From Research to Individualized Practice* and has published in the fields of ADHD, autism, and neuroimaging.

Contributors

Ruth K. Abramson, PhD, Department of Neuropsychiatry, University of South Carolina School of Medicine, Columbia, South Carolina

Simon Baron-Cohen, PhD, Autism Research Centre, University of Cambridge, Cambridge, United Kingdom

Margaret Bauman, MD, LADDERS Program in Wellesley, Massachusetts General Hospital, Boston, Massachusetts

Ayelet Ben-Sasson, ScD, OTR, Department of Psychology, University of Massachusetts, Boston, Massachusetts

April W. Block, PhD, Assessment Choices Team, Department of Psychiatry and Behavioral Sciences, The Children's Hospital, Denver, Colorado

Stephen R. Block, PhD, Denver Options, Inc., and Nonprofit Management Program, Graduate School of Public Affairs, University of Colorado at Denver and Health Sciences Center, Denver, Colorado

Nancy Cason, PsyD, private practice, Denver, Colorado

Sharon A. Cermak, EdD, OTR/L, FAOTA, Department of Occupational Therapy and Rehabilitation Counseling, Sargent College of Health and Rehabilitation Sciences, Boston University, Boston, Massachusetts

Robin L. Gabriels, PsyD, Departments of Psychiatry and Pediatrics, University of Colorado at Denver and Health Sciences Center, and Neuropsychiatric Special Care Program, The Children's Hospital, Denver, Colorado

Eynat Gal, PhD, OTR, Department of Occupational Therapy, University of Haifa, Haifa, Israel

Michele Godwin, PhD, DC Department of Mental Health/ St. Elizabeths Hospital, Forensic Inpatient Pre-Trial Branch, Washington, DC

Ofer Golan, PhD, Autism Research Centre, University of Cambridge, Cambridge, United Kingdom

Edward Goldson, MD, Child Development Unit, The Children's Hospital, Denver, Colorado

Alicia V. Hall, PhD, Department of Neuropsychiatry, University of South Carolina School of Medicine, Columbia, South Carolina

Dina E. Hill, PhD, Department of Psychiatry, University of New Mexico School of Medicine, Albuquerque, New Mexico

Paul G. LaCava, MSEd, Department of Special Education, University of Kansas, Lawrence, Kansas

Sharon Lerner-Baron, PhD, private practice, La Jolla, California

Alan Lincoln, PhD, MSCP, Department of Clinical Psychology, Alliant International University, and Center for Autism Research, Evaluation, and Service, Inc., San Diego, California

Brian R. Lopez, PhD, Center for Development and Disabilities, University of New Mexico, Albuquerque, New Mexico

Gary Mesibov, PhD, Division TEACCH, University of North Carolina, Chapel Hill, North Carolina

Ramona Noland, PhD, NCSP, LSSP, Department of Psychology and Philosophy, Sam Houston State University, Huntsville, Texas

Sandy Shaw, PhD, Applied Interventions and Methodologies, Inc., San Diego, California

Laurie Sperry, PhD, Professional Development in Autism Center, University of Colorado at Denver and Health Sciences Center, Denver, Colorado

Wayne Steedman, JD, LCSW, Callegary & Steedman, PA, Baltimore, Maryland

Diane Twachtman-Cullen, PhD, CCC-SLP, ADDCON Center, LLC, Higganum, Connecticut

Jennifer Twachtman-Reilly, MS, CCC-SLP, ADDCON Center, LLC, Higganum, Connecticut

Mary E. Van Bourgondien, PhD, Division TEACCH, University of North Carolina, Chapel Hill, North Carolina

Harry H. Wright, MD, Department of Neuropsychiatry, University of South Carolina School of Medicine, Columbia, South Carolina

Acknowledgments

We owe endless gratitude to children with autism and their families. They teach us to recognize their unique talents and strengths that can affect positive outcomes, no matter how great the burden.

We also wish to express our gratitude to the chapter authors for their commitment to the vision of this project and willingness to share their insights and expertise.

We would like to thank the following people for their support with this book: Sharon Mann, for giving us a parent's perspective to guide the development of the family-focused chapters; Cathy Malchiodi, for helping us give this book wings; Lisa Boyum, for her valuable clinical editorial suggestions and encouragement; John Agnew, for his technical assistance in getting this book in order; and Geoff McKee, for lending his forensic expertise and advice regardless of where in the world he was at the time.

We give special thanks to our family members: Ronald and Barbara Knight, Curtis Knight, Paul Knight, Priscilla Gabriels, Donald Hill, Denise Hartwell, Darcy Hill, Derek Hill, Flora and Robert Thoma, Kathy Brennan, Annette Brooks, and Kamilla Venner, for their never-ending encouragement and support.

Gillberg, C. (1991). Outcome in autism and autistic-like conditions. *Journal of the American Academy of Child and Adolescent Psychiatry, 30*(3), 375–382.

Happe, F., & Frith, U. (1996). The neuropsychology of autism. *Brain, 119*(Pt. 4), 1377–1400.

Hastings, R. P. (2002). Parental stress and behaviour problems in children with developmental disability. *Journal of Intellectual Disability Research, 27,* 149–160.

Howlin, P., Goode, S., Hutton, J., & Rutter, M. (2004). Adult outcome for children with autism. *Journal of Child Psychology and Psychiatry and Allied Disciplines, 45*(2), 212–229.

Lord, C., & Bailey, A. (2002). Autism spectrum disorders. In M. Rutter & E. Taylor (Eds.), *Child and adolescent psychiatry* (4th ed., pp. 865–882). Oxford: Blackwell Scientific.

Murphy, G. H., Beadle-Brown, J., Wing, L., Gould, J., Shah, A., & Holmes, N. (2005). Chronicity of challenging behaviors in people with severe intellectual disabilities and/or autism: A total population sample. *Journal of Autism and Developmental Disorders, 35*(4), 405–418.

Riley, S. (1994). *Integrative approaches to family art therapy.* Chicago: Magnolia Street Publishers.

ing educational transitions, use of school consultants, treatment and intervention development, and forensic issues specific to this population.

In summary, the goal of this book is to provide professionals with an awareness of the issues pertinent to the individual with autism as he or she enters critical periods of development that include physical and sexual maturity. We hope that having such knowledge will allow professionals to make more useful recommendations for individuals with autism and to more effectively support families. Finally, the importance of developing a community network of support for these individuals as they grow older is reflected in the words of the same father whose words introduced this preface.

"In the early years my son's condition was very isolating. Our family hunkered down—exhausted, afraid of scenes, one big exposed nerve. Over time, we have been able to develop a community, a rarity for many in modern America. It is our community of support made up of our family; other families facing the same challenges; committed friends; caregivers; and dedicated professionals. Parents of children with autism need that community of support. We can't do it alone. Now my burdens are lighter, I trust more, things are easier. I realize there is a community that cares deeply about my son and my family. We are on the same team in an imperfect world in which my son has autism."

REFERENCES

Chakrabarti, S., & Fombonne, E. (2005). Pervasive developmental disorders in preschool children: Confirmation of high prevalence. *American Journal of Psychiatry, 162*(6), 1133–1141.

Cunningham, P. B., & Henggeler, S. W. (1999). Engaging multiproblem families in treatment: Lessons learned throughout the development of multisystemic therapy. *Family Process, 38*(3), 265–281.

DeMyer, M. K., & Goldberg, P. (1983). Family needs of the autistic adolescent. In E. Schopler & G. Mesibov (Eds.), *Autism in adolescents and adults.* New York: Plenum Press.

Emerson, E. (2003). Mothers of children and adolescents with intellectual disability: Social and emotional situation, mental health status and the self-assessed social psychological impact of the child's difficulties. *Journal of Intellectual Disability Research, 47,* 385–399.

Gabriels, R. L., Hill, D. E., Pierce, R. A., Rogers, S. J., & Wehner, B. (2001). Predictors of treatment outcome in young children with autism: A retrospective study. *Autism, 5*(4), 407–429.

PART I: THE INDIVIDUAL WITH AUTISM

The challenging behaviors of individuals with intellectual disabilities, including those with autism, can be an important factor in determining the quality of life for the individual and the levels of caregiver stress (e.g., Emerson, 2003; Hastings, 2002). Chapters 1 through 6 focus on the challenges specific to more severely impaired individuals with autism, with an emphasis on illuminating the multiple ways to explain behavior challenges, along with intervention suggestions to address these challenges. The chapters cover behavioral and medical issues common to this particular group, as well as the important topics of sexuality, communication, sensory–motor issues, and social skills.

PART II: FAMILY AND CAREGIVERS OF THE INDIVIDUAL WITH AUTISM

Chapters 7 through 9 shift the focus from children and adolescents with autism to the needs of their families. Results of a pilot survey of problems reported by families of adolescents with autism revealed that the number one problem was not being able to take family vacations. Additional concerns include the unavailability of respite care, financial pressure, parents' emotional and physical health, and relationships among family members (DeMyer & Goldberg, 1983). The chapters in this section provide clinicians with practical advice on how to help families access services, while considering legal and future planning issues, and enjoy positive vacation and leisure experiences.

PART III: COMMUNITY ASPECTS OF INTERVENTION

The expectations of the community for individuals with autism will change as they enter school age and adolescence. There are also changes in schools, teachers, and other therapeutic support networks. It is likely that these changes contribute in some degree to increased problems in adolescence for this population (Gillberg, 1991). Chapters 10 through 13 go beyond the child and his or her immediate family to consider issues that involve the social community. This section provides a review of relevant clinical and theoretical research in the autism field, as well as offering hands-on suggestions and techniques to assist professionals in addressing child and caregiver needs. The chapters cover topics includ-

estimated 70–75% of this population is also diagnosed with mental retardation, with approximately 50% of individuals lacking functional communicative speech (Happe & Frith, 1996). The heterogeneity of impairment in this population likely contributes in large part to the variability documented in treatment outcome research, with some children making great progress and others making little, regardless of the type and intensity of intervention (e.g., Gabriels, Hill, Pierce, Rogers, & Wehner, 2001; Howlin, Goode, Hutton, & Rutter, 2004). However, research indicates that the most significant predictor of later outcome appears to be the level of intellectual functioning in childhood (e.g., Lord & Bailey, 2002).

The goal of this book is to comprehensively address one of the most challenging aspects of the autism population: the needs of school-age children and adolescents with autism as they prepare for adulthood. Since the majority of individuals with autism are severely impaired and may require lifelong supports, the focus of the following chapters is on this population at a time when professionals can assist families to move beyond the stage of early intervention and consider how the fundamental difficulties of the child's autism diagnosis may interfere with such aspects of their lives as integrated classroom settings, pubescence, and preparation for adulthood.

The individual chapters are organized within the perspective of a multisystemic therapy model derived from family systems theory. This model views a circular process of systems change needed to resolve the problems of the individual and considers the interconnections among the individual, family subsystems, and broader systems of community service (Cunningham & Henggeler, 1999). The onset of adolescence and puberty in individuals with autism is a critical period that brings with it changes in the needs of the individual and family. "As the child [with a disability] grows older, the developmental steps of each member of the family are thrown off balance": parents continue to be tied to a child who requires extensive support and supervision (Riley, 1994, p. 142). Other changes that occur during adolescence, affecting both the individual with autism and the family, are the types and amounts of community services available. Professionals and therapeutic services may no longer be as easy to access or may not consist of a coherent network compared with early intervention services. In response to these issues, the chapters in this book are divided into three major sections, based on the interconnected systems (individual, family, and community) with which professionals are faced when working with the population of more severely impaired school-age children and adolescents with autism.

Preface

"Now, 12 years later, following our son's diagnosis of autism and an endless series of early interventions, our son still speaks in two- to three-word sentences. He still obsessively flips sticks and other objects while pacing the room to control what I think must be a storm in his head. He is, however, a lot bigger."
                    –ROBERT WARD, father of an adolescent with autism

These words reflect the reality that, despite early intervention efforts, some children with autism may require lifelong intervention. The behaviors that were once tolerable in a small child with autism can become more socially intrusive and intolerable as the child matures in age and physical size. Of concern is that individuals with autism can often require lifelong intervention (e.g., Howlin, Goode, Hutton, & Rutter, 2004). This appears to be the case particularly for those individuals with significant impairments in areas such as intelligence, expressive language, and social skills (Gillberg, 1991; Murphy et al., 2005). The behavioral, emotional, and dependency issues of this population are likely to become of paramount concern for communities as the increasing numbers of identified children with autism grow up (Chakrabarti & Fombonne, 2005).

    Children with autism differ in the degree of impairment in core diagnostic symptoms (social, communication, and behavioral) and associated symptom impairments (e.g., intellectual and adaptive ability). An

1

Understanding Behavioral and Emotional Issues in Autism

Robin L. Gabriels

This chapter provides an overview of the core diagnostic features of autism along with the cognitive, sensory, medical, and psychiatric issues that can affect the behavioral presentation of school-age children and adolescents with autism. Clinicians working with this population face challenges in assessing behavioral problems (e.g., irritability, tantrums, aggression, and self-injury) and making accurate comorbid diagnoses. Assessing and diagnosing these behaviors can be particularly difficult, given that many of these children lack the cognitive capacity necessary to report internal physical or emotional experiences and have few or no communication skills. Thus, accurate assessment and diagnosis of behavior problems in this less able population of individuals with autism requires an understanding not only of the core deficits of autism, but how other biological or behavioral problems may be affected by or affect these core diagnostic features.

Within the autism field there is a debate as to whether presenting behavior problems are manifestations of the core diagnostic symptoms of autism or represent distinct comorbid psychiatric diagnoses (American Academy of Child and Adolescent Psychiatry, 1999; Tsai, 1996).

3

Despite these debates, accurately assessing the nature of the presenting behaviors and deciding whether these behaviors are best viewed as part of autism or as an indication of comorbid psychiatric diagnoses can lead to better-targeted intervention (Leyfer et al., 2006). This chapter serves as an introduction to the medical, communication, sensory, and social issues that are discussed more extensively in Chapters 2, 3, 4, and 5. This chapter also provides a framework for assessing the presenting behavior problems in this autism population by integrating the understanding of behavioral and biological symptoms.

BEHAVIOR PROBLEMS AND CORE DIAGNOSTIC FEATURES OF AUTISM

When individuals with autism are referred for assessment of behavior problems, clinicians should consider the contributing role of the core diagnostic features of autism in the areas of social relatedness, communication, and restricted, repetitive, stereotyped behaviors and interests (American Psychiatric Association, 1994; World Health Organization, 1994). These core diagnostic features may be the underlying cause of behavior problems as described in the following sections.

Social Relatedness

Deficits in social relatedness include marked impairments in the use of nonverbal communication to regulate social interactions, impaired peer relationships, impaired sharing of interests or achievements, and impaired social/emotional reciprocity (American Psychiatric Association, 1994). Early autism longitudinal studies (through the 1970s) did not directly address the developmental pattern of social behaviors (Lotter, 1974). Later studies reported improved social functioning as children with autism age, in that they tend to be less aloof (Gillberg, 1991). This finding was supported by more recent longitudinal studies indicating fewer social difficulties (e.g., Piven, Harper, Palmer, & Arndt, 1996), as well as parental endorsement of fewer social impairments as the child moved into adolescence (McGovern & Sigman, 2005). Regardless of the improvements in social functioning, it is the case that the majority of individuals continued to meet criteria for the disorder and, therefore, continued to demonstrate marked impairments in social relatedness compared to typical peers.

The social features by which autism is diagnosed also include difficulties appropriately initiating, maintaining, and terminating social interactions; understanding the thoughts and feelings of others; and perceiving the impact of one's behavior on others ("theory of mind") (e.g., American Psychiatric Association, 1994; Baron-Cohen & Belmonte, 2005; Lord & Paul, 1997; Tager-Flusberg, 1992). For example, an adolescent with autism may insist on discussing odd topics unaware that this may be irritating to others. This adolescent may then become highly agitated, even aggressive, when interrupted or ignored by others. Social conversations can be affected by other autism impairments such as "lack of central coherence," which involves difficulties seeing the "big picture" and a tendency to focus on small, fragmented details (Frith, 1989). For instance, the disjointed descriptions of an event by a school-age child with autism can appear to clinicians unfamiliar with the diagnostic impairments of autism as bizarre and possibly a manifestation of psychosis. An additional problem as children with autism become older and larger in size is that their impairments may become more problematic due to the increased social demands and the expectations of daily life (Lainhart, 1999). Behaviors such as talking loudly or making odd statements or noises in public places might be more easily tolerated or even ignored in a young child with autism, but this behavior becomes more socially unacceptable or even threatening when observed in a physically mature adolescent with autism.

Communication

Impaired communication, also a core feature of autism, includes delayed or lack of functional language, impairment in initiating or sustaining conversations, stereotyped or repetitive use of language, and a lack of varied, spontaneous make-believe play (American Psychiatric Association, 1994). The presence of communicative speech by the age of 5 years has been correlated with improved outcomes (Gillberg, 1991). However, longitudinal studies are mixed in findings related to social communication, with some studies reporting reduced communicative impairments (e.g., Piven et al., 1996) and other studies indicating no substantial changes (e.g., McGovern & Sigman, 2005).

An estimated 50% of the autism population does not develop an ability to communicate effectively (Sturmey & Sevin, 1994). Behavior interventionists have asserted that challenging behaviors such as self-injury, aggression, and tantrums reflect underlying communication difficulties, as evidenced by a reduction in these behaviors when the individual with autism is taught functional communication skills (Carr & Durand, 1985; Dunlap, Johnson, & Robbins, 1990; Durand & Merges, 2001; Reeve, 1996). For example, if a nonverbal adolescent with autism becomes frustrated because he wants something and has limited communication strategies (e.g., slapping or grabbing others), his behaviors may be seen as threatening or aggressive. If caregivers are not able to determine the cause or function of these behaviors, they may be unable to consistently remedy the frustrating situation for the adolescent. Given this dilemma, over time this adolescent might escalate his behaviors to the point of inadvertently causing physical harm to others.

Restrictive, Repetitive, and Stereotyped Behaviors and Interests

The final core feature of autism is restrictive, repetitive, and stereotyped behaviors and interests (RBs), and this includes preoccupation with stereotyped/restricted patterns of interest, adherence to nonfunctional routines, stereotyped/repetitive motor mannerisms, and persistent preoccupation with parts of objects (American Psychiatric Association, 1994). Based on studies of young children with developmental disabilities, it is clear that RBs may have a predictable developmental course (Berkson, 2002; Berkson, Tupa, & Sherman, 2001).There is some evidence to suggest that the onset of puberty may be associated with a worsening of RB symptoms, such as insistence on sameness, aggression, and self-injury (Gillberg & Steffenburg, 1987).

RBs encompass a wide range of behavioral phenomena including stereotyped and repetitive body movements and manipulation of object parts; compulsive or ritualized behaviors or routines; insistence on sameness of the environment and of routines; narrow and circumscribed interests; and self-injurious behaviors (Bodfish, Symons, Parker, & Lewis, 2000; Lewis & Bodfish, 1998; Schultz & Berkson, 1995). Stereotyped behaviors (e.g., body rocking, hand flapping, finger flicking, and object movements like spinning and twirling with a lack of obvious purpose or function) occur in up to 50% of children and adults with nonspecific mental retardation (Bodfish et al., 1995; Rojahn, 1986) and up to 100% of children and adults with autism (Bodfish et al., 2000; Campbell et al., 1990). Self-injury, although less prevalent than stereotypy, occurs in up to a third of children and adults with mental retardation or autism (Bartak & Rutter, 1976; Bodfish et al., 1995, 2000). Regardless of the particular RB subtype, what is of paramount concern for professionals to consider when working with caregivers is the potential disruption of daily life activities caused by the presence of RBs in the child with autism, regardless of cognitive ability level (de Bildt, Sytema, Kraijer, Sparrow, & Minderaa, 2005; Dunlap, Dyer, & Koegel, 1983; Howlin, Goode, Hutton, & Rutter, 2004). An increase in inappropriate behaviors has also been observed in young children with autism when their repetitive behaviors or routines with objects are interrupted (Reese,

Richman, Belmont, & Morse, 2005). For example, a nonverbal adolescent may begin to bang her head when a well-meaning caregiver stops the adolescent's favorite video to rewind it for her. Such behaviors can be a significant source of stress for caregivers. In a study by Konstantareas and Homatidis (1989) of children with autism (age range: 28 months to 12 years, 7 months) and their parents, a child's self-abusive behaviors were the best predictors of parental stress. The child's hyperirritability (defined by self-stimulation, continuous vocalization, and pacing) and increasing age were other predictors of stress particular to mothers (Konstantareas & Homatidis, 1989).

BEHAVIOR PROBLEMS
AND COMORBID DISORDERS

Individuals with autism frequently have clinical symptoms outside of the DSM-IV autism diagnostic criteria, such as mental retardation (Lainhart, 2003); unusual sensory response (Baranek, David, Poe, Stone, & Watson, 2006; Dunn, 1999; Greenspan & Wieder, 1997; Hirstein, Iversen, & Ramachandran, 2001); medical issues including sleep abnormalities (Schreck, Mulick, & Smith, 2004) and seizures (Elia, Musumeci, Ferri, & Bergonzi, 1995; Tuchman, Rapin, & Shinnar, 1991b); and a myriad of psychiatric and behavioral symptoms (Bradley, Summers, Wood, & Bryson, 2004; Leyfer et al., 2006; Sverd, 2003). Comorbidity is defined as the presence of one or more conditions that co-occur with the individual's primary condition (Matson & Nebel-Schwalm, 2006). The determination of which condition is primary or secondary varies. For example, the primary condition can be seen as the one that was first diagnosed or the one that is the focus of the majority of treatment efforts due to its pervasive interference with daily life (Matson & Nebel-Schwalm, 2006). Whether a condition is considered primary or secondary has fueled debates with insurance companies over medical versus psychiatric financial coverage of treatment when individuals diagnosed with autism (often covered as a medical condition) begin to exhibit psychiatric symptoms outside the DSM-IV definition of autism (American Psychiatric Association, 1994).

Cognitive Impairments

A large proportion (70–75%) of the autism population also meets the criteria for a DSM-IV diagnosis of mental retardation (American Psychiatric Association, 1994; Happe & Frith, 1996). Intellectual impairments can contribute to individuals' inability to understand expectations, leading them to become frustrated and to engage in temper tantrums or other problematic behaviors. Another complication is that some individuals with autism present with higher-functioning skills in particular cognitive areas, while at the same time they are lower functioning in other skill areas (Lainhart, 1999). When evaluating individuals with autism referred for "psychiatric problems," it may be necessary to assess whether caregiver demands placed on the individual are realistic, based on the individual's intellectual level and profile of cognitive strengths and weaknesses. Such information can help clinicians determine the role of an individual's cognitive impairment in the presenting "psychiatric problems" and focus intervention on defining appropriate cognitive support strategies such as visual supports. (See Chapters 10, 11, and 12 for information about intervention strategies in school settings.)

Unusual Sensory Response

Abnormal sensory response in individuals with autism has been reported in numerous studies (Baranek, Foster, & Berkson, 1997; Gillberg et al., 1990; Ornitz, Guthrie, & Farley, 1977, 1978; Tecchio et al., 2003; Volkmar, Cohen, & Paul, 1986; Wainwright-Sharp & Bryson, 1993). These abnormal responses to sensory input include over- and/or under-responsiveness, as well as seeking additional sensory stimulation, and involve the auditory, visual, vestibular, tactile, and oral sensory domains (Dunn, 1999). Abnormal sensory responsiveness has been observed to co-occur with RBs in individuals with developmental disabilities and those with autism (e.g., Baranek et al., 1997; Colman, Frankel, Ritvo, & Freeman, 1976; Gal, Dyck, & Passmore, 2002; Grandin, 1992; Willemsen-Swinkels, Buitelaar, Dekker, & van Engeland, 1998). For example, more rigid stereotyped behaviors such as insistence on sameness and repetitive verbalizations were related to tactile defensiveness (i.e., overresponsiveness to tactile stimulation that is not noxious to most people) (Baranek et al., 1997). An increase or decrease in RBs in response to certain sensory environments has been observed. For example, fluorescent lighting conditions have resulted in the display of significantly more RBs in children with autism compared with an incandescent lighting condition (Colman et al., 1976). Specific types of sensory environments (neutral, aversive, and attractive) were related to stereotyped movement behaviors in four children diagnosed with autism and mental retardation (IQ scores < 50) (Gal et al., 2002). The "attractive," or preferred, sensory stimulus condition was consistently related to a reduction in stereotyped movement behaviors, while the child's "aversive" sensory stimulus condition was consistently related to an increase in stereotyped movement behaviors (Gal et al., 2002). In addition to considering the possible impact of the child's sensory environment on the expression of behavior problems, it is also important to assess whether the child has adequate vision and hearing, as this can also influence the child's behavioral response (Baranek, Parham, & Bodfish, 2005).

Medical Problems

There are a myriad of medical problems that may underlie the presentation of behavior problems. This topic is more extensively discussed in Chapter 2; however, a brief discussion of sleep, seizure disorders, and experience of pain in relationship to behavior problems is presented here.

A study comparing children with autism to nonautistic children with mental retardation or other learning disabilities indicates that although children with autism appear to sleep as much as the other groups, their caregivers report significant differences in the *quality* of sleep. This includes behaviors that tended to waken parents in the night (e.g., screaming and sleepwalking), higher frequencies of breathing cessation, and teeth grinding (Schreck & Mulick, 2000). Additionally, there is an indication that the sleep problems exhibited by children with autism may exacerbate autism symptoms (e.g., stereotypic behavior and communication problems) observed during daytime activities (Schreck et al., 2004).

An estimated 30–45% of individuals with autism are also diagnosed with seizures. Seizures in this population usually present prior to age 5 or begin around puberty (Poustka, 1998; Volkmar & Nelson, 1990). A seizure disorder should be considered if individuals exhibit deterioration of functioning from baseline levels of behavior or if they begin to experience psychotic symptoms such as hallucinations (Gillberg, 1991; Tuchman, Rapin, & Shinnar, 1991a; Tuchman et al., 1991b). Individuals with autism who are at higher risk for developing seizures include those who have more severe cognitive, motor, and language impairments, are female, or have a family history of seizures (Elia et al., 1995; Tuchman et al., 1991b). There is evidence to suggest that hyperactivity, aggression, property destruction, self-injury, and insistence on sameness become worse upon entering puberty in the subset of children diagnosed with a combination of autism, seizure disorders, and moderate to severe mental retardation (Gillberg & Steffenburg, 1987).

Finally, the experience of pain in the autism population is rarely discussed in the literature, even though this issue can be of paramount concern for clinicians when attempting to evaluate whether a child with autism, particularly one who has limited communication skills, is experiencing pain. Research in this area has focused on the hypothesis of reduced pain sensitivity in children with autism, specifically examining the opioid system (Gillberg, 1995). In addition, studies of parents' views of pain perception in their children with cognitive impairments indicate that they tend to consider their children as being less sensitive to and reactive to pain than nonimpaired children (Fanurik, Koh, Schmitz, Harrison, & Conrad, 1999). However, a study by Nader and colleagues (2004) of the response to venepuncture procedures found that children with autism did exhibit similar levels of pain sensitivity and even higher levels of behavioral distress compared to typically developing, chronologically aged matched peers, even though parents tended to perceive their children with autism as underresponsive to pain (Nader, Oberlander, Chambers, & Craig, 2004). Additional research is needed in this area to better understand ways to accurately assess the experience of pain in children with autism, particularly in less verbal children.

Psychiatric Symptoms

Currently, the incidence rates of psychiatric comorbidity in individuals with autism are unknown due to a lack of epidemiological studies (Lainhart, 1999; Sverd, 2003; Sverd, Dubey, Schweitzer, & Ninan, 2003). However, compared with nonautistic individuals with mental retardation, individuals with autism appear to have higher rates of psychiatric and behavioral disorders, such as mood, anxiety, and psychotic disorders (Bradley et al., 2004; Dekker & Koot, 2003; Evans, Canavera, Kleinpeter, Maccubbin, & Taga, 2005; Sverd, 2003). There is consistent evidence to suggest an increased rate of depression in individuals diagnosed with an autism spectrum disorder (Abramson et al., 1992; Chung, Luk, & Lee, 1990; Ghaziuddin & Greden, 1998; Leyfer et al., 2006; Tantam, 1991). Reported rates of bipolar disorder in the autism population have been less consistent (Ghaziuddin & Greden, 1998; Leyfer et al., 2006; Wozniak et al., 1997) The limited studies of fears and phobias in the autism population consistently report that children with autism tend to have a distinctly different profile of fears or phobias (e.g., loud noises) compared to typically developing children and children with Down syndrome (Evans et al., 2005; Leyfer et al., 2006; Matson & Love, 1990). Coexisting symptoms of anxiety, obsessive–compulsive, and attention deficit disorders have been reported in the autism population; however, controversy exists as to whether these symptoms indicate psychiatric diagnoses separate and distinct from the features of autistic disorder (Ando & Yoshimura, 1979; Ghaziuddin, Alessi, & Greden, 1995; Ghaziuddin & Greden, 1998; Leyfer et al., 2006; Muris, Steerneman, Merckelbach, Holdrinet, & Meesters, 1998; Rumsey, Rapoport, & Sceery, 1985; Wozniak et al., 1997). Available studies suggest that the incidence of psychotic symptoms or disorders in the autism population is similar to that in the general population (Lainhart, 1999).

The following sections review the literature regarding a variety of psychiatric symptoms that have been observed in the autism population. Of note, some psychiatric conditions (e.g., depression) may be more distinguishable from the core features of autism than other conditions (e.g., attention deficit disorder or obsessive–compulsive disorder). This particular issue makes it challenging for clinicians to determine appropriate intervention directions (e.g., use of psychotropic medications, behavioral therapy, or both).

Mood Disorders

Mood disorders found in children with autism include both depressive and bipolar disorders, and the severity of symptoms can range from mood irritability to psychosis (American Psychiatric Association, 1994). Depressive symptoms have been associated with a change in or exacerbation of the features "typical" of the diagnosis of autism, including an increase in irritability, noncompliance, aggression (Kim, Szatmari, Bryson, Streiner, & Wilson, 2000), social withdrawal or catatonia (Wing & Shah, 2000), obsessive–compulsive behaviors, sleep disturbance, or appetite problems (Ghaziuddin, Ghaziuddin, & Greden, 2002). In addition to these changes, signs of depression in more cognitively impaired and language-impaired individuals with autism can also include a regression in daily living skills (Ghaziuddin et al., 2002). Consideration of these indicators is important when evaluating for the possibility of a mood disorder in individuals with autism, as this population tends to display a lack of emotional expression that can be misinterpreted as the flattening of affect often associated with depression (Capps, Kasari, Yirmiya, & Sigman, 1993).

Risks for a comorbid diagnosis of depression or other mood disorders have been reported in the autism population and include genetic, environmental, and gender factors, additional medical conditions, and other types of psychiatric disorders (Ghaziuddin et al., 2002). As seen in the general population, a genetic risk factor for depression in the autism population includes a family history of depression, particularly major depression (Ghaziuddin & Greden, 1998). Having first-degree relatives with early-onset and recurrent symptoms of major depression appears to increase the risk of comorbid depressive symptoms in children with autism (Bolton, Pickles, Murphy, & Rutter, 1998; Piven et al., 1991).

Environmental factors or negative life events, such as bereavement or family discord, have been associated with the presence of depressive symptoms in the general child and adult population (Kendler, Karkowski, & Prescott, 1999). There is limited information about the relationship between negative life events and the presence of depressive symptoms in the autism population, or consideration of how the level of individuals' mental retardation affects their response to negative life events. One study of children with autism and depression revealed that, compared to children with autism and no depressive symptoms, the children with both conditions experienced significantly more negative life events in the 12 months prior to the onset of depression (Ghaziuddin et al., 1995). In this study, depressive symptoms were defined as any change in specific behaviors including increased crying spells, social withdrawal, irritability, sleep or appetite disturbance, and verbalizations of sadness. Additionally, subjects with autism and depression reported having an excess of negative life events (e.g., changes in living situations or educational placements, family illness, or the death of a family member) (Ghaziuddin et al., 1995).

In the general population, females are more likely to suffer from symptoms of depression with changes in androgen and estrogen levels suggested as a contributing factor (Angold, Costello, Erkanli, & Worthman, 1999). It is unknown whether the same is true in the autism population, given the lack of similar systematic investigations, though a review of published studies of depression and autism revealed a high proportion of females (Lainhart & Folstein, 1994). There are a few case reports of the co-occurrence of menstrual-related mood disorders and severe behavior problems (Douglas & Martin, 2004; Skinner, Ng, McDonald, & Walters, 2005). For example, Skinner and colleagues (2005) discussed a case study of an 18-year-old woman with autism and mild to moderate mental retardation whose menstruation triggered an increase in severe depressive symptoms, including sadness, expressed desires to die, distress evidenced by obsessive–compulsive behaviors related to menstrual hygiene, episodes of agitation, aggressive outbursts, head banging, and self-mutilation, along with damaging family property and possessions.

Medical conditions such as seizure disorders are associated with depression in the general population (Hermann, Seidenberg, & Bell, 2000). The relationship between seizures and symptoms of depression in the autism population is unknown. However, it may be important for clinicians to be mindful of the possibility of comorbid depressive symptoms in individuals with autism, given the high prevalence of seizures in this population (Happe & Frith, 1996; Volkmar & Nelson, 1990). In addition to medical conditions, other psychiatric conditions, such as anxiety disorders, have also been observed to co-occur with mood disorders both in the general population and in the autism population (Ghaziuddin et al., 2002).

Anxiety Disorders

As previously mentioned, several studies investigating types of fears and phobias in children with autism suggest that children with autism may have different types of fears than children without autism (Evans et al., 2005; Leyfer et al., 2006; Matson & Love, 1990). For example, Evans and colleagues (2005) compared a group of 23 children with autism to 43 children with Down syndrome and 37 typically developing, age-matched children. In this study, children with autism had significantly more situational phobias (e.g., being in a theater, busy mall, small room, elevator, or subway) and medical fears (e.g., shots, having blood drawn, or teeth cleaned) than children in the two control groups, and had significantly fewer fears of harm (e.g., death or injury of parent, injury to self, or fear of guns) (Evans et al., 2005). In a study by Leyfer et al. (2006), examining rates of comorbid psychiatric disorders in 109 children with autism (ages 5 to 17), the diagnosis of a specific phobia was the most common (44% of the sample) and 10% of this subgroup had a phobia of loud noises. This study also found low rates of other anxiety disorders (i.e., separation anxiety disorders and social phobias) in the autism sample (Leyfer et al., 2006).

Varied rates (1.5% to 81%) of obsessive–compulsive disorder have been reported in the autism population (Charlop-Christy & Haymes, 1996; Le Couteur et al., 1989; Ghaziuddin, Tsai, & Ghaziuddin, 1992; Leyfer et al., 2006; Muris et al., 1998; Rumsey et al., 1985). This inconsistency is likely due to the variety of measures and criteria employed (Leyfer et al., 2006). Another confounding issue is that many features of autism (e.g., restricted interests, insistence on sameness, or engaging in rituals and routines) overlap with the diagnostic criteria for obsessive–compulsive disorder (American Psychiatric Association, 1994). However, there is some evidence to suggest that, compared to nondisabled individuals, adults with autism exhibit less complex or organized obsessive and compulsive thoughts and behaviors (McDougle et al., 1995).

Attention-Deficit/Hyperactivity Disorder

The findings from several studies suggest that attention-deficit/hyperactivity disorder (ADHD) symptoms in children with autism are observed with rates varying from 29% to 73%, regardless of intelligence level (Ghaziuddin & Greden, 1998; Leyfer et al., 2006; Wozniak et al., 1997). In a study by Leyfer and colleagues (2006), 55% of the children with autism displayed significantly impairing symptoms of ADHD; 31% of this group met DSM-IV criteria for ADHD, with 65% of this subgroup meeting criteria for the inattentive subtype (Leyfer et al., 2006). There is a unique pattern of attention commonly observed in the autism population that involves an ability to focus intensely on things of particular interest to the individual, but an inability to attend to things that are not of interest (Dawson & Levy, 1989).

Psychotic Disorders

Limited research indicates that, unlike previously thought, autism is a clinically distinct disorder from schizophrenia or childhood psychosis, particularly regarding symptoms of language (e.g., poverty of speech), social skills, and ability to adapt to change (Dykens, Volkmar, & Glick, 1991; Matese, Matson, & Sevin, 1994; Rumsey, Andreasen, & Rapoport, 1986). Individuals with autism can develop symptoms of psychosis or schizophrenia (McEachin, Smith, & Lovaas, 1993; Petty, Ornitz, Michelman, & Zimmerman, 1984). A review of available studies reported an average co-occurrence rate of 1.08% for individuals with autism. Although it is a likely underestimate given issues of sample bias, this rate does indicate that the risk of schizophrenia in individuals with autism is not obviously higher than what is expected in the general population (Lainhart, 1999). As previously mentioned, the core features of autism can be confused with some of the negative symptoms of schizophrenia, such as flat or restricted range of emotional expression (Lainhart, 1999), particularly if such symptoms are viewed out of context from other diagnostic features of autism.

Other Diagnoses

There is limited information about the co-occurrence of oppositional defiant disorder (ODD) and autism, and a recent study suggests that this is relatively infrequent (7%) (Leyfer et al., 2006). Given the diagnostic and cognitive features associated with autism (e.g., insistence on sameness and lack of understanding of the thoughts and feelings of others), it does not seem possible that many children with autism, particularly those with more severe cognitive and language impairments, can comprehend the concepts of intentionality inherent in the diagnosis of ODD.

There is minimal research on the experience of posttraumatic stress symptoms in individuals with cognitive disabilities or autism; however, this population is not immune to experiencing abuse or neglect and may in fact have a higher risk of exposure to abusive or neglectful environments (Howlin & Clements, 1995; Turk & Brown, 1993). Individuals with autism and/or other cognitive disabilities may present with new behavior problems, regressions in previous functioning levels, or exacerbations of existing behaviors problems, including symptoms of anxiety, sleep disturbance, aggression, irritability, and self-injury, in response to being exposed to abusive environments, though they may be unable to articulate what has happened to them (Howlin & Clements, 1995; McCarthy, 2001; Turk, Robbins, & Woodhead, 2005). These problem behaviors may be misattributed to issues other than possible abuse or neglect if clinicians fail to take a detailed history from a variety of caregivers, including noting any changes in the individual's behavioral symptom presentation. (See Chapter 13 for a discussion of abuse risk in the autism population.)

COMORBID ASSESSMENT CONSIDERATIONS

To avoid the type of situation described in John Godfrey Saxe's (1889) poem about the six blind men who debated over and never resolved their differing perspectives of what an elephant might be, assessing possible comorbid disorders in children with autism, particularly in those children with more severely impaired cognitive and language abilities, requires the coordinated efforts of a multidisciplinary team of specialists, community providers, and caregivers, along with the use of systematic assessment strategies and instruments. Consider the hypothetical case of a 190-pound adolescent with autism who has limited communication abilities and independent daily living skills. An increase in this adolescent's aggressive and assault behaviors has resulted in harm to family members and suspension from school. It is unclear whether these behaviors are due to (1) frustration over not being able to communicate his needs, (2) exposure to perceived aversive environmental stimuli, (3) the onset of a mood or other psychiatric disorder, (4) the onset of medical problems, or (5) a combination of any or all of these issues. Understanding how to intervene in this case may require the coordinated efforts of professionals from various disciplines including psychology, psychiatry, pediatrics, speech/language pathology, occupational therapy, nutrition, and neurology.

General Considerations

Gardner (2003) urges that clinicians should take a *transactional* view when evaluating and developing interventions for presenting behavior problems. This involves making an attempt to understand the many influences (personal and environmental) that can affect behavior in individuals with developmental disabilities. Bodfish (2006) discusses the importance of understanding the multiple factors likely to be involved in the development and expression of behavior problems (e.g., stereotypy and self-injurious behaviors) in individuals with autism, such as environmental factors, learning processes, neurobiological factors, and genetic factors. Procedures for assessment of presenting problem behaviors recommended by the American Academy of Child and Adolescent Psychiatry (1999) include the following:

- Gather detailed information on the child's (1) early development and medical and pharmacological history, (2) family history of disorders and symptoms, (3) previous diagnostic assessment data, and (4) current home and educational environment status.
- Observe the child's current symptoms of autism involving social interaction, communication/play, and behavioral responses in structured and unstructured settings to obtain mental status information.
- Order any necessary medical evaluations based on information gathered from the child's history. (See Chapter 2 for more information regarding medical concerns and evaluations.)

Gathering Medical, Psychiatric, and Family History

Matson and Nebel-Schwalam (2006) recommend that clinicians determine whether there is a marked change in the child's symptoms or in the contexts in which problem behaviors occur or if there is a change in the intensity of symptoms over days or weeks. Consider the hypothetical case of an adolescent male patient with autism and mental retardation who presents with rapid, often incoherent speech and noise making. When attempts are made by caregivers to redirect him, there is an increase in the frequency and severity of his aggressive behaviors. This same patient has a history of engaging in repetitive verbalizations about idiosyncratic topics and making repetitive sound effects; in the past, however, this behavior has not impaired his ability to complete school and daily living tasks and his vocalizations have not had a distinct rapid, pressured quality. Given the changes in symptom presentation, the possible onset of a manic episode might be hypothesized.

In addition to gathering information about the child's symptom changes, it has been proposed that the assessment process should include a family history of psychiatric symptoms or disorders, particularly when the individual with autism has more severe cognitive and language impairments that might obscure the presentation of psychiatric symptoms (Ghaziuddin et al., 2002; Matson et al., 1999). Along with this, it is important to thoroughly survey the strengths and needs of the child and family to assist in developing individualized intervention hypotheses. One example of such a survey is the Child and Caregiver Information Form (CCIF) codeveloped by Gabriels, Hill, and Goldson (2003) (see Appendix 1.1 at the end of the chapter). The CCIF can be used as part of the intake process in a variety of hospital-based clinic settings for children with autism who are presenting with possible medical and psychiatric problems.

Behavioral Assessment and Observation

Overt problem behaviors such as irritability, tantrums, aggression, and self-injury, particularly in individuals diagnosed with autism and mental retardation, are often addressed by prescribing atypical antipsychotic medications (Langworthy-Lam, Aman, & Van Bourgondien, 2002; Lindsay & Aman, 2003; McCracken et al., 2002), even though the antecedents of these behaviors may be unclear. Although medication may temporarily treat the presenting symptom, this approach does little to address core diagnostic features of autism or any possible coexisting sensory, medical, psychiatric, or environmental problems that may be driving the behavioral expression.

A variety of assessment tools have been developed to specifically assess a range of behavior problems in the developmentally disabled population; however, research is still needed to develop reliable and valid assessment instruments to examine comorbid psychiatric disorders with individuals who have autism (see Leyfer et al., 2006, and Rush, Bowman, Eidman, Toole, & Mortenson, 2004, for a review of assessment instruments). Finding instruments that survey a broad range of directly observable symptoms not dependent on the child's ability to verbalize ideas and experiences is another challenge (Feinstein, Kaminer, Barrett, & Tylenda, 1988; Hellings et al., 2005; Rush et al., 2004). Pharmacological clinical trials have employed caregiver questionnaires that focus on directly observable symptoms (e.g., aggression, irritability) in the autism population (Hellings et al., 2005; Langworthy-Lam et al., 2002; Lindsay & Aman, 2003; McCracken et al., 2002). Two measures frequently used are the Overt Aggression Scale—Modified (OAS-M, Coccaro, Harvey, Kupsaw-Lawrence, Herbert, & Bernstein, 1991; Coccaro & Kavoussi, 1997; Endicott, Tracy, Burt, Olson, & Coccaro, 2002) and the Aberrant Behavior Checklist—Community (ABC-C, Aman, Burrow, & Wolford, 1995). Recently, a new caregiver interview, the Autism

Comorbidity Interview–Present and Lifetime Version (ACI-PL; Leyfer et al., 2006), was developed and piloted as a modified version of the Kiddie Schedule for Affective Disorders and Schizophrenia (KSADS; Kaufman et al., 1997) to assess comorbid psychiatric disorders in children with autism. Although the ACI-PL shows promise as an autism-specific measure of comorbid psychiatric symptoms, reliability and validity data are needed (Leyfer et al., 2006).

Conducting functional behavioral assessments provides a means of examining how the individual's interpersonal and physical environments are related to problem behaviors. A functional behavioral assessment is a technique modeled on applied behavior analysis (ABA) and is useful in helping to define problem behaviors and identify assessment-based remediation strategies (Donnellan, LaVinga, Negri-Shoultz, & Fass-bender, 1998; Dunlap & Fox, 1999). An example of this type of assessment interview with caregivers is the Functional Assessment Interview (FAI; O'Neill et al., 1997). An additional resource for evaluating problem behaviors and developing behavioral support intervention strategies is the book *Antecedent Control: Innovative Approaches to Behavioral Support* by Luiselli and Cameron (1998). Finally, a functional assessment approach can include the integration of assessments or observations by various professionals, interviews with primary caregivers, and direct observation of the child. The goal is to develop a comprehensive description of the problem behavior, its antecedents or triggers, and consequences (Davis & Mohr, 2004).

CONCLUSIONS

The triad of core autism impairments in the domains of social relatedness, communication, and behavior, along with indicators of various co-occurring conditions, presents a challenge to clinicians who are attempting to assess and intervene effectively with individuals diagnosed with autism. The high co-occurrence of mental retardation in individuals with autism, combined with social and communication limitations, puts this subset of the autism population at risk for being difficult to evaluate for medical or environmental issues that may be contributing to the expression of problem behaviors. Assessment methods, such as functional behavioral assessments, that include careful clinical observation and caregiver interviews can provide guidance for clinicians in identifying interventions most appropriate for specific individual needs. Continued diagnostic comparison studies in the autism population along with improved diagnostic measurement tools will assist clinicians in determining whether or not behavior problems presenting in individuals with autism are due to the core features of autism, medical problems, sensory response abnormalities, cognitive disabilities, comorbid psychiatric diagnoses, life experiences, or a combination thereof.

REFERENCES

Abramson, R. K., Wright, H. H., Cuccaro, M. L., Lawrence, L. G., Babb, S., Pencarinha, D., et al. (1992). Biological liability in families with autism. *Journal of the American Academy of Child and Adolescent Psychiatry, 31*(2), 370–371.

Aman, M. G., Burrow, W. H., & Wolford, P. L. (1995). The Aberrant Behavior Checklist—Community: Factor validity and effect of subject variables for adults in group homes. *American Journal of Mental Retardation, 100*(3), 283–292.

American Academy of Child and Adolescent Psychiatry. (1999). Practice parameters for the assessment and treatment of children, adolescents, and adults with autism and other pervasive developmental disorders. *Journal of the American Academy of Child and Adolescent Psychiatry, 38*, 32S–54S.

American Psychiatric Association. (1994). *Diagnostic and statistical manual of mental disorders* (4th ed.). Washington, DC: Author.

Ando, H., & Yoshimura, I. (1979). Effects of age on communication skill levels and prevalence of maladaptive behaviors in autistic and mentally retarded children. *Journal of Autism and Developmental Disorders, 9*(1), 83–93.

Angold, A., Costello, E. J., Erkanli, A., & Worthman, C. M. (1999). Pubertal changes in hormone levels and depression in girls. *Psychological Medicine, 29*(5), 1043–1053.

Baranek, G., David, F. J., Poe, M. D., Stone, W. L., & Watson, L. R. (2006). Sensory Experiences Questionnaire: Discriminating sensory features in young children with autism, developmental delays, and typical development. *Journal of Child Psychology and Psychiatry, 47*(6), 591–601.

Baranek, G. T., Foster, L. G., & Berkson, G. (1997). Tactile defensiveness and stereotyped behaviors. *American Journal of Occupational Therapy, 51*, 91–95.

Baranek, G. T., Parham, L. D., & Bodfish, J. W. (2005). Sensory and motor features in autism: Assessment and intervention. In F. Volkmar, R. Paul, A. Klin, & D. J. Cohen (Eds.), *Handbook of autism and pervasive developmental disorders (3rd ed.): Vol. 2. Assessment, interventions, and policy* (pp. 831–861). Hoboken, NJ: Wiley.

Baron-Cohen, S., & Belmonte, M. K. (2005). Autism: A window onto the development of the social and the analytic brain. *Annual Review of Neuroscience, 28*, 109–126.

Bartak, L., & Rutter, M. (1976). Differences between mentally retarded and normally intelligent autistic children. *Journal of Autism and Childhood Schizophrenia, 6*(2), 109–120.

Berkson, G. (2002). Early development of stereotyped and self-injurious behaviors: II. Age trends. *American Journal of Mental Retardation, 107*(6), 468–477.

Berkson, G., Tupa, M., & Sherman, L. (2001). Early development of stereotyped and self-injurious behaviors: I. Incidence. *American Journal of Mental Retardation, 106*(6), 539–547.

Bodfish, J. W. (2006). Stereotypy, self-injury and related abnormal repetitive behaviors. In J. W. Jacobson, J. A. Mulick, & J. Rojahn (Eds.), *Handbook of mental retardation and developmental disabilities* (pp. 481–505). New York: Springer.

Bodfish, J. W., Crawford, T. W., Powell, S. B., Parker, D. E., Golden, R. N., & Lewis, M. H. (1995). Compulsions in adults with mental retardation: Prevalence, phenomenology, and comorbidity with stereotypy and self-injury. *American Journal of Mental Retardation, 100*(2), 183–192.

Bodfish, J. W., Symons, F. J., Parker, D. E., & Lewis, M. H. (2000). Varieties of repetitive behavior in autism: Comparisons to mental retardation. *Journal of Autism and Developmental Disorders, 30*(3), 237–243.

Bolton, P. F., Pickles, A., Murphy, M., & Rutter, M. (1998). Autism, affective and other psychiatric disorders: Patterns of familial aggregation. *Psychological Medicine, 28*(2), 385–395.

Bradley, E. A., Summers, J. A., Wood, H. L., & Bryson, S. E. (2004). Comparing rates of psychiatric and behavior disorders in adolescents and young adults with severe intellectual disability with and without autism. *Journal of Autism and Developmental Disorders, 34*(2), 151–161.

Campbell, M., Locascio, J. J., Choroco, M. C., Spencer, E. K., Malone, R. P., Kafantaris, V., et al. (1990). Stereotypies and tardive dyskinesia: Abnormal movements in autistic children. *Psychopharmacology Bulletin, 26*(2), 260–266.

Capps, L., Kasari, C., Yirmiya, N., & Sigman, M. (1993). Parental perception of emotional expressiveness in children with autism. *Journal of Consulting and Clinical Psychology, 61*(3), 475–484.

Carr, E. G., & Durand, V. M. (1985). Reducing behavior problems through functional communication training. *Journal of Applied Behavior Analysis, 18*(2), 111–126.

Charlop-Christy, M. H., & Haymes, L. K. (1996). Using obsessions as reinforcers with and without mild reductive procedures to decrease inappropriate behaviors of children with autism. *Journal of Autism and Developmental Disorders, 26*(5), 527–546.

Chung, S. Y., Luk, S. L., & Lee, P. W. (1990). A follow-up study of infantile autism in Hong Kong. *Journal of Autism and Developmental Disorders, 20*(2), 221–232.

Coccaro, E. F., Harvey, P. D., Kupsaw-Lawrence, E., Herbert, J. L., & Bernstein, D. P. (1991). Development of neuropharmacologically based behavioral assessments of impulsive aggressive behavior. *Journal of Neuropsychiatry and Clinical Neurosciences, 3*(2), S44–S51.

Coccaro, E. F., & Kavoussi, R. J. (1997). Fluoxetine and impulsive aggressive behavior in personality-disordered subjects. *Archives of General Psychiatry, 54,* 1081–1088.

Colman, R. S., Frankel, F., Ritvo, E., & Freeman, B. J. (1976). The effects of fluorescent and incandescent illumination upon repetitive behaviors in autistic children. *Journal of Autism and Childhood Schizophrenia, 6,* 157–162.

Davis, R., & Mohr, C. (2004). The assessment and treatment of behavioural problems. *Australian Family Physician, 33*(8), 609–613.

Dawson, D., & Levy, A. (1989). Arousal, attention and the socio-emotional impairments of individuals with autism. In G. Dawson (Ed.), *Autism: Nature, diagnosis and treatment* (pp. 49–74). New York: Guilford Press.

de Bildt, A., Sytema, S., Kraijer, D., Sparrow, S., & Minderaa, R. (2005). Adaptive functioning and behaviour problems in relation to level of education in children and adolescents with intellectual disability. *Journal of Intellectual Disability Research, 49*(Pt. 9), 672–681.

Dekker, M. C., & Koot, H. M. (2003). DSM-IV disorders in children with borderline to moderate intellectual disability: I. Prevalence and impact. *Journal of the American Academy of Child and Adolescent Psychiatry, 42*(8), 915–922.

Donnellan, A. M., LaVinga, G. W., Negri-Shoultz, N., & Fassbender, L. L. (1998). *Progress without punishment: Effective approaches for learners with behavior problems.* New York: Teachers College Press.

Douglas, R. J., & Martin, K. A. (2004). Neuronal circuits of the neocortex. *Annual Reviews of Neuroscience, 27,* 419–451.

Dunlap, G., Dyer, K., & Koegel, R. L. (1983). Autistic self-stimulation and intertrial interval duration. *American Journal of Mental Deficiency, 88*(2), 194–202.

Dunlap, G., & Fox, L. (1999). A demonstration of behavioral support for young children with autism. *Journal of Positive Behavior Interventions, 1,* 77–87.

Dunlap, G., Johnson, L. F., & Robbins, F. R. (1990). Preventing serious behavior problems through skill development and early intervention. In A. C. Repp & N. N. Singh (Eds.), *Current perspectives in the use of non-aversive and aversive interventions with developmentally disabled persons* (pp. 273–286). Sycamore, IL: Sycamore Press.

Dunn, W. (1999). *Sensory profile.* San Antonio, TX: Psychological Corporation.

Durand, V. M., & Merges, E. (2001). Functional communication training: A contemporary behavior analytic intervention for problem behaviors. *Focus on Autism and Other Developmental Disabilities, 16*(2), 110–136.

Dykens, E., Volkmar, F., & Glick, M. (1991). Thought disorder in high-functioning autistic adults. *Journal of Autism and Developmental Disorders, 21*(3), 291–301.

Elia, M., Musumeci, S. A., Ferri, R., & Bergonzi, P. (1995). Clinical and neurophysiological aspects of epilepsy in subjects with autism and mental retardation. *American Journal of Mental Retardation, 100*(1), 6–16.

Endicott, J., Tracy, K., Burt, D., Olson, E., & Coccaro, E. F. (2002). A novel approach to assess inter-rater reliability in the use of the Overt Aggression Scale—Modified. *Psychiatry Research, 112*(2), 153–159.

Evans, D. W., Canavera, K., Kleinpeter, F. L., Maccubbin, E., & Taga, K. (2005). The fears, phobias and anxieties of children with autism spectrum disorders and Down syndrome: Comparisons with developmentally and chronologically age matched children. *Child Psychiatry and Human Development, 36*(1), 3–26.

Fanurik, D., Koh, J. L., Schmitz, M. L., Harnson, R. D., & Conrad, T. M. (1999). Children with cognitive impairment: Parent report of pain and coping. *Journal of Developmental and Behavioral Pediatrics, 20*(4), 228–234.

Feinstein, C., Kaminer, Y., Barrett, R. P., & Tylenda, B. (1988). The assessment of mood and affect in developmentally disabled children and adolescents: The Emotional Disorders Rating Scale. *Research in Developmental Disabilities, 9*(2), 109–121.

Frith, U. (1989). A new look at language and communication in autism. *British Journal of Disorders of Communication, 24*(2), 123–150.

Gabriels, R. L., Hill, D. E., & Goldson, E. (2003). *The Child and Caregiver Information Form (CCIF).* The Children's Hospital, Denver, CO, and The University of New Mexico, Albuquerque, NM. Unpublished manuscript.

Gal, E., Dyck, M. J., & Passmore, A. (2002). Sensory differences and stereotyped movements in children with autism. *Behaviour Change, 4,* 207–219.

Gardner, W. I. (2003). Diagnostically based treatments of biomedical and psychosocial conditions that influence self-injurious behaviors: A multimodal case formulation. *NADD Bulletin, 6*(2), 23–28.

Ghaziuddin, M., Alessi, N., & Greden, J. F. (1995). Life events and depression in children with pervasive developmental disorders. *Journal of Autism and Developmental Disorders, 25*(5), 495–502.

Ghaziuddin, M., Ghaziuddin, N., & Greden, J. (2002). Depression in persons with autism: Implications for research and clinical care. *Journal of Autism and Developmental Disorders, 32*(4), 299–306.

Ghaziuddin, M., & Greden, J. (1998). Depression in children with autism/pervasive developmental disorders: A case-control family history study. *Journal of Autism and Developmental Disorders, 28*(2), 111–115.

Ghaziuddin, M., Tsai, L. Y., & Ghaziuddin, N. (1992). Comorbidity of autistic disorder in children and adolescents. *European Child and Adolescent Psychiatry, 1,* 209–213.

Gillberg, C. (1991). Outcome in autism and autistic-like conditions. *Journal of the American Academy of Child and Adolescent Psychiatry, 30*(3), 375–382.

Gillberg, C. (1995). Endogenous opioids and opiate antagonists in autism: Brief review of empirical findings and implications for clinicians. *Developmental Medicine and Child Neurology, 37*(3), 239–245.

Gillberg, C., Ehlers, S., Schaumann, H., Jakobsson, G., Dahlgren, S. O., Lindblom, R., et al. (1990). Autism under age 3 years: A clinical study of 28 cases referred for autistic symptoms in infancy. *Journal of Child Psychology and Psychiatry, 31*(6), 921–934.

Gillberg, C., & Steffenburg, S. (1987). Outcome and prognostic factors in infantile autism and similar conditions: A population-based study of 46 cases followed through puberty. *Journal of Autism and Developmental Disorders, 17*(2), 273–287.

Grandin, T. (1992). An inside view of autism. In E. Schopler & G. B. Mesibov (Eds.), *High-functioning individuals with autism* (pp. 105–126). New York: Plenum Press.

Greenspan, S. I., & Wieder, S. (1997). Developmental patterns and outcomes in infants and children with disorders in relating and communicating: A chart review of 200 cases of children with autistic spectrum disorder. *Journal of Developmental and Learning Disorders, 1,* 87–141.

Happe, F., & Frith, U. (1996). The neuropsychology of autism. *Brain, 119*(Pt. 4), 1377–1400.

Hellings, J. A., Nickel, E. J., Weckbaugh, M., McCarter, K., Mosier, M., & Schroeder, S. R. (2005). The overt aggression scale for rating aggression in outpatient youth with autistic disorder: Preliminary findings. *Journal of Neuropsychiatry and Clinical Neurosciences, 17*(1), 29–35.

Hermann, B. P., Seidenberg, M., & Bell, B. (2000). Psychiatric comorbidity in chronic epilepsy: Identification, consequences, and treatment of major depression. *Epilepsia, 41*(Suppl. 2), S31–S41.

Hirstein, W., Iversen, P., & Ramachandran, V. S. (2001). Autonomic responses of autistic children to people and objects. *Proceedings of the Royal Society of London, 268*(1479), 1883–1888.

Howlin, P., & Clements, J. (1995). Is it possible to assess the impact of abuse on children with pervasive developmental disorders? *Journal of Autism and Developmental Disorders, 25*(4), 337–354.

Howlin, P., Goode, S., Hutton, J., & Rutter, M. (2004). Adult outcome for children with autism. *Journal of Child Psychology and Psychiatry and Allied Disciplines, 45*(2), 212–229.

Kaufman, J., Birmaher, B., Brent, D., Rao, U., Flynn, C., Moreci, P., et al. (1997). Schedule for Affective Disorders and Schizophrenia for School-Age Children—Present and Lifetime Version (K-SADS-PL): Initial reliability and validity data. *Journal of the American Academy of Child and Adolescent Psychiatry, 36*(7), 980–988.

Kendler, K. S., Karkowski, L. M., & Prescott, C. A. (1999). Causal relationship between stressful life events and the onset of major depression. *American Journal of Psychiatry, 156*(6), 837–841.

Kim, J. A., Szatmari, P., Bryson, S. E., Streiner, D. L., & Wilson, F. J. (2000). The prevalence of anxiety and mood problems among children with autism and Asperger syndrome. *Autism, 4*(2), 117–132.

Konstantareas, M. M., & Homatidis, S. (1989). Assessing child symptom severity and stress in parents of autistic children. *Journal of Child Psychology and Psychiatry, 30*(3), 459–470.

Lainhart, J. E. (1999). Psychiatric problems in autistic individuals and their parents and siblings. *International Review of Psychiatry, 11,* 278–298.

Lainhart, J. E. (2003). Increased rate of head growth during infancy in autism. *Journal of the American Medical Association, 290*(3), 393–394.

Lainhart, J. E., & Folstein, S. E. (1994). Affective disorders in people with autism: A review of published cases. *Journal of Autism and Developmental Disorders, 24*(5), 587–601.

Langworthy-Lam, K. S., Aman, M. G., & Van Bourgondien, M. E. (2002). Prevalence and patterns of use of psychoactive medicines in individuals with autism in the Autism Society of North Carolina. *Journal of Child and Adolescent Psychopharmacology, 12*(4), 311–321.

Le Couteur, A., Rutter, M., Lord, C., Rios, P., Robertson, S., Holdgrafer, M., et al. (1989). Autism diagnostic interview: A standardized investigator-based instrument. *Journal of Autism and Developmental Disorders, 19*(3), 363–387.

Lewis, M. H., & Bodfish, J. W. (1998). Repetitive behavior disorders in autism. *Mental Retardation and Developmental Disabilities Research Reviews, 4*(2), 80–89.

Leyfer, O. T., Folstein, S. E., Bacalman, S., Davis, N. O., Dinh, E., Morgan, J., et al. (2006). Comorbid psychiatric disorders in children with autism: Interview development and rates of disorders. *Journal of Autism and Developmental Disorders, 36*(7), 849–861.

Lindsay, R. L., & Aman, M. G. (2003). Pharmacologic therapies aid treatment for autism. *Pediatric Annals, 32*(10), 671–676.

Lord, C., & Paul, R. (1997). Language and communication in autism. In D. J. Cohen & F. Volkmar (Eds.), *Handbook of autism and pervasive developmental disorders* (2nd ed., pp. 195–225). New York: Wiley.

Lotter, V. (1974). Factors related to outcome in autistic children. *Journal of Autism and Childhood Schizophrenia, 4*(3), 263–277.

Luiselli, J. K., & Cameron, M. J. (1998). *Antecedent control: Innovative approaches to behavioral support.* Baltimore: Brookes Publishing.

Matese, M., Matson, J. L., & Sevin, J. (1994). Comparison of psychotic and autistic children using behavioral observation. *Journal of Autism and Developmental Disorders, 24*(1), 83–94.

Matson, J. L., & Love, S. R. (1990). A comparison of parent-reported fear in autistic and nonhandicapped age-matched children and youth. *Australia and New Zealand Journal of Developmental Disabilities, 16,* 349–357.

Matson, J. L., & Nebel-Schwalm, M. S. (2006). Comorbid psychopathology with autism spectrum disorder in children: An overview. *Research in Developmental Disabilities, 28*(2), 109–118.

Matson, J. L., Rush, K. S., Hamilton, M., Anderson, S. J., Bamburg, J. W., Baglio, C. S., et al. (1999). Characteristics of depression as assessed by the Diagnostic Assessment for the Severely Handicapped–II (DASH-II). *Research in Developmental Disabilities, 20*(4), 305–313.

McCarthy, J. (2001). Post-traumatic stress disorder in people with learning disability. *Advances in Psychiatric Treatment, 7,* 163–169.

McCracken, J. T., McGough, J., Shah, B., Cronin, P., Hong, D., Aman, M. G., et al. (2002). Risperidone in children with autism and serious behavioral problems. *New England Journal of Medicine, 347*(5), 314–321.

McDougle, C. J., Kresch, L. E., Goodman, W. K., Naylor, S. T., Volkmar, F. R., Cohen, D. J., et al. (1995). A case-controlled study of repetitive thoughts and behavior in adults with autistic disorder and obsessive–compulsive disorder. *American Journal of Psychiatry, 152,* 722–777.

McEachin, J. J., Smith, T., & Lovaas, O. I. (1993). Long-term outcome for children with autism who received early intensive behavioral treatment. *American Journal of Mental Retardation, 97*(4), 359–372; discussion 373–391.

McGovern, C. W., & Sigman, M. (2005). Continuity and change from early childhood to adolescence in autism. *Journal of Child Psychology and Psychiatry and Allied Disciplines, 46*(4), 401–408.

Muris, P., Steerneman, P., Merckelbach, H., Holdrinet, I., & Meesters, C. (1998). Comorbid anxiety symptoms in children with pervasive developmental disorders. *Journal of Anxiety Disorders, 12*(4), 387–393.

Nader, R., Oberlander, T. F., Chambers, C. T., & Craig, K. D. (2004). Expression of pain in children with autism. *Clinical Journal of Pain, 20*(2), 88–97.

O'Neill, R. E., Homer, R. H., Albin, R. W., Sprague, J. R., Storey, K., & Newton, J. S. (1997). *Functional assessment and program development for problem behavior.* Pacific Grove, CA: Brooks/Cole.

Ornitz, E. M., Guthrie, D., & Farley, A. H. (1977). The early development of autistic children. *Journal of Autism and Childhood Schizophrenia, 7*(3), 207–229.

Ornitz, E. M., Guthrie, D., & Farley, A. H. (1978). The early symptoms of childhood autism. In G. Serban (Ed.), *Cognitive defects in the development of mental illness* (pp. 24–42). New York: Brunner/Mazel.

Petty, L. K., Ornitz, E. M., Michelman, J. D., & Zimmerman, E. G. (1984). Autistic children who become schizophrenic. *Archives of General Psychiatry, 41*(2), 129–135.

Piven, J., Chase, G. A., Landa, R., Wzorek, M., Gayle, J., Cloud, D., et al. (1991). Psychiatric disorders in the parents of autistic individuals. *Journal of the American Academy of Child and Adolescent Psychiatry, 30*(3), 471–478.

Piven, J., Harper, J., Palmer, P., & Arndt, S. (1996). Course of behavioral change in autism: A retrospective study of high-IQ adolescents and adults. *Journal of the American Academy of Child and Adolescent Psychiatry, 35*(4), 523–529.

Poustka, F. (1998). Neurobiology of autism. In F. Volkmar (Ed.), *Autism and pervasive developmental disorders* (pp. 130–168). Cambridge, UK: Cambridge University Press.

Reese, R. M., Richman, D. M., Belmont, J. M., & Morse, P. (2005). Functional characteristics of disruptive behavior in developmentally disabled children with and without autism. *Journal of Autism and Developmental Disorders, 35*(4), 419–428.

Reeve, C. E. (1996). *Prevention of severe behavioral problems in children with developmental disabilities.* Unpublished dissertation, State University of New York at Stony Brook.

Rojahn, J. (1986). Self-injurious and stereotypic behavior of noninstitutionalized mentally retarded people: Prevalence and classification. *American Journal of Mental Deficiency, 91*(3), 268–276.

Rumsey, J. M., Andreasen, N. C., & Rapoport, J. L. (1986). Thought, language, communication, and affective flattening in autistic adults. *Archives of General Psychiatry, 43*(8), 771–777.

Rumsey, J. M., Rapoport, J. L., & Sceery, W. R. (1985). Autistic children as adults: Psychiatric, social, and behavioral outcomes. *Journal of the American Academy of Child Psychiatry, 24*(4), 465–473.

Rush, K. S., Bowman, L. G., Eidman, S. L., Toole, L. M., & Mortenson, B. P. (2004). Assessing psychopathology in individuals with developmental disabilities. *Behavior Modification, 28*(5), 621–637.

Saxe, J. G. (1889). The blind men and the elephant. In *Poetical Works* (pp. 135–136). Boston: Houghton Mifflin.

Schreck, K. A., & Mulick, J. A. (2000). Parental report of sleep problems in children with autism. *Journal of Autism and Developmental Disorders, 30*(2), 127–135.

Schreck, K. A., Mulick, J. A., & Smith, A. F. (2004). Sleep problems as possible predictors of intensified symptoms of autism. *Research in Developmental Disabilities, 25*(1), 57–66.

Schultz, T. M., & Berkson, G. (1995). Definition of abnormal focused affections and exploration of their relation to abnormal stereotyped behaviors. *American Journal of Mental Retardation, 99*(4), 376–390.

Skinner, S. R., Ng, C., McDonald, A., & Walters, T. (2005). A patient with autism and severe depression: Medical and ethical challenges for an adolescent medicine unit. *Medical Journal of Australia, 183*(8), 422–424.

Sturmey, P., & Sevin, J. A. (1994). Defining and addressing autism. In J. L. Matson (Ed.), *Autism in children and adults: Etiology, assessment and intervention* (pp. 13–36). Pacific Grove, CA: Brooks/Cole.

Sverd, J. (2003). Psychiatric disorders in individuals with pervasive developmental disorder. *Journal of Psychiatric Practice, 9*(2), 111–127.

Sverd, J., Dubey, D. R., Schweitzer, R., & Ninan, R. (2003). Pervasive developmental disorders among children and adolescents attending psychiatric day treatment. *Psychiatric Services, 54*(11), 1519–1525.

Tager-Flusberg, H. (1992). Autistic children's talk about psychological states: Deficits in the early acquisition of a theory of mind. *Child Development, 63*(1), 161–172.

Tantam, D. (1991). Asperger syndrome in adulthood. In U. Frith (Ed.), *Autism and Asperger syndrome* (pp. 147–183). Cambridge, UK: Cambridge University Press.

Tecchio, F., Benassi, F., Zappasodi, F., Gialloreti, L. E., Palermo, M., Seri, S., et al. (2003). Auditory sensory processing in autism: A magnetoencephalographic study. *Biological Psychiatry, 54*(6), 647–654.

Tsai, L. Y. (1996). Brief report: Comorbid psychiatric disorders of autistic disorder. *Journal of Autism and Developmental Disorders, 26*(2), 159–163.

Tuchman, R. F., Rapin, I., & Shinnar, S. (1991a). Autistic and dysphasic children: I. Clinical characteristics. *Pediatrics, 88*(6), 1211–1218.

Tuchman, R. F., Rapin, I., & Shinnar, S. (1991b). Autistic and dysphasic children: II. Epilepsy. *Pediatrics, 88*(6), 1219–1225.

Turk, V., & Brown, H. (1993). The sexual abuse of adults with learning disabilities: Results of a two year incidence survey. *Mental Handicap Research, 6,* 193–216.

Turk, V., Robbins, I., & Woodhead, M. (2005). Post-traumatic stress disorder in young people with intellectual disability. *Journal of Intellectual Disability Research, 49*(2), 872–875.

Volkmar, F. R., Cohen, D. J., & Paul, R. (1986). An evaluation of DSM-III criteria for infantile autism. *Journal of the American Academy of Child Psychiatry, 25*(2), 190–197.

Volkmar, F. R., & Nelson, D. S. (1990). Seizure disorders in autism. *Journal of the American Academy of Child and Adolescent Psychiatry, 29*(1), 127–129.

Wainwright-Sharp, J. A., & Bryson, S. E. (1993). Visual orienting deficits in high-functioning people with autism. *Journal of Autism and Developmental Disorders, 23*(1), 1–13.

Willemsen-Swinkels, S. H., Buitelaar, J. K., Dekker, M., & van Engeland, H. (1998). Subtyping stereotypic behavior in children: The association between stereotypic behavior, mood, and heart rate. *Journal of Autism and Developmental Disorders, 28*(6), 547–557.

Wing, L., & Shah, A. (2000). Catatonia in autistic spectrum disorders. *British Journal of Psychiatry, 176,* 357–362.

World Health Organization. (1994). *The international statistical classification of diseases and health problems* (10th ed.). Geneva, Switzerland: Author.

Wozniak, J., Biederman, J., Faraone, S. V., Frazier, J., Kim, J., Millstein, R., et al. (1997). Mania in children with pervasive developmental disorder revisited. *Journal of the American Academy of Child and Adolescent Psychiatry, 36*(11), 1552–1559; discussion 1559–1560.

APPENDIX 1.1

Child and Caregiver Information Form (CCIF)

Name of Interviewer: _____ Date: _____

Name of Responder: _____ Relationship to Child: _____

I. Child and Family Demographics

Child's Name: _____

Date of Birth: __ / __ / __ Age: _____

If child is adopted, check here: _____

Child's Diagnoses:

Developmental _____

Medical _____

Psychiatric _____

Father's Name: _____

Work Phone: _____

Occupation: _____

Mother's Name: _____

Work Phone: _____

Occupation: _____

Home Phone: _____

List all persons living at home with the child.

Name	Age	Sex	Relationship

Address: _____

          Street

_____

City   State   ZIP

II. Behavior Problems

A. *What brought your child to the hospital/clinic now and how are the child's symptoms or behaviors affecting other people involved in the child's care?*

_____

_____

_____

_____

_____

_____

_____

_____

(continued)

B. *Types of problematic behaviors the child demonstrates:*

☐ Hitting? ☐ Property Destruction ☐ Crying ☐ Biting

☐ Self-Injury ☐ Yelling/Screaming ☐ Kicking ☐ Other _____

C. *Specifically describe what the child actually does for each of the problem behaviors indicated:* _____

_____

_____

D. *How long has your child had these behaviors or when did these behaviors increase?* _____

_____

_____

E. *How often do these behaviors occur in a week?* _____

_____

F. *What do you think is the purpose of these behaviors and/or is there a pattern to these behaviors?* _____

_____

_____

G. *Does your child have any known fears, anxieties, or sensory sensitivities? What situations might agitate your child?* _____

_____

_____

H. *Behavior Intervention Strategies: What strategies do you use to address the child's behavior problems?*

☐ Time Out ☐ Consequences ☐ Visual Cues

☐ Ignoring ☐ Token System ☐ Physical Prompts

☐ Redirection ☐ Positive Praise ☐ Physical Holding

Explain: _____

_____

_____

_____

I. *Self-Regulation (Calming) Strategies and Reinforcements: Please list any calming strategies, special interests/characters, activities, toys, or food items that calm your child or assist with their behavior management.* _____

_____

_____

(continued)

III. Communication Ability

A. *How does your child communicate his or her needs (check all that apply)?*

☐ Tantrums/Crying   ☐ Picture/Symbols   ☐ Vocalizations (grunts/
                                                           babbling)

☐ Sign Language*   ☐ Object symbols

☐ Gestures (pointing,   ☐ Phrases/Sentences   ☐ Other communication
    leads by the hand)   ☐ Single Words   device—specify: _____

*If you checked sign language, please indicate if your child <u>understands</u> and/or <u>uses</u> signs (circle) and indicate which signs these include.

_____

_____

B. *Structured visual systems the child uses during the day:*

<u>Daily Schedule:</u> ☐ Object ☐ Picture-Word ☐ Word ☐ Other _____

<u>Work Systems:</u> Workbaskets ☐ Work Notebooks ☐ Other _____

IV. Medical Health: *Please indicate all issues that are of concern and include more information where indicated.*

A. *List current medications your child is taking.*

Medication	Dosage	Symptoms medication is addressing

B. *Medication compliant?* Yes ☐ No ☐ Explain: _____

C. *Vision and Hearing*

Has your child had <u>vision screening</u> Yes ☐ No ☐ Date _____

Has your child had a <u>hearing screening</u>? Yes ☐ No ☐ Date _____

Indicate any concerns regarding your child's vision or hearing: _____

_____

D. *Seizures*

1. Has your child been formally diagnosed with a seizure disorder? Yes ☐ No ☐
   If your child does have seizures, please describe the symptoms:

_____

_____

_____

(continued)

2. If your child has not been diagnosed with a seizure disorder, do you have concerns that your child may have seizures? Yes ☐ No ☐ If yes, please explain why you have these concerns:

_____

_____

3. Has your child seen a neurologist (if yes, list doctor's name)? _____

4. Has your child had an MRI? Yes ☐ No ☐ If yes, date of MRI: _____

   Has your child had an EEG? Yes ☐ No ☐ If yes, date of EEG: _____

E. *Dental Issues*

1. Does your child see a dentist on a regular basis? Yes ☐ No ☐

   If, no, do you have any concerns about your child's dental health at this time? Yes ☐ No ☐

   Explain: _____

   _____

2. Does your child grind his or her teeth? Yes ☐ No ☐

   If yes, when does your child engage in this behavior and are there times or circumstances when this behavior occurs more frequently? _____

F. *Puberty* Has your child entered puberty? Yes ☐ No ☐

   For girls: Breast development, pubic hair, axillary (underarm) hair

   For boys: Enlarged penis, enlarged scrotum, pubic hair, axillary (underarm) hair

G. *Adaptive Devices:* Please check all adaptive devices that your child uses:

   ☐ Glasses   ☐ Hearing Aids   ☐ Helmets   ☐ Wheel chair

   ☐ Other: _____

H. *Other Current Medical Problems/Concerns?* _____

   _____

   _____

I. *Family Medical History:* Please indicate if there is any history of the following on either side of the child's biological parents' family. Indicate father or mother's side and specify who (uncle, etc.)

Description	No	Yes	Father's side	Mother's side	Specific remarks
Genetic disorders (e.g., Down syndrome, fragile X)					
Mental retardation					
Learning disabilities					
Slow development					
Speech problems					

(continued)

Description	No	Yes	Father's side	Mother's side	Specific remarks
Difficulty with social interaction					
Extreme shyness					
Autistic disorder					
Asperger disorder					
Pervasive developmental disorder NOS (PDD NOS)					
Tics or Tourette disorder					
Obsessive–compulsive disorder					
Schizophrenia					
Mood swings					
Depression					
Bipolar disorder (manic–depression)					
Hyperactivity or overactivity					
Attention problems or short attention problem					
Birth defects					
Seizures/convulsions					
Tuberculosis					
Neurological disease					
Diabetes					
Cancer					
Allergies/asthma					
Gland disorder/thyroid					
Hearing impairments					
Vision impairments					
Miscarriages					
Substance abuse problems (drugs, alcohol, tobacco)					
Other:					

(continued)

J. Child's Medical History: Has your child ever been treated for or had a history of the following:

Description	No	Yes	If yes, explain further
Abdominal pain/bowel issues			
Allergies			
Birth defects			
Concussion/head injury			
Dental problems			
Ear infections			
Eating issues/gagging/ choking/drooling			
Headaches			
Hearing loss			
Heart condition			
Blood disorders/anemia			
Hormone problems			
Ingesting poisons or other non-nutritive substances (pica)			
Joint or bone problems			
Lung or breathing problems			
Muscular problems			
Suffered high prolonged fever			
Surgeries			
Seizures or convulsions			
Significant accidents			
Skin diseases			
Sleep problems			
Tics or repetitive movements			
Urinary problems/infections			
Visual/eye problems			
Other medical concerns, hospitalizations			

(continued)

K. *Current Dietary Issues (check all that apply).*

Description	No	Yes	If yes, please explain
Picky eater			
Special diet			
Poor weight gain			
Food refusal			
Food intolerance			
Pica (eating of nonnutritive substances, e.g., chalk, wood, grass)			
Food allergy			

L. *Current Gastrointestinal Symptoms (check all that apply).*

Description	No	Yes	If yes, please explain
Bloating			
Belching			
Passing gas (flatus)			
Pain with bowel movement			
Diarrhea (frequent loose stools; > 3 times/day)			
Abdominal pain			
Constipation			
Encopresis: the passage of feces (stool) into inappropriate places (clothing, floor), with or without constipation and/or overflow diarrhea.			

M. *Current medical insurance (list all types)*: _____

_____

V. Psychological Health

☐ *Check here if there is a history of abuse or neglect.* If checked, please specify, including type of abuse, when abuse occurred, and actions taken to address the abuse issues: _____

_____

_____

☐ *Check here if there is a history of recent loss or change in the child's environment.* If checked, explain any changes in behaviors or skills (e.g., increase, decrease, loss of, etc.): ____

_____

_____

(continued)

VI. **Daily Living/Self-Care Skills** *Check all that apply, and include written comments in the spaces provided.*

A. *Sleep Issues and Routines*

Bedtime routine	Bedtime behaviors	Other
Time to bed: ____ P.M. ☐ Requires certain activities before going to sleep: _____ _____ _____ ☐ Wakes up/gets up during night. Behaviors: _____ _____ Time wakes up: ____ A.M.	☐ Requires picture or verbal schedule of bedtime routine ☐ Requires picture or verbal cue of time to bed ☐ Needs nightlight ☐ Needs door open or closed ☐ Has toys/blankets/other objects for sleep: _____ ☐ Wets or soils bed	

B. *Eating and Drinking Behaviors*

Eating	Drinking	Favorite foods and drinks	Disliked foods and drinks	Other
☐ Food allergies or sensitivities ☐ Eats independently ☐ Requires verbal cues and monitoring ☐ Requires physical prompts/assistance ☐ Chokes on foods ☐ Eats nonfood items (consider lead screen)	☐ Allergies or sensitivities to drinks ☐ Drinks independently ☐ Requires verbal cues and monitoring ☐ Requires physical prompts/assistance ☐ Needs sippy/covered cup			

List any other food-related issues: _____

_____

C. *Toileting*

Use of toilet during the day	Use of toilet at night	Behavioral problems	Other issues
☐ Independent ☐ Will ask to use the toilet ☐ Needs verbal reminders ☐ Needs assistance with clothes/ wiping self ☐ Wears diapers or Depends	☐ Independent ☐ Needs to be awakened during the night ☐ Wears diapers or Depends	☐ No behavioral problems with toileting ☐ Will refuse to use toilet ☐ Problems with flushing toilet/playing with toilet paper/playing with feces	

(continued)

D. Daily Living Skills

Dressing	Bathing	Hair washing/care	Tooth brushing
☐ Dresses self independently ☐ Undresses self independently ☐ Requires verbal cues to dress/undress ☐ Requires physical assistance to dress/undress ☐ Needs assistance selecting clothes ☐ Ties shoes independently ☐ Needs assistance to tie shoes ☐ Fastens zippers, buttons, snaps independently ☐ Requires assistance with fasteners	☐ Takes bath or shower independently ☐ Bathes in A.M./P.M. ☐ Requires verbal cues for steps of bathing ☐ Requires physical assistance to bathe ☐ Requires supervision due to behaviors or safety issues	☐ Washes hair independently ☐ Brushes/combs hair independently ☐ Requires verbal cues for steps for hair washing ☐ Requires verbal cues for steps for combing hair ☐ Requires physical assistance to wash hair ☐ Requires physical assistance for combing hair ☐ Resists hair washing or combing	☐ Brushes teeth independently ☐ Requires verbal cues for steps for brushing teeth ☐ Requires physical assistance for brushing teeth ☐ Resists tooth brushing ☐ Requires supervision due to lack of follow-through

List any other self-care considerations: _____

_____

VII. Community Resources

Check all that apply	Service provider	Provider's name	Phone #
	Family therapist/case coordinator		
	Behavioral specialist/consultant		
	Paraprofessional/home trainer		
	Speech therapist		
	Occupational therapist		
	Physical therapist		
	Physician/pediatrician		
	Psychiatrist		
	Neurologist		
	Dentist		

(continued)

Check all that apply	*Service provider*	*Provider's name*	*Phone #*
	Advocate		
	Community service case manager		
	Respite care		
	School-based special education coordinator		
	Other:		

Indicate state/federal funding currently received or on wait list for: _____

_____

Indicate any services needed that might be helpful to your child and family: _____

_____

VIII. Academic Interests and Abilities

A. *Does your child have an individualized education plan (IEP)?* No ☐ Yes ☐ (If yes, please provide copy of IEP.) If your child has an IEP, what is the child's educational label? _____

_____

B. *Is your child currently in a school program (name of school) or home-schooled?* _____

_____

C. *Has your Child had an IQ assessment?* No ☐ Yes ☐ *If yes, please give date of assessment, test name, and IQ score if known:* _____

_____

D. *Academic Skills: Please check your child's current independent/mastered skills in all areas.*
Attending

  ☐ Sits at a table and completes tasks   ☐ Plays with toys independently

  ☐ Looks at pictures in books   ☐ Plays with toys with others prompting

Gross motor/play	**Matching and sorting**	**Visual–motor coordination/sequencing patterns**	
☐ Jumps	☐ Objects	☐ Pull apart or take off tasks	☐ Cutting
☐ Runs	☐ Colors		☐ 1-inch strips
☐ Throws	☐ Shapes	☐ Put/push together tasks	☐ 2-inch strips
☐ Swings	☐ Pictures		☐ across line
☐ Other	☐ Pictures to objects	☐ Turn/twist tasks	☐ shapes (1-, 2-, 3-sided)
		☐ Open/close tasks	☐ Imitates patterns
	☐ Size (big/little)	☐ Imitates 2- to 4-step block designs from demo/picture model	☐ Color, shape, color–shape, picture, bead patterns (ABA, ABBA, ABC)
	☐ Functional categories		

(continued)

Chores/office skills		Social/play skills
Office	**Chores**	☐ Engages in a variety of sensory mediums in play
☐ Folds paper	☐ Gathers trash	☐ Returns greeting
☐ Stuffs envelopes	☐ Sets and clears table	☐ Takes turn w/ simple action toys/ sensory materials
☐ Collates	☐ Sweeps	☐ Engages in toy play imitation
☐ Files	☐ Puts toys away	☐ Sits in group for up to ____ minutes
☐ Alphabetizes	☐ Sorts silverware	☐ Imitates simple body movements
☐ Stamps ink pad	☐ Empties dishwasher	☐ Passes objects to peers when asked
☐ Addresses labels	☐ Loads dishwasher	☐ Plays in same area with others (parallel play)
☐ Staples	☐ Folds shirts	☐ Takes turns in simple board games
☐ Punches holes	☐ Waters plants	☐ Engages in familiar dramatic play routines
☐ Operates a computer	☐ Sorts lights and darks	☐ Assists younger peers
☐ Delivers/sorts mail	☐ Assists with cooking	
☐ Picks up recycling bins	☐ Follows picture/word sequence to prepare food item	
	☐ Wipes tables	
	☐ Other: _____	

Math		Writing	
☐ Counts rotely	☐ Understands more/ less	☐ Imitates simple drawings (lines, square, circle, triangle, and variations of these, such as circle within a circle, meaningful forms)	☐ Writing
☐ Counts 1:1 correspondence	☐ Addition		☐ Letters
☐ Recognize/identify/ match numbers	☐ Subtraction		☐ Numbers
☐ Sequences numbers (dot-to-dot/puzzles)	☐ Money skills (value, name)		☐ Name
	☐ Time skills		☐ Words
	☐ Measurement: (length, weight, quantity)	☐ Coloring	☐ Sentences
☐ Matches numbers to quantities	☐ Calculator	☐ Trace paths	☐ On unlined paper
☐ Responds to "How many?"		☐ Trace or copy	☐ On lined paper
☐ Gives correct number of objects		☐ Letters	☐ Types words/ sentences on computer
		☐ Numbers	
		☐ Name	
		☐ Words	

Reading		
☐ Matches letters (upper/ lower case)	☐ Sight words	☐ Community:
☐ Identifies letters	☐ Follows instructions	☐ Menu
☐ Sequences ABCs	☐ Pictured	☐ Telephone book
☐ Match	☐ Written	☐ Dictionary
☐ Word to word	☐ Sequences social story cards	☐ Public transportation
☐ Word to object	☐ Answers who, what, when, and where questions about story paragraphs	☐ Textbooks
☐ Word to picture		
☐ Recognize name		

2

Medical Health Assessment
and Treatment Issues in Autism

Edward Goldson
Margaret Bauman

This chapter reviews medical disorders that frequently affect older children and adolescents with autism; many may be overlooked or go unsuspected. This is of great concern to parents and a challenge to the primary care physician. Primary care physicians must be careful not to simply attribute changes in behavior or the appearance of signs and symptoms of illness to the idea that "this is just autism"; rather, physicians must take responsibility for the careful review of presenting symptoms in a child with autism and reduce their exclusive reliance on specialists. The goal of this chapter is to provide clinicians, particularly primary care physicians, with the background to better understand some of the atypical symptoms encountered in children with autism. In addition, this chapter provides a systematic framework for the evaluation and treatment of this population of children. Particular emphasis will be on the recognition of significant medical problems in the face of often unusual modes of presentation in nonverbal or hypoverbal children who cannot indicate their discomfort to others and may also have difficulty localizing pain. Finally, this chapter reviews plans for the development of national guidelines to ensure high-quality, comprehensive health care for complex, often difficult to examine children and adolescents with special needs.

Over the years, the field of medicine has moved into a managed care format, making it increasingly challenging for primary care physicians and specialists to devote the time within a busy daily practice to delve into the presentation of perplexing symptoms in children who are not cooperative or cannot speak, or whose office behavior may be difficult. A further complication is the fact that many of these symptoms may have causes that are not immediately apparent. This situation is of significant concern, given the fact that the American Academy of Pediatrics has estimated that approximately 10–15% of the pediatric population in the United States consists of children with special health care needs. It is now known that a significant number of them are children with autism spectrum disorders, which are evident in one of every 166 to 250 children worldwide (Fombonne, 2003).

While it is important that all children have access to health care, it is similarly important that this care be of good quality in order to ensure opportunities for optimal developmental progress. However, the meaning of "quality" in health care, as well as what constitutes "optimal health," can be difficult to define and measure. Quality health care involves a clear definition of the patient population of concern, a delineation of effective and efficient strategies for diagnosis and treatment, and a good understanding of potential outcomes assuming the provision of appropriate therapeutic interventions. In order to achieve these goals, it is necessary to have in place a systematic approach to evaluation and treatment as well as access to multidisciplinary, community-based diagnostic and therapeutic resources and, most importantly, coordination of care.

Although children with autism share the core symptoms of impaired social skills, delayed, disordered language, and stereotyped behaviors and isolated areas of interest, they are a heterogeneous group both etiologically and clinically (Kanner, 1943, 1949). These children can present with a broad range of cognitive and functional skills, behavioral disorders, unusual talents, and neurodevelopmental trajectories. Interventions that prove effective for one child may be ineffective for another. Some children with autism will be symptomatic almost from birth, while others may not show signs of developmental disturbances until well into the second year of life. Thus, the medical and educational approach to the child with autism must be individualized in order to give each child the opportunity to achieve maximum good health and developmental potential.

While health care management for children with autism is important throughout life, this chapter focuses on medical issues that frequently emerge during middle childhood through adolescence, a period of life that can be challenging even in typically developing children. These challenges can be compounded when the child is nonverbal or has severe developmental delays. Further, obtaining an accurate and meaningful medical history and conducting an informative physical examination can also be difficult. However, despite these inherent problems, it must be recalled that these children have many of the same health issues as those encountered in their typically developing peers. Thus, the same "rules" of assessment and diagnosis should apply. The clinical presentation of medical disorders in children with autism may be atypical and, therefore, unfamiliar to the average physician; however, significant changes in behavior should be considered as a "red flag," especially in nonverbal children. Alternatively, the child may be able to provide some indication of discomfort but have trouble localizing that discomfort, or parents may suspect or describe a change in their child's routine or behavior that is otherwise unexplained. Under these circumstances, it is important for the physician to take the time necessary to consider a variety of medical possibilities, gather a detailed history including timing of events, and obtain further diagnostic assessments as indicated.

THE MEDICAL HOME

Children with autism can present with a complex variety of behavioral and medical disorders and require a wide array of therapeutic interventions. Therefore, the availability of a site in which this care can be coordinated in a cohesive fashion is essential. The "medical home" concept has the potential to achieve this goal in a cost-effective and comprehensive manner. The medical home is defined as the setting in which "health care services are accessible, family centered, continuous, comprehensive, coordinated and compassionate" (American Academy of Pediatrics, 1992, p. 774). Thus, within this medical home, the primary care physician can provide care in partnership with allied health care professionals and the family. The medical home also can provide staff that are sensitive to the challenges of children with special needs, establish a forum for problem solving and advocacy, and be available for all children. The result of health care provision within a medical home is improved coordination and efficacy of diagnosis and treatment, more efficient use of limited resources, and increased professional satisfaction.

MEDICAL ISSUES OF CONCERN

It is the responsibility of the primary care physician to diagnose, or at least be alert to, developmental delays and medical disorders in children of all ages, including those with any disorder, including autism. It is now recognized that children with autism comprise a heterogeneous group of patients in terms of cognitive, functional, and behavioral characteristics. Like typically developing children, patients with autism can be impacted by a number of childhood illnesses, but their behavior, atypical communication skills, and altered sensory processing may make these illnesses difficult to diagnose. Thus, the primary care physician must maintain a high level of vigilance with these children, most especially with the recognition that the presentation of some of these illnesses may be atypical. In some cases, the definitive diagnosis and ultimate treatment may require a team of professionals with varying expertise. The fact that the child has autism does not rule out the possibility that he or she may have one or more other illnesses or disorders. These potential associations introduce the concept of "double syndromes" (Gillberg & Coleman, 1996, 2000a, 2000c), namely the existence of a potentially recognizable syndrome in the presence of autism spectrum disorders. This concept should enable the physician to think more broadly with respect to the management of children with autism.

Seizure Disorders

Since Kanner's original paper on infantile autism, published in 1943, the association of autism and seizure disorders has been recognized and reported. Current data suggest that approximately one-third of individuals with autism are known to have seizures at some time during their lives, with peak risk periods in early childhood and during the adolescent years (Volkmar & Nelson, 1990; Gillberg & Coleman, 2000b). No one seizure type has been reported to be specifically associated with autism, and most known electroencephalographic (EEG) patterns and clinically expressed seizure types have been observed in the autism population. As is the case with typically developing children, if seizures are suspected, physicians should implement the appropriate diagnostic procedures, including the performance of an EEG, identify the type(s) of seizures, and begin treatment. The involvement of a neurologist is desirable in most cases, especially if the seizure management becomes complex. In some cases, the onset of a seizure may signal the need for more extensive evaluations and referrals to specialists to rule out the possibility of underlying metabolic disorders, syndromes, degenerative disorders, or head trauma or mass lesions, previously unsuspected. Although there is a general consensus that most clinical seizure disorders of childhood should be treated, there is less agreement with regard to the diagnosis and management of "subclinical" seizures. A child is considered by some experts to have "subclinical" seizures if that child presents with a change in behavior or developmental progression or new unusual mannerisms, and the EEG demonstrates abnormal paroxysmal electrographic events, usually without clinical accompaniment. There is disagreement reported in the literature with regard to the concept of subclinical seizures and, further, if they are a true phenomenon, how they should be best managed. Some reports detail behavioral, cognitive, and/or linguistic improvement following the initiation of anticonvulsant therapy. However, many of these reports should be interpreted with caution since some of the anticonvulsants used to treat seizures, most notably valproic acid and carbamazepine, are known to have mood-stabilizing effects, and the apparent clinical improvement in some cases may have little to do with seizure control. The fact that there has been clinical improvement reported in some children with autism is, however, of interest and more carefully designed research studies are warranted.

Atypical behavioral patterns can often be observed in children with autism, further complicating the diagnosis of a potential seizure disorder. While it may be stating the obvious, it is worth noting that not all unusual movements or mannerisms seen and reported in children with autism are seizure related. Some in fact may be related to other medical disorders such as otitis media, gastroesophageal reflux disorder (GERD), or other gastrointestinal disturbances (Niehus & Lord, 2006; Valicent-McDermott et al., 2006). Thus, it is critical to carefully analyze the behaviors of concern in order to target the most appropriate and therefore effective treatment. Since more often than not, the child does not exhibit the concerning behaviors during the office visit, asking the family to videotape the behavioral events at home or school can be very informative and frequently lead to a diagnosis.

Approximately one-third of parents of children with autism report a history of developmental regression in their child, most commonly around 18 to 24 months of age (Rapin, 1995). These regressions may either be acute or may occur over weeks to months. In some cases, there has been a level of spontaneous recovery, rarely back to baseline, but, more commonly, functional improvement follows the implementation of intensive therapeutic interventions both at home and at school. Numerous hypotheses have been offered to explain the phenomenon of regression with little consensus at this time. Suggested causes have included emotional stress secondary to an otherwise benign intercurrent illness, trivial physical trauma, the sudden absence of a significant adult figure in the child's life, moving a household or other significant change in the daily environment, and, in recent years, vaccinations. In a small portion of children with autistic regression, the developmental deterioration has seemed to coincide with the advent of clinical seizures or be associated with paroxysmal activity on an EEG obtained at or near the time of the regression. However, there continues to be a debate within the research community as to whether or not there is a direct association between EEG abnormalities and autistic regression. Although it is believed that there is a higher incidence of seizures and regression among mentally retarded autistic children than in those of higher cognitive ability, there is no evidence that autistic regression is a risk factor for seizures (Tuchman & Rapin, 1997).

One additional disorder that may be difficult to distinguish from seizure disorders in autism is the Landau–Kleffner syndrome (LKS; Landau & Kleffner, 1957). LKS is a known epileptic syndrome in which there is an association between an acquired aphasia and the presence of a specific epileptiform pattern on the EEG associated with spike and spike and slow wave discharges over the temporal and parietal regions of the brain. The onset and clinical course of LKS are very different from those of epilepsy in children with autism or autistic regression. In LKS, language regression is often dramatic and occurs well after 3 years of age, typically after a period of normal development. Affected children usually retain their social awareness, use of gestures, interest in toys, imaginary play, and cognitive abilities, all skills that are impaired in childhood autism (Mantovani, 2000; Rapin, 1995; Tuchman, 2000). The EEG pattern in LKS is characterized by centrotemporal spike waves, whereas in autism, EEG patterns tend to be more variable and diffuse (Mantovani, 2000; Tuchman, 2000). Thus, there should be little confusion between LKS and childhood autism, and treatment approaches to LKS should not be generalized to the treatment and management of autistic regression (Mantovani, 2000; Tuchman, 1997).

Sleep Disorders

Disturbances of sleep are said to occur in approximately 30% of typically developing children. Although relatively common across the age span, sleep disruptions are more common in early childhood and decrease in frequency with age (Ferber, 1996; Richdale, 1999). Sleep disorders have been categorized into three subtypes: (1) trouble getting to sleep and staying asleep, (2) sleeping too much, and (3) events that interfere with sleep, such as nightmares or night terrors. The first two subtypes are considered "dyssomnias" and the third type is called "parasomnias" (Stores & Wiggs, 2001).

The physiology of sleep is complex and involves both rapid-eye-movement (REM) sleep and non-rapid-eye-movement (NREM) sleep. In theory, sleep is said to provide physical and psychological restoration, energy conservation, consolidation of memories, discharge of emotions, brain growth, and other biological functions, such as secretion of growth hormone and cortisol production (Stores, 2001). REM sleep is associated with "active sleep" and makes up approximately 20–25% of the sleep state in children and adolescents. NREM sleep is divided into four stages according to electrographic patterns observed on the EEG, with Stages 3 and 4 being associated with the deepest level of sleep. REM and NREM sleep patterns alternate throughout the night, with NREM sleep decreasing and REM sleep increasing as the night progresses (Mindel & Owens, 2003; Stores, 2001).

During any 24-hour cycle, there are normally periods of maximum alertness and maximum sleepiness. These periods are influenced by social cues, ambient temperature, mealtime, noise level, and the tasks at hand. These circadian rhythms are also influenced by environmental factors called "zeitgebers," the most powerful of which is the light–dark cycle. During these cycles, light is transmitted to the "circadian clock" located in the suprachiasmatic nucleus (SCN) of the hypothalamus via the circadian photoreceptor system in the retina, which is separate from the visual system. This mechanism then influences the production of melatonin in the pineal gland. Melatonin is activated in darkness and is turned off during periods of light. The secretion of melatonin also varies with age, nighttime levels peaking between 1 and 3 years, after which point it declines. Thus, infants generally sleep approximately 18 hours during a 24-hour period, while 4-year-olds sleep an average of 12 hours, 10-year-olds sleep 8–10 hours and adolescents 7–8.5 hours per day.

Sleep disruptions appear to be common among children with autism and have an impact on the well-being of the entire family (Allik, Larsson, & Smedje, 2006; Honomichl, Goodlin-Jones, Burnham, Gaylor, & Anders, 2002; Patzold, Richdale, & Toue, 1998; Richdale, 1999). These disturbances are more common in very young children but can persist into adolescence and adulthood. In an analysis of the sleep patterns of 44- to 152-month-old children with autism in comparison with age-matched, typically developing children, Patzold and colleagues (1998) noted that children with autism had shorter sleep duration, longer sleep latencies, and more frequent nighttime awakenings followed by prolonged periods of wakefulness than control children. In addition, children with autism displayed more unusual bedtime rituals, such as the need to sleep with their parents until they fell asleep, the need for all family members to go to bed at the same time, or the refusal to get into bed. The researchers also looked at daytime behaviors and noted that the children with autism demonstrated more energy and periods of overarousal, and more difficult daytime behaviors than the control children. The researchers suggested that some of the impaired social relatedness and disruptive behaviors exhibited by the children with autism might be related to their inefficient sleep patterns.

Limoges and colleagues (2005) examined sleep patterns in adults with high-functioning autism and Asperger disorder without sleep complaints in comparison to age- and sex-matched controls. Sleep questionnaires suggested evidence of insomnia and/or a tolerable phase advance of the sleep–wake cycle among the participants with autism spectrum disorder. Electromyographic (EMG) and EEG studies on a subset of these participants revealed prolonged sleep latency, more frequent nocturnal awakenings, lower sleep efficiency, increased duration of Stage 1 sleep, decreased non-REM sleep (Stages 2, 3, and 4) and slow-wave sleep (Stages 3 and 4), fewer Stage 2 EEG sleep spindles, and a lower number of rapid eye movements in REM sleep. The researchers concluded that adults with autism spectrum disorders demonstrated atypical sleep patterns by EEG and EMG and that these findings would be consistent with the concept of an atypical organization of neural networks subserving the macro- and microstructure of sleep architecture in individuals with autism.

Using parental report, sleep patterns have been compared in children with mental retardation, autism, learning disabilities, and typical development (Honomichl et al., 2002). In this study, children with autism and typically developing children were found to have the same quantity of sleep as did children with mental retardation (MR) and learning disabilities (LD). But the parents of the children with autism reported more dyssomnias and parasomnias in their children, as well as issues such as talking in their sleep, environmental sensitivities, disoriented awakenings, and the need for comfort measures such as a nightlight or a transitional object, as compared to the children with MR and LD (Honomichl et al., 2002).

Additional sleep-related events, including nocturnal enuresis, head banging and rocking behavior, nightmares, night terrors, and bruxism (grinding of the teeth), have been reported in typically developing children as well as in children with a variety of disabilities, including autism (Hering, Epstein, Elroy, Iancu, & Zelnick, 1999; Schreck &

Mullick, 2000; Wiggs & Stores, 2004; Williams, Sears, & Allard, 2004). One of the more serious concerns among the autism population is nighttime wanderings, which can pose a serious safety concern, especially when wandering occurs at night without parental observation or supervision. Thus, it is imperative that parents and physicians work together to ensure the child's safety within the home environment. (See Chapter 13 for more information about safety issues for children with autism.)

The causes of sleep disturbances can be many and may often be obscure. Causes may include seizures, maltreatment and abuse, or undetected injuries or fractures. While relatively rare, these should be considered in the face of persistent sleep disturbances and in the absence of other health-related disorders. There are several medical conditions that can negatively affect sleep, both in typically developing children and in children with autism. One such condition is GERD, in which gastric contents reflux from the stomach into the esophagus, frequently exacerbated by lying in the supine position, causing discomfort, retching, vomiting, or throat irritation, and thus resulting in nighttime awakenings. A trial of antacids may be both therapeutic and diagnostic. If more conservative interventions prove ineffective, a referral to a gastroenterologist may lead to a more specific diagnosis and more specific treatment modalities. Another condition that could negatively impact sleep is sleep apnea. This disorder is frequently associated with nocturnal snoring, irregular breathing with prolonged apneic spells, restlessness, and "twitchy" leg movements. Apnea may be caused by central nervous system dysregulation of arousal and/or respiratory control (central apnea) or by enlarged tonsils and/or adenoids (obstructive apnea). An all-night sleep study may be useful in distinguishing between the two should there be any question of etiology. A referral to an otolaryngologist (ear, nose, and throat specialist) may also be useful. In considering other medical conditions that might impact on sleep, one must also take into account the possibility of a urinary tract infection or bladder spasticity, both of which can be associated with nocturnal enuresis. Bedwetting can often be associated with sleep disturbances and merits careful medical investigation. Thus, medical conditions should be ruled out before assuming that the sleep disorder exhibited by the child with autism is simply a behavioral aspect of the child's diagnosis of autism.

Treatment of disordered sleep onset can include behavioral strategies and improved bedtime "hygiene" (Stores, 1996). Melatonin has been helpful in many cases, as well as some prescription medications such as clonidine or trazodone. However, all medications should be used with caution and with careful monitoring for potential side effects.

Gastrointestinal Disorders

There has been much discussion in the lay press, online, and, to a lesser extent, in the medical literature regarding a possible relationship between gastrointestinal (GI) dysfunction and autism. Parents frequently report flatus, eructation, chronic constipation, recurrent diarrhea, dietary selectivity, and general GI discomfort in their autistic children. In 1999, Horvath and colleagues (Horvath, Papadimitriou, Rabsztyn, Drachenberg, & Tildon, 1999) evaluated a group of children with autism who presented with complaints of abdominal pain, chronic diarrhea, gas/bloating, and unexplained nighttime awakening. The researchers noted that a significant number of these children demonstrated reflux esophagitis, disaccharide malabsorption, and gastric and duodenal inflammation. Since many of these conditions have also been reported in children with other neurological disorders, these disorders do not appear to be specific to autism. In the past, celiac disease was considered to be a possible cause of autism, but more recent research has failed to show an association between the two disorders. Steatorrhea/autism syndrome, in which the child presents with fatty, foul-smelling diarrhea, has also been considered causative of autism, but no clear etiology for this association has been found and no growth failure in this disorder has been reported. Lastly, Wakefield, Anthony, & Murch (2000) have described lymphoid nodular hyperplasia in the GI tracts of a number of children with autism and have suggested that this finding is specific to autism. However, research from other groups has not supported this contention (e.g., Quigley & Hurley, 2000 and Kuddo & Nelson, 2003). Nevertheless, the debate continues and a final answer to this question remains for future research.

When present, GI symptoms should be taken seriously and deserve to be investigated and therapeutically addressed inasmuch as they can be associated with discomfort, behavioral disruptions, and reduced quality of life. Many children with autism, especially those who are low-functioning and/or nonverbal, may present with aggression and/or self-injurious behaviors and, in some cases, without obvious GI symptoms. It is likely that at least some of these children do not have the language with which to express their discomfort or to accurately localize their pain and, therefore, they may be demonstrating their discomfort through behavioral means. Elimination diets have been attempted with variable results. At this time, in the face of our current lack of knowledge, in the presence of these symptoms, a referral to a GI specialist is warranted. Well-designed research is needed to clarify the prevalence and types of GI disorders within the autism population and the symptoms with which the child with autism may present (some of which may be atypical), as well as the development of evidence-based, effective treatments (Erickson et al., 2005).

Hearing Impairment

The incidence of hearing impairment appears to be increased among children with autism as compared to the general population. In a study of 1,150 children assessed at a school for the deaf, 46 children also met the criteria for autism. Of this group, 50% had known causes for the hearing loss, including congenital rubella, preterm birth, bacterial meningitis, and malformation syndromes. The cause in the remainder of the children with autism was genetic in 13% and unknown in 37% (Jure, Rapin, & Tuchman, 1991). In Sweden another study of 199 children with autism found mild to moderate sensorineural hearing loss in 7.9% of the children, unilateral hearing loss in 1.9%, and pronounced to profound hearing loss in 3.5% of individuals, with a total of 13.3% of the population having some form of sensorineural hearing loss (Rosenhall, Nordin, Sandstrom, Ahlsen, & Gillberg, 1999). In addition, 23.5% of this population had serous otitis media, of which 18.3% had conductive hearing loss.

Hearing abilities in children with autism can be difficult to evaluate. Often, the usual behavioral measures employed to assess hearing cannot be performed. Regardless of this difficulty, all children with autism should have their hearing tested, as early as possible. The most effective and reliable measure is the auditory brainstem response (ABR) examination. In this procedure, children are presented with several distinct tones. Their response to these tones is reflected in an electrical pattern in the brain, which is measured using an EEG. The nature and degree of hearing loss can be quite accurately determined with this method and appropriate interventions can then be instituted. If the hearing loss is significant, then hearing aids may be used.

Sensory Processing Disorders

There has been much discussion about sensory processing in children with autism, and sensory processing disorders have recently been defined (Interdisciplinary Council on Developmental and Learning Disorders, 2005; Zero to Three, 2005). Sensory processing disorders are generally characterized by difficulties processing internal and external sensory information, thus preventing the child from functioning adaptively in the environment. The major central processes that seem to be affected include vestibular (gravity and movement), proprioceptive (muscles and joints), and tactile (touch) senses, along with vision and hearing. Because many of the behaviors observed in children with autism are similar to those encountered among nonautistic children with sensory processing disorders, it can be difficult to distinguish between the two. There is nothing to suggest, however, that a child with autism cannot have a sensory processing disorder. If a sensory processing disorder is suspected, the child should be referred to an occupational therapist who is trained in the evaluation and treatment of children with this disorder. (See Chapter 5 for a review of sensory issues in autism.)

Attention-Deficit/Hyperactivity Disorder

The exact incidence of attention-deficit/hyperactivity disorder (ADHD) behaviors among children with autism is unknown. Aman, Van Bourgondien, Wolford, and Sarphare (1995) reviewed the literature and found that about 12% of children with autism spectrum disorders were treated with stimulant medications, suggesting that this constellation of symptoms is frequently identified and treated with psychotropic medications. However, there is a paucity of research about the efficacy of these medications in ameliorating ADHD symptoms in this population (King, 2000).

Puberty and Sexuality

Children and youths with autism have sexuality needs and considerations. The impairment specific to the diagnosis of autism can present challenges to their ability to establish and maintain emotional and sexual intimacy (Murphy & Elias, 2006). For the general population, puberty in children in the United States starts between 8.5 and 13 years of age in girls and between 9 and 14 years of age for boys, and this also appears to be the case for children with autism (Murphy & Elias, 2006). In addition, as is the case with typically developing children, several medical issues should be considered as children enter puberty, including nutrition (either poor nutrition, weight gain, or obesity), scoliosis, skin problems (e.g., acne), hypertension, and fatigue, which may be associated with hypothyroidism or infectious mononucleosis (Volkmar & Wiesner, 2004).

Teaching any child about sexuality can be challenging. This is even more the case for children with autism, due in part to the problems of communication and social understanding, intellectual disability, and the constellation of behavioral problems specific to the autism population. The parent or teacher must be sure that the child understands what is being communicated, and appropriate behavior needs to be taught and encouraged. That is to say, one needs to teach the concepts of privacy and modesty and to model what is appropriate and inappropriate behavior, recognizing the contexts in which sexual behaviors take place. For example, masturbation is a normal and acceptable behavior for both girls and boys, but it is not acceptable or appropriate when it takes place in public.

Girls, depending on the degree of their impairment, may have to be taught about breast development as well as menstruation. Some girls may be able to care for themselves independently but may not understand what is happening with their bodies and will need much reassurance, guidance, and support. All girls deserve appropriate gynecological care. If a young woman is not sexually active, a pelvic examination is not indicated during the first 2 years of menarche. But, an external examination should be performed by a trusted clinician who is accompanied by a trusted parent or caretaker. As with other aspects of the physical examination (see the following section), the child must be alerted to what will take place and should be reassured that no harm or pain will befall her.

Unfortunately, there are no accepted general guidelines for how to address puberty with all of its physical, psychological, and emotional ramifications. A sensitive, individualized approach to addressing this developmental transition is best. (See Chapter 3 for a review of sexuality issues in autism.)

APPROACHES TO THE MEDICAL EVALUATION
OF THE CHILD WITH AUTISM

Access to quality medical care for children with autism is a unique challenge for their parents and families. Attempting to provide that care to a frequently anxious, nonverbal, often impulsive, and noncompliant child can be equally challenging for the practicing physician. Patient anxiety is likely to be exacerbated by the novel, often busy and overstimulating environment of a hospital setting or pediatric waiting room. While it could be argued that examining such children in the comfort and familiarity of their home would be optimal, this arrangement is largely impractical. However, several approaches have proven useful. Planning physician visits after hours when the office is likely to be less busy and there is a shorter wait to see the doctor can often be helpful. However, this timing runs the risk of having the child seen at the end of a very tiring school day when fatigue could be a potential negative factor. Another option is to allow the child to bring a favored toy, portable video player, or Game Boy. A third approach is to desensitize the child to the office visit experience through repeated trips to the office, usually after hours, and behavioral techniques such as explaining to the child exactly where the child will go and what will happen. No medical encounter actually takes place. In this way, the child is familiarized with making the trip to the clinic, via car or public transportation, and then going into the office. While this latter plan may take longer, it is ultimately likely to have a longer-lasting effect.

It is often helpful for physicians to arrange the office so that there is space in which the child can move about and have a variety of toys available. The physician should plan to speak with the parent before approaching the child, thus giving the child time to accommodate to the environment. If the child resists being placed on the examining table, he can be comfortably examined in a chair or in his mother's lap. The child should be allowed to play with some of the medical instruments prior to their use. Visually demonstrating the use of each instrument can also be useful. The child should always be given advance verbal and visual warning when approached for any procedure and parents should always be available to the child for assurance. (See Chapter 9 for a discussion of ideas regarding how to best prepare a child with autism for novel experiences.)

While the examination itself is a challenge, there is the equally difficult task of recognizing significant health concerns in a nonverbal or hypoverbal child who is unable to accurately convey or localize pain or discomfort. Thus, physicians must use their powers of observation and clinical instinct in order to consider reasonable diagnoses in the face of few traditionally recognizable clues. For example, some children with autism may present with episodes of aggressive or self-injurious behavior. Despite the complete absence of gastrointestinal symptoms, many of these children have been found to have disorders such as colitis, gastroesophageal reflux, or esophagitis (Buie, 2005). When the underlying medical condition is recognized and treated, the behaviors subside or disappear completely. Thus, to assume that such negative behaviors are "just part of the autism" could be a significant disservice to the child, who will continue to experience pain, be poorly responsive to medical or behavioral management, experience poor quality of life, and be too uncomfortable to adequately benefit from therapeutic and educational programs. Therefore, even though there may be no overt symptoms to suggest a specific diagnosis, disorders such as ear infections, dental pain, gastrointestinal disorders, appendicitis, joint pain, or unrecognized injury should be considered. No matter how difficult the child may be to examine, the physician must always remember that children with autism can and do have the same range of illnesses as those seen in typically developing children, and that these illnesses need to be investigated, diagnosed, and treated. Failure to actively pursue underlying medical disorders in children with autism is not only poor medical care, it could be life threatening.

CONCLUSIONS

Children with autism present many challenges when it comes to providing their medical care. Setting aside the issue of insurance coverage, the challenge of providing comprehensive, coordinated, family-focused, and sensitive care is paramount to the well-being of this population of children. In this chapter we have discussed the concept of a medical home and identified some of the more common medical problems identified in the school-age child and adolescent with autism. Physicians must be mindful not to simply attribute all symptoms to the diagnosis of autism, as this can place the child in danger of not being adequately treated.

In addition, we have put forth an approach to the examination of the child with autism. There are no "shortcuts" or "pat" answers to the care of these individuals. One needs to be mindful that children with autism have the same medical and surgical problems that typically developing children may experience. Thus, it behooves the physician to be even more attentive to these children and to listen to and collaborate with the parent, since the ability of the child to provide a comprehensible medical history is frequently compromised. It is critical that parents trust and have confidence in their child's physician and are able to establish a partnership with the physician. This relationship can extend beyond the purely medical aspects of the child's care in the form of advocacy and can serve to optimize the child's outcome and ability to access services, thus enabling the child to function more autonomously.

The care of the child with autism is challenging. At the same time, when there is truly comprehensive care, the rewards for the physician, child, and family can be enormous. This is an exciting, yet somewhat difficult group of children to care for. Our challenge as physicians is to serve them well.

FUTURE DIRECTIONS

The provision of quality medical care to children with autism is extremely variable throughout the United States. In general, children living in urban areas, often in the shadows of large academic centers, receive more appropriate health care and have more therapeutic and educational options than those children living in more rural communities where fewer resources may be available. However, even in the best medical centers, the quality of care can vary. In large part, this situation reflects assumptions about what autism is and who autistic children are. In addition, as has been discussed, the child with autism is frequently very difficult to examine, cannot verbally relate or accurately localize discomfort, and may not present with symptoms that the average physician has been taught to recognize as being significant. This situation places the health, and in fact the very life of the child with autism in serious jeopardy. Given the growing prevalence rates for autism spectrum disorders, there is a real urgency to remedy this situation. First, pediatric training programs should begin to incorporate exposure of interns, residents, and fellows to the complexity of the autistic population and to the "language" of pain and distress in nonverbal children. Currently, the American Academy of Pediatrics has taken these concerns under advisement and is in the process of proposing guidelines for improved medical management for children with special needs, including children with autism. In addition, the Autism Treatment Network (ATN), a collaboration by five medical centers in the United States, has been established to formally investigate a number of medical disorders in autistic children and to establish evidence-based standards of best practices. Thus, it is likely that national standards of care for autistic children will be established within the next 3 to 5 years and, with the availability of such standards, the quality of life, longevity, and developmental outcomes for these children will improve substantially in the years to come.

REFERENCES

Allik, H., Larsson, J. O., & Smedje, H. (2006). Insomnia in school-age children with Asperger syndrome or high-functioning autism. *BMC Psychiatry, 6,* 18.

Aman, M. G., Van Bourgondien, M. E., Wolford, P., & Sarphare, G. (1995). Psychotropic and anticonvulsant drugs in subjects with autism: Prevalence and patterns of use. *Journal of the American Academy of Child and Adolescent Psychiatry, 34,* 1672–1681.

American Academy of Pediatrics. (2001). The pediatrician's role in the diagnosis and management of autistic spectrum disorder in children. *Pediatrics, 107,* 1221–1226.

American Academy of Pediatrics, Ad Hoc Task Force on Definition of the Medical Home. (1992). The medical home. *Pediatrics, 90,* 774.

Erickson, C. A., Stigler, K. A., Corkins, M. R., Posey, D. J., Fitzgerald, J. F., & McDougle, C. J. (2006). Gastrointestinal factors in autistic disorder. *Journal of Autism and Developmental Disorders, 35,* 713–727.

Ferber, R. (1996). Childhood sleep disorders. *Neurologic Clinics, 14,* 493–511.

Fombonne, E. (2003). The prevalence of autism. *Journal of the American Medical Association, 289,* 87–89.

Gillberg, C., & Coleman, M. (1996). Autism and medical disorders: A review of the literature. *Developmental Medicine and Child Neurology, 3,* 191–202.

Gillberg, C., & Coleman, M. (2000a). Diagnosis in infancy. In C. Gillberg & M.

Coleman (Eds.), *The biology of the autistic syndromes.* (pp. 53–62). London: MacKeith Press.

Gillberg, C., & Coleman, M. (2000b). Epilepsy and electrophysiology. In C. Gillberg & M. Coleman (Eds.), *The biology of the autistic syndromes.* (pp. 185–196). London: MacKeith Press.

Gillberg, C., & Coleman, M. (2000c). The disease entities of autism. In C. Gillberg & M. Coleman (Eds.), *The biology of the autistic syndromes.* (pp. 118–135). London: MacKeith Press.

Greenspan, S. I., & Wieder, S. (2005). *Diagnostic manual for infancy and early childhood: Mental health, developmental, regulatory-sensory processing and language disorders and learning challenges.* Bethesda, MD: Interdisciplinary Council on Developmental and Learning Disorders.

Hering, E., Epstein, R., Elroy, S., Iancu, D. R., & Zelnick, N. (1999). Sleep patterns in autistic children. *Journal of Autism and Developmental Disorders, 29,* 143–147.

Honomichl, R. D., Goodlin-Jones, B. L., Burnham, M., Gaylor, M., & Anders, T. F. (2002). Sleep patterns of children with pervasive developmental disorders. *Journal of Autism and Developmental Disorders, 32,* 553–561.

Horvath, K., Papadimitriou, J. C., Rabsztyn, A., Drachenberg, C., & Tildon, J. T. (1999). Gastrointestinal abnormalities in children with autistic disorder. *Journal of Pediatrics, 135,* 559–563.

Jure, R., Rapin, I., & Tuchman, R. F. (1991). Hearing-impaired autistic children. *Developmental Medicine and Child Neurology, 33,* 1062–1072.

Kanner, L. (1943). Autistic disturbances of affective contact. *Nervous Child, 2,* 217–250.

Kanner, L. (1949). Problems of nosology and psychodynamics of early infantile autism. *American Journal of Orthopsychiatry, 19,* 416–426.

King, B. H. (2000). Pharmacological treatment of mood disturbances, aggression, and self-injury in persons with pervasive developmental disorders. *Journal of Autism and Developmental Disorders, 30,* 439–445.

Kuddo, T., & Nelson, K. (2003). How common are gastrointestinal disorders in children with autism? *Current Opinion in Pediatrics, 15,* 339–343.

Landau, W. M., & Kleffner, F. (1957). Syndrome of acquired aphasia with convulsive disorder in children. *Neurology, 7,* 523–530.

Limoges, E., Mottron, L., Bolduc, C., Berthiaume, C., & Godbout, R. (2005). Atypical sleep architecture and the autism phenotype. *Brain, 128,* 1049–1061.

Mantovani, J. F. (2000). Autistic regression and Landau-Kleffner syndrome: Progress or confusion. *Developmental Medicine and Child Neurology, 42,* 349–353.

Mindel, J. A., & Owens, J. A. (2003). *A clinical guide to pediatric sleep: Diagnosis and management of sleep problems.* Philadelphia: Lippincott Williams & Wilkins.

Murphy, N. A., & Elias, E. R. (2006). Sexuality of children and adolescents with developmental disabilities. *Pediatrics, 118,* 398–403.

Niehus, R., & Lord, C. (2006). Early medical history of children with autism spectrum disorders. *Journal of Developmental and Behavioral Pediatrics (Supplement), 27,* S120–S127.

Patzold, L. M., Richdale, A. L., & Tone, B. J. (1998). An investigation into sleep characteristics of children with autism and Apserger's Disorder. *Journal of Paediatrics and Child Health, 34,* 528–533.

Quigley, E. M., & Hurley, D. (2000). Autism and the gastrointestinal tract. *American Journal of Gastroenterology, 95,* 2154–2156.

Rapin, I. (1995). Autistic regression and disintegrative disorder: How important is the role of epilepsy. *Seminars in Pediatric Neurology, 24,* 278–285.

Richdale, A. L. (1999). Sleep problems in autism: Prevalence, cause and intervention. *Developmental Medicine and Child Neurology, 41,* 60–66.

Rosenhall, U., Nordin, V., Sandstrom, M., Ahlsen, G., & Gillberg, C. (1999). Autism and hearing loss. *Journal of Autism and Developmental Disorders, 29,* 349–357.

Schreck, K. A., & Mulick, J. A. (2000). Parental report of sleep problems in children with autism. *Journal of Autism and Developmental Disorders, 30,* 127–135.

Stores, G. (1996). Practitioner review: Assessment and treatment of sleep disorders in children and adolescents. *Journal of Child Psychology and Psychiatry, 37,* 907–925.

Stores, G. (2001). Normal sleep including developmental aspects. In G. Stores & L. Wiggs (Eds.), *Sleep disturbance in children and adolescents with disorders of development: Its significance and management.* (pp. 10–14). London: MacKeith Press.

Stores, G., & Wiggs, L. (2001). Sleep problems and sleep disorders: General. In G. Stores & L. Wiggs (Eds.), *Sleep disturbance in children and adolescents with disorders of development: Its significance and management* (pp. 15–23). London: MacKeith Press.

Tuchman, R. (1997). Acquired epileptiform aphasias. *Seminars in Pediatric Neurology, 4,* 93–101.

Tuchman, R. (2000). Treatment of seizure disorders and EEG abnormalities in children with autism spectrum disorders. *Journal of Autism and Developmental Disorders, 30,* 485–489.

Tuchman, R., & Rapin, I. (1997). Regression in pervasive developmental disorders: seizures and epileptiform electroencephalogram correlates. *Pediatrics, 99,* 560–566.

Valicenti-McDermott, M., McVicar, K., Rapin, I., Wershil, B. K., Cohen, H., & Shinar, S. (2006). Frequency of gastrointestinal symptoms in children with autism spectrum disorders and the association with family history of autoimmune disease. *Journal of Developmental and Behavioral Pediatrics (Supplement), 27,* S128–S136.

Volkmar, F. R., & Nelson, D. S. (1990). Seizure disorders in autism. *Journal of American Academy of Child and Adolescent Psychiatry, 29,* 127–129.

Volkmar, F. R., & Wiesner, L. A. (2004). *Healthcare for children on the autism spectrum: A guide to medical, nutritional, and behavioral issues.* Bethesda, MD: Woodbine House.

Wakefield, A. J., Anthony, A., & Murch, S. H. (2000). Enterocolitis in children with developmental disorders. *American Journal of Gastroenterology, 95,* 2285–2295.

Wiggs, L., & Stores, G. (2004). Sleep patterns and sleep disorders in children with autistic spectrum disorders; insights using parent report and actigraphy. *Developmental Medicine and Child Neurology, 46,* 372–380.

Williams, P. G., Sears, L. L., & Allard, A. (2004). Sleep problems in children with autism. *Journal of Sleep Research, 13,* 265–268.

Zero to Three. (2005). *Diagnostic classification of mental health and developmental disorders of infancy and early childhood, revised* (DC:0-3R). Washington, DC: Zero to Three Press.

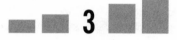

3

Sexuality and Autism

Individual, Family, and Community Perspectives
and Interventions

Robin L. Gabriels
Mary E. Van Bourgondien

The terms *adolescence* and *puberty* are often used interchangeably when referring to the transition period from childhood to adulthood. This transition includes sexual maturation of physical characteristics, such as skeletal growth, development of reproductive organs, and secondary sexual characteristics (e.g., pubic hair growth and breast development), as well as changes in cognitive, psychological, and social maturity (Dalldorf, 1983). In typically developing adolescents, the cognitive changes involve an increased capacity for abstract thought, reflection, and social understanding of what others think and feel, while at the same time psychological and social changes are reflected in the increased involvement of the adolescent in developing friendships, dating, and working, all of which help typical adolescents make sense of their physical changes and urges (Harris, Glasberg, & Delmolino, 1998). Therefore, puberty is not only defined by various physical changes, but brings with it changes in family and societal expectations, including the appropriate expression of sexual needs, which can be more challenging with less able individuals with autism (Adams & Sheslow, 1983; Holmes, Isler, Bott, & Markowitz, 2005).

Individuals with autism enter the physical maturation aspects of puberty at roughly the same time period as the general population (Murphy & Elias, 2006), though the nature of the core autism impairments impedes the cognitive and psychosocial developmental progress that typically coincides with physical maturation, thus creating unique challenges for individuals with autism. As Gillberg and Coleman (1992, p. 65) noted, "The growth of sexual drive, as a rule, is not accompanied by corresponding growth in the field of social 'know-how,' and this often leads to embarrassing behavior." For this reason, it is imperative that professionals working with school-age children and adolescents with autism be alert to sexuality issues in this population so preparations to address and teach appropriate social boundaries and personal self-care can be made long before the child with autism enters puberty. For example, sexuality issues such as masturbation, menstruation, pregnancy, and sexual interests can present health and safety risks if they are not addressed directly by professionals working with this population. The sexuality behaviors and interests of individuals with autism, along with their difficulty understanding social expectations and the complexities involved in sexuality, make them particularly vulnerable to being misunderstood or possibly victimized by others. This chapter will provide a review of general sexuality issues as they pertain to the more cognitively and language-impaired individuals with autism, their caregivers, and the communities in which they live. (See Chapter 2 for a discussion of medical needs in puberty.)

SEXUALITY AND INDIVIDUALS WITH AUTISM

Although the topic of sexuality and individuals with autism is understudied, it should not be assumed that this population does not experience issues of sexuality. Of the few available studies, it is clear from caregiver report and direct interview of individuals with autism that both high- and low-functioning individuals are aware of and interested in sexuality issues, and that this population engages in a variety of sexual behaviors (Haracopos & Pendersen, 1992; Konstantareas & Lunsky, 1997; Ousley & Mesibov, 1991; Ruble & Dalrymple, 1993; Van Bourgondien, Reichle, & Palmer, 1997).

A study by Konstantareas and Lunsky (1997) is of particular interest for the purposes of this chapter, because these researchers attempted to directly question a group of individuals with autism (age range 16–46 years) with mild, moderate, or severe mental retardation and compare their responses to those of a group of nonautistic individuals with mental retardation/developmental delay (DD). Of note, several of the participants had limited verbal skills and either employed signs or used simple words. Given these limitations, pictures were used to enhance comprehension of all aspects of the study interview measure: the Socio-Sexual Knowledge, Experience, Attitudes, and Interests (SSKEAI) questionnaire, a measure adapted from Ousley and Mesibov (1991). This measure involved four types of questions: (1) receptive and expressive sexual vocabulary, (2) sociosexual experiences, (3) sociosexual attitudes, and (4) interest in engaging in sexual activities. Results indicated that almost all participants understood gender labels and the term *pregnancy*, but it was of concern that only 56% had an awareness of how a woman becomes pregnant. Issues specific to the autism group involved use of preservative responses (e.g., "I don't know" or repeated use of the same word), idiosyncratic responses (e.g., diaphragm = frying pan), or concrete/literal interpretation responses to questions requiring knowledge of sexual terms (e.g., "a man's explanation of a drawing depicting intercourse [simply] as two people lying on a towel") (Konstantareas & Lunsky, 1997, p. 410). The two groups did not differ significantly in regards to the types of sexual experiences reported, though there was considerable variability in the experiences reported. The sexual experiences of both male and female individuals with autism included: going on a date (73.3%), holding hands (100%), putting arms around another (73%), kissing (86.7%), petting (46.7%), heavy kissing (46.7%), naked with a partner (13.3%), masturbation (60%), and intercourse (26.7%). However, the autism group was less able than the DD group to define sexual activities, perhaps due to the significantly lower communication and social skills that are particular to the diagnosis of autism. The authors of the study urged caution when, for example, interpreting the responses of an individual with autism who referred to "intercourse" (by saying he was "masturbated" by someone [p. 406]). Finally, sexual attitudes about what is right and wrong to do reflected what individuals had been taught by caregivers, and the sexual interests of individuals with autism were similar to those in the DD groups and included interests in getting married and having children. The anecdotal elements of this study highlight the issue that the core impairments in autism (social and communication skills, along with behavioral features) can hinder sexuality development in this population. These issues need to be taken into account when identifying appropriate sexuality interventions for individuals with autism.

Social Issues

Social dysfunction has been recognized as a particular area of difficulty for individuals with autism, and one that uniquely differentiates them from nonautistic individuals with mental retardation or other developmental disabilities, such as communication disorders (e.g., Gillham, Carter, Volkmar, & Sparrow, 2000; Volkmar, Carter, Sparrow, & Cicchetti, 1993). Ongoing dysfunction in social interactions and social understanding in this population has foundational roots in the early developmental delays or deviances observed in infants and young children with autism such as absent or abnormal use of eye gaze (e.g., Volkmar & Mayes, 1990), impoverished joint attention exchanges with caregivers (e.g., Mundy, Sigman, & Kasara, 1990), problems with imitation and lack of or delays in social play skills (e.g., Stone, Lemanek, Fishel, Fernandez, & Altemeier, 1990), failure to socially engage others or take others' point of view into account (Volkmar & Cohen, 1985), and difficulties recognizing emotions in others (e.g., Ozonoff, Pennington, & Rogers, 1990).

The lack of social understanding in the autism population can present serious problems with the onset of puberty (Gillberg, 1984). The social deficits in autism can interfere not only with the obvious area of an individual's ability to develop friendships and romantic relationships but also in an individual's ability to use social judgment to determine what should be done in private versus public settings, how and why to manage personal hygiene, and how to avoid sexual exploitation by others. The lack of ability to surmise that others may not have good intentions has resulted in individuals with autism being involved in unsolicited sexual contacts with others (Haracopos, 1988). For more impaired individuals with autism, the routine of having physical assistance for activities such as dressing and toileting can not only blur boundaries about nudity, but can also make them more vulnerable to unsolicited sexual contacts (Cole & Cole, 1993).

Communication Issues

Most children with autism have significant delays in the development of speech and language skills, and a large proportion of individuals with autism never acquire communicative language (Tager-Flusberg, Paul, & Lord, 2005). One aspect of communication often observed in individuals with autism is a tendency to engage in echolalia, that is, the repetition of words or phrases in immediate or delayed contexts (Tager-Flusberg et al., 2005). Other areas of communication impairment observed in autism include pronoun reversal (e.g., Lee, Hobson, & Chiat, 1994), odd intonation or voice qualities (e.g., Rutter, Mawhood, & Howlin, 1992), and significant delays in the comprehension of language compared to the ability to produce language (Chairman, Drew, Baird, & Baird, 2003).

Implications of these communication abnormalities for sexuality development in individuals with autism include having the ability to label or talk about sexuality terms while having little to no understanding of their meaning, having an inclination to simply repeat or echo sexuality terms previously heard regardless of the social context, or speaking in an odd tone of voice that does not appropriately reflect the sexual nature of the topic being discussed. All of these possibilities can put the individual with autism at risk for being misunderstood by others, sometimes even to the point of requiring involvement by the legal system. (See Chapter 13 for a discussion of legal vulnerabilities in autism and Chapter 4 for a review of communication features in autism.) Of additional concern, is the fact that adolescent girls with autism who have weaker receptive language abilities may not understand the pain and discharge associated with menses, thus making it difficult to teach hygiene skills or even how to cope with this new physical development (Harris et al., 1998). Limited expressive communication can also prevent individuals from informing others about pain or the discomfort they may be experiencing from the body changes of puberty (aches in the joints or limbs, or cramps). Communication difficulties, along with the social deficits, also limit these adolescents' ability to appropriately initiate an interaction with someone they find attractive.

Behavior Issues

In addition to the social and communication deficits in autism, the third area of diagnostic impairment is the tendency of this population to engage in restrictive, repetitive, stereotyped behaviors and/or to have circumscribed interests of unusual intensity (American Psychiatric Association, 1994). Individuals with autism tend to have a limited behavioral repertoire, particularly those who have more severe cognitive and language impairments. Therefore, engaging in self-stimulating activities, like masturbation, can be one of the few activities an individual with autism knows how to perform, and this can impact time spent on other activities. However, time spent masturbating can be reduced by teaching other activities of interest to the individual (Gillberg & Coleman, 1992). For example, there is evidence that teaching children, adolescents, and adults with autism to engage in aerobic exercise can reduce self-stimulatory behaviors and increase productive on-task behaviors (Elliot, Dobbin, Rose, & Soper, 1994; Kern, Koegel, & Dunlap, 1984; Powers, Thibadeau & Rose, 1992; Rosenthal-Malek & Mitchell, 1997; Watters & Watters, 1980).

Individuals with autism are observed to perseverate on odd topics or objects or to be preoccupied with engaging in "fixed" rituals or routines (Bodfish, Symons, Parker, & Lewis, 2000). Odd objects, including "shoes, shampoo bottles, coupons or paper, and body parts such as legs" (Van Bourgondien et al., 1997, p. 119), have been reported to lead to sexual arousal in adolescents and adults with autism, even without using them for direct stimulation. However, both Haracopos and Pedersen (1992) and Van Bourgondien and colleagues (1997) reported that one-third to one-fourth of the individuals in their study samples used objects to directly stimulate themselves sexually.

CAREGIVER PERSPECTIVES AND INTERVENTIONS

As previously mentioned, although adolescents with autism experience the same physical sexual development as their typical peers, they lack the social and cognitive skills to understand their new sexual interests and desires (Harris et al., 1998). Raising a child who appears to be developing into a physically normal adolescent and yet may not understand even the basic nature of social relationships can be quite confusing for parents (Cairns, 1986; DeMyer, 1979). Caregivers of children with autism identify major concerns regarding their child's sexuality and sexual behaviors. Ruble and Dalrymple (1993) surveyed 100 caregivers of individuals with autism (ages 9 to 35) regarding their views of their child's sexual and social awareness, sexual education, and sexual behaviors, and their parental concerns regarding their child's sexuality. (Of note, 84% of the children with autism in this sample also had mental retardation.) Results from this survey indicated that these children engaged in a variety of inappropriate sexual behaviors, including touching private parts (65%) or removing clothing in public settings (28%), masturbating in public (23%), touching the opposite sex inappropriately (18%), and masturbating with odd objects (e.g., socks; 14%). Overall, the major concerns of parents involved worries that their child's odd or inappropriate behaviors might be misinterpreted as sexual when they were not or that their child's sexual behaviors would be misunderstood by others. Parents of females were concerned about issues including pregnancy (61%) and the possibility that their daughter might be taken advantage of by the opposite sex (80%), or that she would need birth control (50%). Parents of males were concerned about issues including sexual violation of their sons by another male (80%) and controlling masturbation (81%). Of importance, this study found no relationship between verbal ability levels in individuals with autism and their display of inappropriate sexual behaviors. These researchers noted that, given this finding, "the need for sex education is best determined by the behaviors of the person rather than by the functioning or verbal levels" (p. 238).

Van Bourgondien (2006) reported the results of a values clarification exercise conducted with parents and professionals throughout the United States and Europe (see Tables 3.1 and 3.2). This exercise involved asking parents and professionals about the sexual behaviors they were comfortable considering in individuals with autism. In general, results were more reflective of the interests of typical adults than those of the person with autism. For example, compared to results from studies of individuals with autism suggesting that a sizable number (24–31%) of individuals diagnosed with autism and mental retardation find the use of objects sexually stimulating (Haracopos and Pedersen, 1992; Van Bourgondien et al., 1997) and become sexually aroused from just looking at objects (9%; Van Bourgondien et al., 1997), the professionals and parents surveyed indicated less comfort with these behaviors (interest in objects: professionals = 39%; parents = 14%) than with intercourse (professionals = 43%; parents = 63%). Also reflecting a typical perspective is the increased comfort of parents and professionals with individuals with autism being sexually aroused by looking at a whole person (professionals = 63%; parents = 49%), rather than parts of the person (professionals = 41%; parents = 33%). However, a cognitive characteristic of individuals with autism is that they tend to pay more attention to the parts of objects than to the whole. Overall, as parents and professionals come together to plan educational interventions for individuals with autism, it is important to keep in mind the different perspectives of these individuals.

Parents of children with autism and autism professionals have debated whether or not, as well as how, to teach individuals with autism about sexuality issues (Elgar, 1985; Money, 1985; Torisky & Torisky, 1985). Sexual education even for typically developing children is a very controversial topic where one's opinions are influenced by one's values. These values are derived from many sources—one's upbringing, one's religious views, societal views, and even the current political and legal climate. As a team comes together to develop an intervention plan in the area of sexuality, it is important to ensure that all members of the team

TABLE 3.1. Survey Results for Professionals: United States/Sweden/Canada/England/Germany

Behavior	Yes	Percent
Engaging in masturbation	253	74
Teaching to masturbate	174	51
Engaging in fondling or kissing	172	51
Sexual interests in objects	132	39
Sexual interests in photographs of people	215	63
Sexual interests in body parts	138	41
Sexual interests in someone	240	71
Dating	196	58
Marriage	141	41
Intercourse	147	43
Having a child	77	23

take the time to reflect on their own values so as to ensure that decisions are made (as much as possible) from the perspective of the person with autism.

For most adolescents and adults with autism, the starting place in sexuality education is teaching the person both how to do specific self-care activities and how to be safe. Shea and Gordon (1991), in their book *Growing Up,* provide a sexuality education curriculum for individuals with general developmental disabilities that is also appropriate to adapt for individuals diagnosed with autism and mental retardation. The book is designed as a loose-leaf binder so parents and professionals can individualize and use the exercises or materials that fit their individual needs. The line drawings are helpful for individuals who need concrete visual cues to learn concepts. The curriculum areas range from social behavior and personal safety to sexual anatomy and puberty. Menstrual hygiene, sexual behavior, pregnancy, and birth control are also included. The following is a list of sexuality-related topic areas that should be taught using autism-specific teaching strategies, including the use of visual cues.

- *Safety.* Individuals with autism should be taught who can or cannot touch them, as well as what to do if someone touches them inappropriately. These individuals should be taught how to say "no" to other people who make them uncomfortable, either through verbal means or physical actions.

TABLE 3.2. Survey Results for Parents: United States/Sweden/Canada/Germany

Behavior	Yes	Percent
Engaging in masturbation	62	75
Teaching to masturbate	26	31
Engaging in fondling or kissing	42	51
Sexual interests in objects	12	14
Sexual interests in photographs of people	41	49
Sexual interests in body parts	27	33
Sexual interests in someone	61	73
Dating	55	66
Marriage	51	61
Intercourse	52	63
Having a child	31	37

• *Personal hygiene.* Individuals with autism must be taught proper hygiene, including teaching females how to handle their menstrual cycle. It may be helpful to teach such hygiene issues just prior to the onset of menses, when the individual may be less distracted or distressed by the emotional and physical issues that coincide with the onset of menses.

• *Tension release activities.* Some families may be comfortable with their child engaging in masturbation, whereas others may not. Regardless, all adolescents and adults with autism need to have a tension reduction activity that helps them to deal with life's stresses. Those individuals who masturbate will need a more appropriate activity to do when they are stressed at school, at work, or in the community. Groden, Baron, and Groden (2006) and Cautela and Grodin (1978) describe relaxation activities that can be taught to individuals with autism and other developmental disabilities. These techniques generally involve breathing exercises coupled with muscle tensing and relaxation. For some individuals with autism, having time to pursue their special interest or, as previously mentioned, engage in aerobic exercise may be a way for them to reduce tension.

• *Social behaviors.* With adolescence comes an increased interest in social interactions (Mesibov, 1983). Thus, it continues to be important to teach adolescents with autism appropriate ways of engaging with others. Koller (2000) suggests that social skills training should focus on improving adolescents' ability to understand more subtle social cues and interactions, as well as teaching empathy.

• *Sexuality.* The most common teaching goal is to teach where and when individuals can and cannot masturbate. Strategies that have been found to be helpful include teaching individuals that there are certain places, such as their bedroom or bathroom at home, where it is appropriate to masturbate. For more concrete learners, families or staff members can use an object or picture cue that uniquely symbolizes masturbation or private time. For example, an individual with autism may find a particular object such as a stuffed animal arousing, and caregivers can use this object as a schedule cue item to indicate when it is appropriate to masturbate and then remove this item from view during work activities when it is not appropriate. For those individuals who understand pictures, line drawings can also be used to indicate "private time."

COMMUNITY PERSPECTIVES AND INTERVENTIONS

Sexuality issues in the low-functioning autism population that are of relevance to the community include forensic and legal issues (described in more detail in Chapter 13), the prevalence of sexual behaviors in community residential settings, and sexuality education. This section reviews research regarding the prevalence of sexual behaviors in community settings (group homes) and the necessary components of sexuality education for application by schools and community-based therapists.

There are very few studies examining the prevalence of sexual behaviors in community settings outside the family environment, such as in residential settings. Haracopos and Pederson (1992) conducted an extensive survey in Denmark on 81 adolescents and adults with autism (57 males and 24 females) living in residential facilities. Results revealed that 68% of this sample masturbated and 53% of the sample had masturbated in public places. Another survey of the sexual behaviors of 89 individuals diagnosed with autism and mental retardation (ages 16 to 59 years), in 35 community-based group homes in North Carolina, found that a large proportion of this sample (76%) engaged in some type of sexual behavior, the most common behavior being masturbation (68%); Van Bourgondien et al., 1997). In contrast to the high incidence of sexual behaviors in this sample, a majority of the staff had not been trained in how to address sexuality issues with these residents. These researchers stressed that "given the high frequency of sexual behaviors in individuals with autism at all levels of cognitive functioning, it is important for residential programs to provide systematic training to their staff members of how and when to provide training to their residents to facilitate the appropriate expression of sexual feelings" (p. 124).

Koller (2000) reviewed components of sexuality education for adolescents with autism, noting the importance of adapting teaching methods to meet each individual's learning style, interests, and needs, as well as individualizing the learning environment. Basic components of instruction included being concrete, brief, specific, and clear when presenting material (e.g., using visual cues, imitation, role play, repetition, and teaching in real-life settings) to match cognitive learning styles and to increase generalization of learning. Shea and Mesibov (2005) described topics to consider when teaching sexuality to individuals with adequate receptive language skills. Essential topics included information about body parts, appropriate hygiene, concepts of privacy, relationship differences (e.g., differences between family members, friends, and romantic partners), public and private behaviors appropriate for various relationships, masturbation, and sexual intercourse.

In addition to providing sexuality education to individuals with autism, staff in residential homes should be taught strategies to ensure that appropriate physical boundaries are maintained. Staff should also be taught to recognize possible signs of sexual abuse. Changes in behaviors, including increased negative behaviors or decreased adaptive behaviors, may signal sexual abuse.

An example of a community-based sexuality education program is the Sexuality and Social Awareness program developed by Melone and Lettick (1983) for individuals with autism (ages 14 to 21 years) at Benhaven day and residential school. This program developed out of their staff–student policies, which included (1) the need to teach socially appropriate behaviors, (2) the need to teach students appropriate places to masturbate, and (3) the need to teach appropriate friendship behaviors. This program was developed with the goal of promoting "behavioral and social growth in the area of sexuality" (p. 175). The program was adapted for individuals with autism who had more severe language impairments or behavioral problems. Parent involvement was an important component of the program, so that concepts and vocabulary could be generalized to and reinforced at home. A total of six units were taught including "identification of body parts, menstruation, masturbation, physical examinations, personal hygiene, and social behavior" (p. 176). The menstruation and physical/gynecological examination units were taught exclusively to females and involved a variety of activities to demonstrate and practice the procedures involved in these events. For those female students who had not yet experienced menstruation, prerequisite skills were taught, including learning how to count to 31, the days of the week, months of the year, and number of days in a month. The social behavior unit included teaching "when" and "where" certain behavior could take place. For example, skills such as teaching students to maintain appropriate social distance, when and where to wear pajamas, and inappropriate times for being nude, partially dressed, or fully dressed were taught. Teaching strategies included the use of role play with materials (e.g., sanitary napkins, paper exam gowns, urine cups), picture cues, categorizing pictures of body parts, games (e.g., "Simon Says"), and art activities (e.g., body tracing, filling in missing body parts, or coloring body parts). The study results, from participants' pre- and postintervention test scores and observations of their behaviors, indicated that the participants had some degree of "behavioral and social growth in the area of sexuality" (p. 185). For example, students demonstrated improved knowledge about the "when" and "where" of sexual behaviors. These authors stressed the importance of practice and follow-through in teaching the skills learned in these units so as to promote generalization of concepts learned.

Other curricula are also available. For example, Koller (2000) reviewed programs that developed autism-specific sexuality education such as the Devereux Centers program that uses parents as sexuality educators and regards sexual expression as normal and natural. Topics of instruction, as well as methods, reflect those at Benhaven that were previously described (Melone & Lettick, 1983). Also, a program instituted in Denmark was reviewed. This program was founded on the rights of individuals with autism to have knowledge of and to engage in appropriate sexual behaviors. Thus, from Koller's perspective, "The goal of sexuality education should be to protect the individual from sexual exploitation, teach healthy sex habits, and increase self-esteem through systematic, individualized approaches" (2000, p. 131).

CONCLUSION

Like typically developing adolescents, individuals with autism experience the physical maturation, sexual urges, and interests that accompany the stages of puberty, though the core impairments of autism can impede the ability of this population to develop the social understanding necessary to adequately meet the challenges of this important developmental stage. Specific intervention considerations should incorporate the following to adequately address this stage of development in the autism population: (1) identifying sexuality needs and issues specific to the child and in reference to family values, (2) proactively teaching general issues related to appropriate social boundaries and hygiene *before* the child enters puberty, and (3) educating caregivers and other community providers about how to better understand and address the sexuality needs of adolescents with autism.

REFERENCES

Adams, W. V., & Sheslow, D. V. (1983). A developmental perspective of adolescence. In E. Schopler & G. B. Mesibov (Eds.), *Autism in adolescents and adults* (pp. 11–36). New York: Plenum Press.

American Psychiatric Association. (1994). *Diagnostic and statistical manual of mental disorders* (4th ed.). Washington, DC: Author.

Bodfish, J. W., Symons, F. J., Parker, D. E., & Lewis, M. H. (2000). Varieties of repetitive behavior in autism: Comparisons to mental retardation. *Journal of Autism and Developmental Disorders, 30*(3), 237–243.

Cairns, A. (1986). Social development: Recent theoretical trends and relevance for autism. In E. Schopler & G. Mesibov (Eds.), *Social behavior in autism* (pp. 15–33). New York: Plenum Press.

Cautela, J., & Grodin, G. (1978). *Relaxation: A comprehensive manual for adults, children, and children with special needs.* Champaign, IL: Research Press.

Chairman, T., Drew, A., Baird, C., & Baird, G. (2003). Measuring early language development in preschool children with autism spectrum disorder using the MacArthur Communication Development Inventory (Infant Form). *Journal of Child Language, 30,* 213–236.

Cole, S. S., & Cole, T. M. (1993). Sexuality, disability, and reproductive issues through the lifespan. *Sexuality and Disability, 11,* 189–205.

Dalldorf, J. S. (1983). Medical needs of the autistic adolescent. In E. Schopler & G. B. Mesibov (Eds.), *Autism in adolescents and adults* (pp. 149–168). New York: Plenum Press.

DeMyer, M. (1979). *Parents and children in autism.* New York: Wiley.

Elgar, S. (1985). Sex education and sexual awareness building for autistic children and youth: Some viewpoints and considerations. *Journal of Autism and Developmental Disorders, 15,* 214–216.

Elliot, R. O., Jr., Dobbin, A. R., Rose, G. D., & Soper, H. V. (1994). Vigorous aerobic exercise versus general motor training activities: Effects on maladaptive and stereotypic behaviors of adults with both autism and mental retardation. *Journal of Autism and Developmental Disorders, 24,* 565–576.

Gillberg, C. (1984). Autistic children growing up: Problems during puberty and adolescence. *Developmental Medicine and Child Neurology, 26,* 125–129.

Gillberg C., & Coleman, M. (1992). *The biology of the autistic syndromes* (2nd ed.). New York: Mac Keith Press.

Gillham, J. G., Carter, A. S., Volkmar, F. R., & Sparrow, S. S. (2000). Toward a developmental operational definition of autism. *Journal of Autism and Developmental Disabilities, 30*(4), 269–278.

Groden, J., Baron, M. G., & Groden, G. (2006). Stress and autism: Assessment and coping strategies. In M. G. Baron, J. Groden, G. Groden, & L. P. Lipsitt (Eds.), *Stress and coping in autism* (pp. 15–51). New York: Oxford University Press.

Haracopos, D. (1988). *What about me?: Autistic children and adults.* Copenhagen, Denmark: Andonia.

Haracopos, D., & Pendersen, L. (1992). *Sexuality and autism: A nationwide sur-*

vey in Denmark. Preliminary report, Copenhagen. Unpublished manuscript.

Harris, S. L., Glasberg, B., & Delmolino, L. (1998). Families and the developmentally disabled adolescent. In V. B. Van Hasselt & M. Hersen (Eds.), *Handbook of psychological treatment protocols for children and adolescents* (pp. 519–548). Mahwah, NJ: Erlbaum.

Holmes, D. L., Isler, V., Bott, C., & Markowitz, C. (2005, Winter). Sexuality and individuals with autism and developmental disorders: A three-part series. *Autism Spectrum Quarterly*, 30–33.

Kern, L., Koegel, R. L., & Dunlap, G. (1984). The influence of rigorous versus mild exercise on autistic stereotyped behaviors. *Journal of Autism and Developmental Disorders, 14*, 57–67.

Koller, R. (2000). Sexuality and adolescents with autism. *Sexuality and Disability, 18*, 125–135.

Kontstantareas, M. M., & Lunsky, Y. J. (1997). Sociosexual knowledge, experience, attitudes, and interests of individuals with autistic disorder and developmental delay. *Journal of Autism and Developmental Disorders, 27*, 397–413.

Lee, A., Hobson, R. P., & Chiat, S. (1994). I, you, me, and autism: An experimental study. *Journal of Autism and Developmental Disorders, 24*, 155–176.

Melone, M., & Lettick, A. L. (1983). Sex education at Benhaven. In E. Schopler & G. B. Mesibov (Eds.), *Autism in adolescents and adults* (pp. 169–186). New York: Plenum Press.

Mesibov, G. B. (1983). Current perspectives and issues in autism and adolescence. In E. Schopler & G. B. Mesibov (Eds.), *Autism in adolescents and adults* (pp. 37–53). New York: Plenum Press.

Money, J. (1985). Response to Sybil Elgar. *Journal of Autism and Developmental Disorders, 15*, 217–218.

Mundy, P., Sigman, M., & Kasara, C. (1990). A longitudinal study of joint attention and language disorders in autistic children. *Journal of Autism and Developmental Disorders, 20*, 115–123.

Murphy, N. A., & Elias, E. R. (2006). Sexuality of children and adolescents with developmental disabilities. *Pediatrics, 118*, 398–403.

Ousley, O., & Mesibov, G. B. (1991). Sexual attitudes and knowledge of high-functioning adolescents and adults with autism. *Journal of Autism and Developmental Disorders, 21*, 471–482.

Ozonoff, S., Pennington, B., & Rogers, S. (1990). Are there specific emotion perception deficits in young autistic children? *Journal of Child Psychology and Psychiatry, 31*, 343–361.

Powers, S., Thibadeau, S., & Rose, K. (1992). Antecedent exercise and its effects on self-stimulation. *Behavioral Residential Treatment, 7*, 15–22.

Rosenthal-Malek, A., & Mitchell, S. (1997). Brief report: The effects of exercise on the self-stimulatory behaviors and positive responding of adolescents with autism. *Journal of Autism and Developmental Disorders, 27*(2), 193–202.

Ruble, L. A., & Dalrymple, N. J. (1993). Social/sexual awareness of persons with autism: A parental perspective. *Archives of Sexual Behavior, 22*(3), 229–240

Rutter, M., Mawhood, L., & Howlin, P. (1992). Language delay and social development. In P. Fletcher & D. Hall (Eds.), *Specific speech and language disorders in children: Correlates, characteristics, and outcomes* (pp. 63–78). London: Whurr.

Shea, V., & Gordon, B. N. (1991). *Growing up: A social and sexual education picture book for young people with mental retardation* (rev. ed.). Chapel Hill, NC: Clinical Center for the Study of Development and Learning.

Shea, V., & Mesibov, G. B. (2005). Adolescents and adults with autism. In F. Volkmar, R. Paul, A. Klin, & D. J. Cohen (Eds.), *Handbook of autism and pervasive developmental disorders: Vol. 2. Interventions and policy* (3rd ed., pp. 288–311). Hoboken, NJ: Wiley.

Stone, W., Lemanek, K., Fishel, P., Fernandez, M., & Altemeier, W. (1990). Play and imitation skills in the diagnosis of autism in young children. *Pediatrics, 86,* 267–272.

Tager-Flusberg, H., Paul, R., & Lord, C. (2005). Language and communication in autism. In F. R. Volkmar, R. Paul, A. Klin, & D. Cohen (Eds.), *Handbook of autism and pervasive developmental disorders* (3rd ed., pp. 335–364). New York: Wiley.

Torisky, D., & Torisky, C. (1985). Sex education and sexual awareness building for autistic children and youth: Some viewpoints and considerations. *Journal of Autism and Developmental Disorders, 15,* 213, 221–223.

Van Bourgondien, M. E. (2006, May 19). *Sexuality in adolescents and adults with autism.* Presentation at the 27th annual TEACCH Conference, Autism in Adolescents and Adults, Chapel Hill, NC.

Van Bourgondien, M. E., Reichle, N. C., & Palmer, A. (1997). Sexual behavior in adults with autism. *Journal of Autism and Developmental Disorders, 27,* 113–125.

Volkmar, F. R., Carter, A., Sparrow, S. S., & Cicchetti, D. V. (1993). Quantifying social development in autism. *Journal of Child and Adolescent Psychiatry, 32,* 627–632.

Volkmar, F. R., & Cohen, D. J. (1985). A first person account of the experience of infantile autism by Tony W. *Journal of Autism and Developmental Disorders, 15,* 47–54.

Volkmar, F. R., & Mayes, L. C. (1990). Gaze behavior in autism. *Developmental Psychopathology, 2,* 61–70.

Watters, A. M., & Watters, W. E. (1980). Decreasing self-stimulatory behavior with physical exercise in a group of autistic boys. *Journal of Autism and Developmental Disorders, 10,* 379–387.

4

Communication and Language Issues in Less Able School-Age Children with Autism

Diane Twachtman-Cullen
Jennifer Twachtman-Reilly

While there are many factors that distinguish between more and less able children with autism, the most significant of these is arguably that of language functioning. The importance of this cannot be overstated, since language functioning is considered a strong prognosticator of outcome in autism (Venter, Lord, & Schopler, 1992) and a necessary component of academic and social success. This chapter reviews critical precursors to communication and language development as a foundation for discussion of intervention approaches tailored to the needs of less able individuals with autism. Our use of the term *less able* encompasses impairment in cognition, socialization, and language and may include significant challenges in other areas of functioning as well. That said, while there are commonalities that apply to children with significant challenges, we acknowledge that each child is an individual with strengths, weaknesses, and needs that are unique to him or her. Finally, from a language development perspective, the focus of this chapter is on those children with autism who are either nonverbal or minimally verbal. The theoretical framework underlying this chapter is transactional in nature and takes its lead from the language research literature. It is based upon the notion that each communicative partner influences the other and that both partners are, in turn, influenced by variables within the environment (Sameroff, 1987; Sameroff & Friese, 1990). This perspective recognizes the dynamic interplay among variables and respects the neuropsychological compromises that children with autism bring to the table.

We support an informed, developmental approach to communication and language intervention that is customized to this population by taking into account the developmental discontinuities associated with autism. Finally, the overarching premise of this chapter is that *all* children with autism—regardless of level of severity—are capable of and entitled to a communication system that is functional, reliable, individualized to their needs, and consistently available to them.

OVERVIEW OF LANGUAGE DEVELOPMENT

At the risk of stating the obvious, it is crucial to understand normal language development in order to fully appreciate the ways in which disordered development deviates from it. We begin by distinguishing between the terms *communication* and *language* since, notwithstanding that the terms are often used interchangeably, they are indeed different, albeit related, parameters.

Communication

Characterized by Muma (1978) as the "primary function of language" (p. 118), communication is at once dynamic, social, and reciprocal. Unlike language (which is defined later), communication requires at least two people—a sender and a receiver. It is important to note that communication can and does occur in the absence of verbal language—although it realizes its finest hour when intertwined with it. Lastly, communication not only comes before language, but also sets the stage for its development.

An example so mired in the ordinary as to obscure its far from trivial significance is illustrative here. Consider the human infant—completely dependent upon his parents for life-sustaining support. Absent language, infants obtain what they need by crying, hence signaling the parents that they are in a state of disequilibrium due to hunger or some other type of discomfort. The parents interpret this cry as a "request," that is, as a plea for something to alleviate the child's discomfort. The important point to keep in mind is that even though infants do not *intend* to summon their parents, the parents act *as if* they had, and do what is needed to satisfy the child's need. Hence, even though the infants are preintentional, their cry has message value. Kaye (1982) refers to this precursor of communication as an "asymmetrical process of interpretation" in which the parent does the "work" of reading in meaning and responding in kind. It is easy to see how infants come to connect their cries with parental response, given the number of times this type of transaction takes place in the first several months of the infants' lives. Stated in behavioral terms, infants learn that their voice has message value because it is continuously reinforced. Enter: *the spoiled cry.*

At approximately 8 to 10 months of age something quite remarkable happens, although its actual significance is "under the radar screen" of most parents. There are qualitative changes in the type and duration of the infants' cry. Where in the first several months of life, babies cry inconsolably, quieting only after their immediate need(s) are met, at approximately 8–10 months of age infants typically quiet upon the parents' mere entrance into the room. After a while, the parents begin to suspect that the infants do not really *need* them, but rather simply *want* them. This is a major milestone that is more fully addressed in a later section of this chapter.

Fortunately, parents are slow enough learners to give babies time to make the connection that their voices are a powerful tool for sending messages and getting needs met, for parents typically do respond to this more purposeful crying, at least for a while. Over time, parents begin to recognize this cry as the baby's *spoiled cry*—that which is *socially* as opposed to *need* based. It is at this time that parents "pull back" (i.e., stop responding to this qualitatively different cry), teaching infants another very important lesson—that if they continue to "cry wolf," eventually Mommy and Daddy will stop tending to their needs.

This age-old, deceptively commonplace scenario is anything but mundane. Indeed, it's actually a developmental extravaganza, for it signals the infant's entry into *intentional communication*—the gateway into the world of two-way socio-communicative interaction. Hence, according to Kaye (1982), infants become intentional when their *undifferentiated* cries are reinforced through *differentiated* parental response and rich interpretation (the *as if* phenomenon).

Language

Historically, while language impairment was recognized early on as a symptom of autism (Kanner, 1943), it was not until the mid-1980s that researchers began to recognize the contributions of social impairment in autism (Fein, Pennington, Markowitz, Braverman, & Waterhouse, 1986). Coincidentally, this period paralleled the so-called *pragmatics revolution,* a term coined by Duchan (1984) to underscore the dramatic shift in focus and clinical practice in the field of speech–language pathology from the form/structure (syntax and phonology) and content (semantics) of language to the function (pragmatics) of language and its use in social interactive contexts (Bloom & Lahey, 1978). This paradigm shift ushered in changes affecting virtually all aspects of our understanding of and approach to language development. It also changed the theoretical framework on which language development rests and influenced both the type and focus of intervention for children with communication and language impairments, including children with autism.

Where earlier the burden of language impairment rested solely on the child with the disability, the pragmatic orientation required a more transactional focus, in which the contribution of both partners in a communicative exchange was given preeminence. Likewise, where earlier conceptualizations of language focused on decontextualized, static elements of word and sentence production, the pragmatic focus emphasized the dynamic, purpose-driven *use* of language in a social interactive context.

In deference to this pragmatic focus, speech–language pathologists began to work on the functions of communication such as *requesting, protesting,* and *commenting* (Dore, 1974, 1975; Halliday, 1975). These pragmatic functions were conceptualized as communicative intents, a view that paved the way for the analysis of both unconventional verbal and nonverbal behavior in children with autism. For example, Prizant and Duchan (1981), in their classic study of the functions of immediate echolalia, found that children with autism use echolalia to convey specific intents (e.g., affirmation, request). Prizant and Rydell (1984) found similar results for delayed echolalia. Similarly, a study by Donnellan, Mirenda, Mesaros, and Fassbender (1984) put a pragmatic "spin" on behavioral analysis by characterizing aberrant behaviors in terms of their pragmatic intents. Carr and Durand (1985) took this notion a step further by teaching children with autism to communicate for the specific purpose served by the undesirable behavior (e.g., requesting attention and assistance) in each of their participants. They reported reductions in problem behaviors following this training.

Nowhere did the implications of this paradigmatic shift in language development and the changes that it brought carry more significance, or hold greater promise, than in the field of autism. Indeed, it might be said that pragmatics offered a perfect fit for children with autism. For one thing, it helped to explain some of the idiosyncratic communicative behaviors associated with the disorder, while at the same time it acknowledged the direct link between communication and behavior that other approaches seemed to gloss over or ignore. For another, it recognized the critical role of the communicative partner and the shared responsibility of both participants in a communicative exchange. Pragmatics also offered an intervention approach that seemed ideally suited to the contours of the child's needs—a way to learn language in contexts that not only promoted sense making but also provided natural reinforcements to facilitate learning. Finally, pragmatics also helped to promote the generalization of skills, since intervention typically took place in the contexts in which the skills were needed.

The definition of language that highlights those elements that are particularly important to take into account when dealing with less able children with autism comes from Owens (1988), who states that language is a "socially shared code or conventional system for representing concepts through the use of arbitrary symbols and rule-governed combinations of those symbols" (p. 453). The important components of this definition are that language is:

- A *socially shared, conventional code:* speakers need to understand (i.e., share) the meanings of the words they use or meaningful communication cannot occur.
- *Representational, though arbitrary:* while speakers use words to stand for things (e.g., *chair* refers to something one sits on), the particular configuration of the word itself is strictly arbitrary. Hence, *chair* might just as well have been called *slook*.
- *Rule-governed:* language operates according to certain (grammatical and syntactical) rules that speakers abide by in using it. For example, one says, "Have a nice day," not "Nice have day a."

Owens's definition of language takes into account two of its three critical features—*form* (rules) and *content* (semantics). There is another feature of language, however, that is essential. This feature is that of *function,* or the *use* of language for communication purposes. Sacks (1989) captures the essence of this feature by stating that language is the "symbolic currency, to exchange meaning" (p. 39). By characterizing language in this manner—as the tender by which *communication* is rendered—Sacks not only underscores the dynamic, reciprocal, and social nature of language use but also gives preeminence to the exchange of meaning. He also highlights the interconnectedness of language and communication.

Of all the elements of language that could be impaired, disordered pragmatic development is "pathognomonic" of the language impairment in autism (Twachtman-Cullen, 1998). There is a very simple explanation for this that has its roots in the developmental events that precede spoken language and constitute the underpinnings of pragmatic communication ability. In the next section, we describe the role and importance of three prelinguistic skills in the development of effective symbolic communication: *joint attention, affect sharing,* and *intention reading.* Discussion of how these develop in typical children will be juxtaposed with a discussion of how they are impaired in children with autism.

INTERRELATED SOCIAL-COGNITIVE PRECURSORS TO SYMBOLIC COMMUNICATION DEVELOPMENT

Joint Attention

Effective communication requires coordinated attention (i.e., joint attention) between communication partners, a referent (object), and word(s) or other symbolic means of communication (manual sign, picture) (Adamson & Chance, 1998). Moreover, joint attention may be broken down into *responding to joint attention* and *initiating joint attention.* While both types are associated with language development in children with autism (Charman et al., 2003; Loveland & Landry, 1986; Mundy, Sigman, Ungerer, & Sherman, 1986; Sigman & Ruskin, 1999), initiating joint attention may be considered the more purely social of the two types of joint attention. Hence, when an individual initiates joint attention to share his or her interest with another, it is considered *a protodeclarative act* in that it serves a social, as opposed to an instrumental, function. According to Mundy and Thorp (2006), "less pronounced deficits" are seen in coordinating social attention for instrumental purposes (i.e., initiating a behavioral request). This is referred to as a *protoimperative act* in that it serves a behavioral regulation, as opposed to social, function. It is important to note that whereas in less impaired children with autism difficulty in responding to joint attention may abate over time, problems in initiating joint attention remain robust in both more and less able individuals with autism over time (Mundy & Thorp, 2006).

The importance of joint attention cannot be overstated. In order to "connect up" a linguistic symbol with its communicative intent, the child must engage in what Tomasello (2003) refers to as a "dual-level social-cognitive process" (p. 65). According to Tomasello:

[The child] must first establish some form of common ground with an adult, in the context of a joint attentional frame, and then within this frame be able to read the adult's specific communicative intention in using a particular linguistic item [word]—by both extracting its form and isolating its [pragmatic] functional role within the adult's [communicative] intention as a whole. (p. 65)

Tomasello (2003) refers to joint attention (between adult and child) and intention reading by the child as "foundational" in the development of two-way, conventional communication, a position that Bruner (1983) held and supported with evidence even earlier. Expanding upon Bruner's work, Tomasello and Todd (1983) and Tomasello, Mannle, and Kruger (1986) investigated the degree to which joint attention between mother and child influences early language development. In both studies a relationship was found between vocabulary size and the amount of time the children spent in joint attention with their mothers.

It is important to note that there is a growing body of research demonstrating the same trend in autism. Specifically, joint attention and vocabulary size are related in children with autism in the *same* manner in which they are related in typically developing children, suggesting that the *same* principles governing language acquisition in typically developing children also govern language acquisition in children with autism (Loveland & Landry, 1986; Mundy, Sigman, & Kasari, 1990). Furthermore, Siller and Sigman (2002) found that for children with autism, joint attention in their early years had predictive value for language development in their adolescent years. Hence, the following conclusions can be drawn from studies of joint attention and language development:

- Joint attention is the "common ground" in which communication takes root and language blossoms.
- Since joint attention and language development bear the same relationship to each other in autism as they do in typical development, the establishment of joint attention has important implications for language intervention in autism, a point that will be elaborated below.

Affect Sharing

Another social-cognitive precursor to symbolic communication, and one that contributes to the capacity for joint attention, is that of affect sharing, or the expression of emotional states. Such expressions can be positive, as, for example, when a person directs attention in order to share with someone else that which is of interest to him. Or, affect sharing can occur with the expression of negative emotions, as when the individual shares her distress with someone for the purpose of obtaining comfort. Sharing affect also enables children to learn how to interpret the emotions expressed by others as they experience the individual's reactions to their own affective states (Wetherby, 2006). Several studies have demonstrated that children with autism have pronounced deficits in affect sharing (Dawson, Hill, Spencer, Galpert, & Watson, 1990; Snow, Hertzig, & Shapiro, 1987) and these deficits are recognized in the DSM-IV (American Psychiatric Association, 1994). A relationship between affect sharing and joint attention has been posited. According to Wetherby (2006), "Evidence suggests that the deficit in the capacity for sharing positive affect among children with ASD [autism spectrum disorder] may be associated with the deficit in initiating and responding to joint attention" (p. 10). Wetherby goes on to state that this may be so because deficits in both joint attention and sharing affect involve the dispersion of attention between persons and objects.

Intention Reading

Another important social-cognitive precursor to the development of communication and language is the ability of the child to "read" the adult's intentions and eventually predict the adult's responses—both of which are by-products of joint attention and affect sharing. The rudiments of intention reading can be seen in early infancy. For example, Legerstee, Barna, and DiAdamo (2000) found that by the age of 6 months, infants had already developed expectations regarding the behavior of adults. Specifically, they expected adults to talk to people rather than to objects and to reach for objects rather than people. Expectation was evidenced by the infants' tendency to gaze longer at an unexpected event than an expected one. According to these researchers, this demonstrated an emerging understanding of the intentions and viewpoints of others.

Intention Reading and Word Learning

Intention reading, like joint attention, is an essential part of word learning. According to Tomasello (2001), "learning new words is dependent on young children's ability to perceive and comprehend adult intentions, and they do this using a wide array of social-pragmatic cues" (p. 114). Tomasello and his colleagues carried out a number of experimental studies that support this contention (Akhtar & Tomasello, 1996; Tomasello & Barton, 1994; Tomasello, Strosberg, & Akhtar, 1995). These studies were designed to specifically preclude the use of the word-learning constraints that other researchers have hypothesized to support their theories of word learning (e.g., predilection toward naming the whole object, syntactic bootstrapping, and mutual exclusivity). In addition, specific precautions were also taken against the use of eye gaze as a clue to the adult's referential intention. These precautions were taken to ensure that intentionality judgments were not confounded by other variables.

All of the outcomes of these studies support the notion that word learning "is a process of skill learning that builds upon a deep and pervasive understanding of other persons and their intentional actions (i.e., social cognition in general) that is available to children by the time language acquisition begins" (Tomasello, 2001, p. 123). What is exceptional about this conclusion is that it answers a very important question that other theories of language development (e.g., accounts based on learning theory) have been unable to answer: Why does language acquisition begin when it does—around the time of, or shortly after, the child's first birthday, rather than much earlier in the child's development? According to Tomasello (2003), "Language acquisition begins when it does because it depends on the ability to share attention with other human beings communicatively and so to form symbols, an ability that emerges near the end of the first year of life" (p. 91). Thus, the emergence of first words and the ability to share attention are not merely coincidental. Rather, they are both interdependent and integral to the process of language acquisition itself. Finally, this is not to dispute that some of the principles of other word-learning theories may apply—indeed some do—but rather to convey that they are limited in their ability to account for the richness and nuances involved in the acquisition of symbolic communication.

Implications of Research Findings for Individuals with Autism

How do the findings regarding the preeminence of joint attention and intention reading in the acquisition of language square with what is known about autism? It is our contention that they help to explain many of the communication and language deficits that are seen in autism. Joint attention deficits are indisputable in children with autism (Lewy & Dawson, 1992; Mundy et al., 1986; Wetherby, Prizant, & Hutchinson, 1998), although the level of impairment varies from mild impairment in some children to severe impairment in others. Furthermore, as noted earlier, higher-level joint attention skills, such as those found in more able children, are associated with increased linguistic ability, while lower-level joint attention skills, such as those found in less able children, are associated with decreased linguistic ability (Loveland & Landry, 1986; Mundy et al., 1990; Siller & Sigman, 2002).

Likewise, deficits in theory of mind—the ability to understand the intentions and viewpoints of others—are also not only associated with autism (Baron-Cohen, 1995; Frith, 1989), but also more apparent in less able than in more able individuals. Moreover, as in the case of joint attention, Tager-Flusberg (1993, 1997) posits a direct link between theory of mind and language acquisition, noting that they are integrated with each other and progress according to similar timetables. Taking all of this information into account, it seems reasonable to conclude that the foundational skills of joint attention and intention reading play similar roles in language acquisition in children with autism and in typically developing children, since those with autism who have higher-level skill development in these areas also have higher-level linguistic ability and vice versa.

To summarize, the prelinguistic skills of joint attention, affect sharing, and intention reading constitute the social roots of pragmatics and are crucial to the development of verbal language. Compromises in these important precursors to symbolic communication in less able children with autism set up a kind of domino effect of pragmatic impairment that severely impacts their ability to understand and use language.

PRAGMATICS AND CHILDREN WITH SEVERE COMMUNICATION AND LANGUAGE IMPAIRMENTS

According to Twachtman-Cullen (1998), "Pragmatics (i.e., the use of language for communication purposes) is best conceptualized as that critical feature of human interaction that represents the intrinsic blending of social, emotional, cognitive, and linguistic factors in the sending and receiving of messages" (pp. 205–206). There are several aspects of pragmatics, including the ability to make judgments, that enable the speaker to regulate the style and content of speech and to apply the rules of discourse in conversational exchanges. Given our focus on children who are either nonverbal or minimally verbal, however, we will confine our discussion to the most basic aspect of pragmatics—the use of speech acts, signs, and/or gestures to accomplish an intended purpose.

It is important to note that there is a complementary relationship between communicative intentions and pragmatic functions, such that when a person uses language to express a specific intent, that piece of language is said to serve a particular function (Tomasello, 2003). For example, if one intends to obtain a cookie by saying "cookie," that word serves the function of *requesting*. If, however, one says "cookie" intending to demarcate a dessert option, the word in that context serves an *informing* function. Simply stated, the pragmatic functions of communication express our intents and are the reasons why we use language. Besides requesting and informing, one can use language to refuse unwanted items, to ask questions, to give answers, and so forth and so on. There is a wide range of pragmatic functions, extending from those that are very basic, such as requesting, protesting, asking, or informing, to those that are more complex, such as negotiating and using sarcasm.

It is also important to note that there are significant differences in the way the pragmatic functions of communication develop in typical children versus those with autism, since this has implications for intervention. In a groundbreaking study, Wetherby and Prutting (1984) found that children with autism developed pragmatic functions in a sequential hierarchy that was not observed in their typically developing counterparts. Specifically, individuals with autism communicated for behavioral regulation purposes (e.g., requesting, protesting) first, followed by social interaction functions (e.g., greeting, obtaining attention), and finally by joint attention functions (e.g., commenting, informing). These researchers further noted that many less able individuals with autism never developed communication for joint attention purposes (Wetherby & Prutting, 1984). In contrast, typically developing children learn the pragmatic functions of communication in a more amalgamated fashion and, indeed, spend countless hours sharing affect and attention with caregivers through the games of infancy (e.g., pat-a-cake and peekaboo) long before they learn to communicate intentionally for behavior regulation purposes.

INTERVENTION CONSIDERATIONS

Setting the Stage for Joint Attention

As discussed earlier, the ability to use symbols—whether words, manual signs, pictures, objects, or computerized devices—depends upon the integrity of the interrelated, social-cognitive precursors to symbolic development: joint attention, affect sharing, and intention reading. Since these precursors are interdependent, disruption in any one of them will affect the others, which, together, will have a deleterious, domino-like effect on language development in general. Given the importance of these processes to communication and language development, when one considers intervention, the question to ask is: If joint attention is a critical precursor to symbolic development, and the vehicle within which affect sharing and intention reading occur, can it be "trained up" in autism?

Kasari (2005) investigated joint attention and symbolic play skills. Fifty-eight children with autism between the ages of 3 and 4 were randomized to a joint attention intervention, a symbolic play intervention, or a control group. Interventions were conducted for a period of 5 to 6 weeks for 30 minutes per day. Results of this study indicate that children with autism can learn to initiate joint attention and symbolic play. Furthermore, a follow-up at 1 year showed that joint attention skills generalized to other individuals and were maintained over a long period of time.

The findings of this study are critically important to communication and language development and to intervention in autism. Lending further credence to approaches that target the two types of joint attention, Yoder and McDuffie (2006) state, "There is theoretical and empirical support for the hypothesis that responding to joint attention and initiating joint attention have developmental and diagnostic importance for children with autism. Therefore, it is surprising that so few interventions target responding to joint attention and initiating joint attention in this population" (p. 121). Very often language intervention with individuals with autism begins with adult-determined instructional targets (e.g., the expression of specific words), to the detriment of shared interest and joint attention. In addition, these interventions may fail to take into account the importance of motivation to successful communication, particularly in less able individuals, for whom motivation is typically problematic.

Another common practice in language intervention with the less able population is that of insistence on verbal language. When this occurs with individuals where problems in praxis (motor planning) or other internal processes compromise verbal language development, two things typically occur: valuable time helping the individual to communicate is lost and the stage is inadvertently set for disruptions in behavior that serve as "compensatory adaptations" for the purpose of communicating one's needs (Damico & Nelson, 2005). We believe that insisting on verbal language to the exclusion of all other forms of expression actually sabotages communication. In contrast, a focus on communication can help to facilitate verbal language if the mechanical transmission processes needed for spoken language are intact. Furthermore, a communication-first approach in this population not only mirrors the normal language-learning process, as articulated earlier in this chapter, but may also help to reduce or eliminate problem behaviors that are used as compensatory adaptations.

The Importance of Initiation in Communication and Language Intervention

Those attempting to teach communication to the less able individual with autism often face a long and difficult journey. Not only can there be severe delays in the development of verbal language—or worse yet, a lack of development of verbal language—but there are also often delays in the development of intentional and symbolic communication of any kind. Individuals who are at a presymbolic and/or preintentional level require specialized intervention that meets them at their developmental level and gradually builds upon previously learned communication skills.

Autism intervention is replete with cases of individuals who, despite years of specialized programming and the best efforts of professionals, are unable to consistently communicate their basic needs independently. This is clearly troubling, given the importance of basic communication for quality of life and the large amount of programming time typically expended on its behalf. Interestingly, the communication training techniques found to be unsuccessful in autism are often successful with individuals who have other developmental disabilities, prompting one to ask whether the most appropriate intervention methods are being employed to teach this specific population. More to the point, could it be that interventionists are overlooking (and hence, neglecting) intervention targets that are critical to successful communication training in this population?

One possible explanation for the frequent failure of less able individuals to develop functional communication skills is that interventionists often take the wrong "road" to communicative success. Specifically, in many communication intervention programs, emphasis is first on the teaching of a symbolic *means* of communication (e.g., spoken words, sign language, pictures, etc.), rather than on the *process* of communication itself (J. L. Twachtman, 1996). It is our opinion that the road leading to functional communication skills in this population is not that of vocabulary development, but rather that which leads to the development of intentional, independently initiated communication onto which vocabulary may be mapped. Significantly, this type of intervention approach incorporates the critical precursors to symbolic communication—joint attention, affect sharing, and intention reading.

Twachtman (1996) proposed a multicomponent intervention methodology that emphasized the development of a reliable communication system that "[the individual] can use immediately, easily, and independently to initiate communicative interactions for all targeted [communicative] functions" (p. 214). This methodology involves several components, including developmental readiness, from the perspective of the discontinuities with which the child with autism presents, and a respect for the individual's role in "designing" his or her own communication system. Here, communication training centers around the individual's communicative initiations, even when these are not intentional communicative acts, but rather reactions that the individual has based upon his or her needs, discomforts, and desires. In the preintentional communicator, and in intentional communicators who are limited in their knowledge of the communicative means available to them, initiations often consist of undesirable behavior. While this behavior is, on its face, problematic, it nevertheless has message value, and can be shaped to more appropriate communicative behavior. For example, less able individuals who are not aware of appropriate means of requesting may simply take food items that they desire. The knowledgeable interventionist, viewing this behavior through the lens of initiation, would likely see that the behavior represents the individual's motivation to obtain something. This is critical, since such motivation is often lacking in communication programs that attempt to teach a preset vocabulary that may not be useful to the individual who lacks a fundamental understanding of the process of communication. The interventionist would then follow the individual's lead and set about shaping the inappropriate communicative means (taking food items) to more appropriate communicative means (requesting through the use of object, picture, manual sign, etc.). It is through this type of process that idiosyncratic communicative behavior becomes more conventional.

A focus on the initiations that the child is currently producing respects the developmental pragmatic hierarchy that has been found to exist in individuals with autism (Wetherby & Prutting, 1984). Thus, the child who communicates only for behavioral regulation functions will receive training that is focused on improving and refining his or her communication at this level. Furthermore, synchronizing language targets to the focus of the child's attention has been shown to improve language outcomes for children with autism spectrum disorder (Siller & Sigman, 2002).

A key component of teaching the preintentional child that his or her initiations have message value is the encouragement of eye-gaze shifts from object of attention to the communication partner. This helps to establish the required component of joint attention (between communication partners and desired object) and provides opportunities for affect sharing and intention reading. It is important to note that intention reading is developed by teaching the individual with autism that his or her communication partner did not know what the individual's need was before the child communicated this to the adult. Hence, the individual learns that he or she must do something to provoke a response in the adult to get a particular need met.

Once intentional communication is established, the interventionist may then attempt to map one or more symbolic means of communication onto the child's initiations. It is important to note here that an individual's communication system will consist of many different means of communication (Vanderheiden & Yoder, 1986). Thus, interventionists using this approach do not (and should not) choose one specific means of communication (e.g., speech *or* sign language *or* pictures) to train the child to use. Rather, they should follow the child's lead in his or her own selection of communicative means, onto which they map language and shape initiations to more conventional communicative behavior. More specific information on how this is done is given in the section below on joint action routines. Finally, we recommend that communication training for less able individuals begin low on the symbolic "ladder" and very gradually proceed upward, based upon the individual's ability to initiate communication.

Considerations Regarding Level of Symbolic Development

Support for proceeding with caution vis-à-vis level of symbolic development is found in the picture-recognition literature, summarized by Troseth, Pierroutsakos, & DeLoache (2004). These researchers note that while young children recognize that a picture represents an object (i.e., its *referent*), typical children below the age of 2 have difficulty recognizing the *relationship* between picture and object. Specifically, toddlers will often attempt to manipulate pictures as if they were the actual objects represented (discussed by DeLoache and colleagues, as cited in Troseth et al., 2004).

Troseth et al. (2004) also described an interesting study by Harris, Kavanaugh, and Dowson that concluded that there was a "dramatic failure by children below the age of 2 years to relate a picture to what it depicts" (p. 18). In this study, neurotypical children witnessed an experimenter squirting a toy pig with ketchup. They were then presented with three pictures—one depicting a clean pig, one in which the pig was covered with ketchup, and one in which the pig had a white spot on its neck. The children were asked to choose the picture that correctly depicted the action they had witnessed. To eliminate difficulties with scanning, the experimenter pointed to each picture and asked the child, "Does the pig look like this?" Despite the fact that the object remained in front of the child during the picture selection process, children below age 2 performed no better than at the level of chance on this task. Of significance here is that the participants in this study were being asked to use a picture to communicate regarding an event and that below the age of 2 they were unable to do this, despite previously established abilities of children this age to recognize that pictures represent objects (Troseth et al., 2004).

This study has important implications for the selection of intervention materials appropriate to less able individuals with autism. Clearly, the ability to *label* a picture with the correct name of the object it represents does not mean that the individual can *use* that picture to communicate. A possible explanation for this result may be found in the autism literature. Specifically, Minshew, Meyer, and Goldstein (2002) found that there is dissociation between concept *formation* and concept *identification* in more able individuals with autism such that these individuals demonstrate greater competence in identification tasks than in concept formation tasks. Similarly, Brown, Solomon, Bauminger, and Rogers (2005), in their study of concept formation versus concept identification, found that children with autism performed about as well as typically developing children on identification tasks, but less well on concept formation tasks. Hence, it appears that the ability to label (i.e., identify) a picture is at a simpler cognitive level than that which is required to actually use that picture to convey communicative intent, an act that clearly requires formation of the concept. That said, using pictures as a means of communication for children with autism who present with language skills below age 2 would seem to be inadvisable—a position that is clearly relevant to less able individuals with autism.

An approach that we have found to be successful for this population is one that employs the use of small objects that clearly depict the actual items they represent. The key issue is iconicity. In other words, the more the small object actually looks like the item it represents, the greater the chance that it will have symbolic value for the less able individual with autism. For example, refrigerator magnets or other small objects representing a hamburger and a hot dog can be used by the individual to request the desired food choice. Similarly, a small plastic glass or cup can be used to request a beverage. By using small objects first, it may be possible for some individuals with autism to later move to the use of pictures. Whether this is possible or not is predominantly dependent upon the individual's functioning level.

AN INTERVENTION APPROACH TAILORED
TO THE NEEDS OF LESS ABLE INDIVIDUALS
WITH AUTISM: THE JOINT ACTION ROUTINE

Naturalistic therapeutic intervention embedded within the environmental setting in which performance of the task would normally occur is particularly important for individuals with more significant challenges, as the context can help to support sense making. This is particularly true from the point of view of generalization, since the context for skill development is also the context for skill use. Consider, for instance, the joint action routine (Snyder-McLean, Solomonson, McLean, & Sack, 1984) as a vehicle that provides communication and language intervention within a joint attention, highly motivating, and naturally reinforcing framework. It is well established that routines provide an important context for learning language (Bruner, 1983; Snow, 1981). Joint action routines can be set up around normally occurring routines such as snack, play, household chores, or shopping (Twachtman, 1995). For example, in a joint action snack routine individuals with autism are presented with an out-of-immediate-reach tray of three or four snack items, the majority of which are preferred, with one or two nonpreferred items available to work on the pragmatic function of protesting (i.e., refusing). Individuals who do not yet exhibit conventional intentional communication may use eye gaze to indicate their preferences. The interventionist would then act *as if* the individual had intentionally communicated and grant the "requested" food item (or support the refusal—perhaps a push-away gesture—of the nonpreferred item). Through such occurrences, over time, even the nonverbal, preintentional individual can learn that gaze shifts between desired items and interventionist (gradually shaped to pointing, object/picture exchange, manual sign, or spoken word) have message value.

In addition to being an excellent vehicle for the establishment of functional vocabulary, the joint action snack routine has many other advantages. Specifically, because it involves desirable food and beverage items, it is naturally motivating. Moreover, this intervention activity also provides in-kind reinforcement. For example, if the individual requests *apple,* he or she is reinforced by receiving a piece of apple. Clearly, this is a direct and logical consequence of the request, making the establishment of meaning more likely. Contrast this with pointing to a picture of an apple and receiving a piece of candy as reinforcement for the correct response. The joint action snack routine also provides an excellent milieu within which to learn important concepts (e.g., requesting *more*; indicating that one is *finished*) and prosocial skills such as sharing.

Finally, the overarching advantage to this intervention approach is that it is an excellent vehicle within which to establish a reliable, functional, and conventional communication system that is particularly well suited to the communication needs that individuals with significant challenges bring to the table.

To summarize, in addition to providing rich opportunities for joint attention, affect sharing, and intention reading, joint action routines also provide:

- A motivating, low-stress setting that promotes sense making
- Need- and usage-based opportunities to develop *functional* communication
- A predictable sequence of events
- Natural reinforcements embedded in the language-learning process
- A commonsense context for learning vocabulary and concepts
- Opportunities for repetition and expansion of language-learning targets
- A vehicle for demonstrating the power of communication to exert control over one's life

It should be obvious that few language intervention techniques offer all of the advantages that joint attention routines offer with respect to naturalistic, in-context communication and language intervention for less able individuals. Clearly, it is a technique that fits the multifaceted needs of this population.

CONCLUSION

Less able individuals with autism present profound challenges with respect to communication and language development. We acknowledge that verbal language may not be feasible for some of the more significantly impaired individuals. Nevertheless, it is our contention that all individuals with autism—regardless of degree of impairment—have the right to a functional, conventional, and reliable communication system. Furthermore, we believe that this goal is achievable when interventionists work within a motivating context to shape the individual's current communicative repertoire to more conventional need- and usage-based forms. Even within this framework, however, for some individuals, communication will be very basic—confined to communicating for behavioral regulation purposes. For others, varying degrees of interactive communication will be possible. Toward this end, we have examined the often overlooked, but critically important social–cognitive precursors to communication and language development—joint attention, affect sharing, and intention reading. Taking our lead from the language research literature, we have drawn the conclusion that a lack of attention to these critical precursors may be at the root of failed efforts in language intervention with less able individuals with autism and attention to them provides a necessary foundation for communication and language skill development. Finally, we have argued that a pragmatically based intervention approach that takes into account both the developmental discontinuities in autism and the precursors to communicative development provides a treatment milieu that precisely fits the needs of this population.

REFERENCES

Adamson, L. B., & Chance, S. E. (1998). Coordinating attention to people, objects, and language. In A. M. Wetherby, S. F. Warren, & J. Reichle (Eds.), *Transitions in prelinguistic communication*. Baltimore: Brookes.

Akhtar, N., & Tomasello, M. (1996). Twenty-four-month-old children learn words for absent objects and actions. *British Journal of Developmental Psychology, 14*, 79–93.

American Psychiatric Association. (1994). *Diagnostic and statistical manual of mental disorders* (4th ed.). Washington, DC: Author.

Baron-Cohen, S. (1995). *Mindblindness: An essay on autism and theory of mind*. Cambridge, MA: MIT Press.

Bloom, L., & Lahey, M. (1978). *Language development and language disorders*. New York: Wiley.

Brown, J., Solomon, M., Bauminger, N., & Rogers, S. (2005). Concept formation and concept identification in high functioning children with autism spectrum disorders [Abstract]. *International Meeting For Autism Research Abstracts, S6(3)*.

Bruner, J. (1983). *Child's talk*. New York: Norton.

Carr, E. G., & Durand, V. M. (1985). Reducing behavior problems through functional communication training. *Journal of Applied Behavior Analysis, 18*, 111–126.

Charman, T., Baron-Cohen, S., Swettenham, J., Baird, G., Drew, A., & Cox, A. (2003). Predicting language outcome in infants with autism and pervasive developmental disorder. *International Journal of Language and Communication Disorders, 38*, 265–285.

Damico, J. S., & Nelson, R. L. (2005). Interpreting problematic behavior: Systematic compensatory adaptations as emergent phenomena in autism. *Clinical Linguistics & Phonetics, 19(5)*, 405–417.

Dawson, G., Hill, D., Spencer, A., Galpert, L., & Watson, L. (1990). Affective exchanges between young autistic children and their mothers. *Journal of Abnormal Child Psychology, 18*, 335–345.

Donnellan, A., Mirenda, P., Mesaros, R., & Fassbender, L. (1984). Analyzing the communicative functions of aberrant behavior. *Journal of the Association for Persons with Severe Handicaps, 9*, 202–212.

Dore, J. (1974). A pragmatic description of early language development. *Journal of Psycholinguistic Research, 3*, 343–350.

Dore, J. (1975). Holophrases, speech acts, and language universals. *Journal of Child Language, 2*, 21–40.

Duchan, J. (1984). Language assessment: The pragmatics revolution. In R. Naremore (Ed.), *Language science: Recent advances.* San Diego, CA: College-Hill Press.

Fein, D., Pennington, B. F., Markowitz, P., Braverman, M., & Waterhouse, L. (1986). Toward a neuropsychological model of infantile autism: Are the social deficits primary? *Journal of the American Academy of Child and Adolescent Psychiatry, 25*(2), 198–212.

Frith, U. (1989). *Autism: Explaining the enigma.* Cambridge, MA: Blackwell.

Halliday, M. A. K. (1975). *Learning how to mean: Explorations in the development of language.* London: Edward Arnold.

Kanner, L. (1943). Autistic disturbances of affective contact. *Nervous Child, 2*, 217–250.

Kasari, C. (2005). Growth in joint attention and symbolic play [Abstract]. *International Meeting For Autism Research Abstracts, S6*(3).

Kaye, K. (1982). *The mental and social life of babies: How parents create persons.* Chicago: University of Chicago Press.

Legerstee, M., Barna, J., & DiAdamo, C. (2000). Precursors to the development of intention at 6 months: Understanding people and their actions. *Developmental Psychology, 36*(5), 627–634.

Lewy, A. L., & Dawson, G. (1992). Social stimulation and joint attention in young autistic children. *Journal of Abnormal Child Psychology, 20*, 555–566.

Loveland, K., & Landry, S. (1986). Joint attention in autism and developmental language delay. *Journal of Autism and Developmental Disorders, 16*, 335–349.

Minshew, N. J., Meyer, J., & Goldstein, G. (2002). Abstract reasoning in autism: A dissociation between concept formation and concept identification. *Neuropsychology, 16*, 327–334.

Muma, J. (1978). *Language handbook.* Englewood Cliffs, NJ: Prentice-Hall.

Mundy, P., Sigman, M., & Kasari, C. (1990). A longitudinal study of joint attention and language development in autistic children. *Journal of Autism and Developmental Disorders, 20*, 115–128.

Mundy, P., Sigman, M., Ungerer, J., & Sherman, T. (1986). Defining the social deficits of autism: The contribution of nonverbal communication measures. *Journal of Child Psychology and Psychiatry and Allied Disciplines, 27*, 657–669.

Mundy, P., & Thorp, D. (2006). The neural basis of early joint-attention behavior. In T. Charman & W. Stone (Eds.), *Social and communication development in autism spectrum disorders: Early identification, diagnosis, and intervention* (pp. 296–336). New York: Guilford Press.

Owens, R. E., Jr. (1988). *Language development: An introduction.* Columbus, OH: Merrill.

Prizant, B., & Duchan, J. (1981). The functions of immediate echolalia in autistic children. *Journal of Speech and Hearing Disorders, 46,* 241–249.

Prizant, B. M., & Rydell, P. J. (1984). An analysis of the functions of delayed echolalia in autistic children. *Journal of Speech and Hearing Research, 27,* 183–192.

Sacks, O. (1989). *Seeing voices: A journey into the world of the deaf.* Los Angeles: University of California Press.

Sameroff, A. (1987). The social context of development. In N. Eisenburg (Ed.), *Contemporary topics in development* (pp. 273–291). New York: Wiley.

Sameroff, A., & Friese, B. (1990). Transactional regulation and early intervention. In S. Meisels & J. Shonkoff (Eds.), *Early intervention: A handbook of theory, practice, and analysis* (pp. 119–149). New York: Cambridge University Press.

Sigman, M., & Ruskin, E. (1999). Continuity and change in the social competence of children with autism, Down syndrome, and developmental delays. *Monographs of the Society for Research in Child Development, 64*(1).

Siller, M., & Sigman, M. (2002). The behaviors of parents of children with autism predict the subsequent development of their children's communication skills. *Journal of Autism and Developmental Disorders 32*(2), 77–89.

Snow, C. (1981). The uses of imitation. *Journal of Child Language, 3,* 205–212.

Snow, M. E., Hertzig, M. E., & Shapiro, T. (1987). Expressions of emotion in young autistic children. *Journal of the American Academy of Child and Adolescent Psychiatry, 27,* 647–655.

Snyder-McLean, L., Solomonson, B., McLean, J., & Sack, S. (1884). Structuring joint action routines: A strategy for facilitating communication and language development in the classroom. *Seminars in Speech and Language, 5,* 213–228.

Tager-Flusberg, H. (1993). What language reveals about the understanding of minds in children with autism. In S. Baron-Cohen, H. Tager-Flusberg, & D. J. Cohen (Eds.), *Understanding other minds: Perspectives from autism* (pp. 138–157). New York: Oxford University Press.

Tager-Flusberg, H. (1997). Language acquisition and theory of mind: Contributions from the study of autism. In L. B. Adamson & M. A. Romski (Eds.), *Communication and language acquisition: Discoveries from atypical development* (pp. 135–160). Baltimore: Brookes.

Tomasello, M. (2001). Perceiving intentions and learning words in the second year of life. In M. Tomasello and E. Bates (Eds.), *Language development: The essential readings* (pp. 111–128). Malden, MA: Blackwell Publishers.

Tomasello, M. (2003). *Constructing a language: A usage-based theory of language acquisition.* Cambridge, MA: Harvard University Press.

Tomasello, M., & Barton, M. (1994). Learning words in non-ostensive contexts. *Developmental Psychology 30,* 639–650.

Tomasello, M., Mannle, S., & Kruger, A. (1986). Linguistic environment of one to two year old twins. *Developmental Psychology, 22,* 169–176.

Tomasello, M., Strosberg, R., & Akhtar, N. (1995). Eighteen-month-old children learn words in non-ostensive contexts. *Journal of Child Language, 22,* 1–20.

Tomasello, M., & Todd, J. (1983). Joint attention and lexical acquisition style. *First Language 4*, 197–212.

Troseth, G. L., Pierroutsakos, S. L., & DeLoache, J. S. (2004). From the innocent to the intelligent eye: The early development of pictorial competence. In R. V. Kail (Ed.), *Advances in child development and behavior* (Vol. 32, pp. 1–35). Boston: Elsevier Academic Press.

Twachtman, D. (1995). Methods to enhance communication in verbal children. In K. A. Quill (Ed.), *Teaching children with autism: Strategies to enhance communication and socialization* (pp. 133–162). Albany, NY: Delmar.

Twachtman, J. L. (1996). Improving the human condition through communication training in autism. In J. R. Cautela & W. Ishaq (Eds.), *Contemporary issues in behavior therapy: Improving the human condition* (pp. 207–231). New York: Plenum Press.

Twachtman-Cullen, D. (1998). Language and communication in HFA and AS. In E. Schopler, G. B. Mesibov, and L. J. Kunce (Eds.), *Asperger syndrome or high-functioning autism?* (pp. 199–225). New York: Plenum Press.

Vanderheiden, G. C., & Yoder, D. (1986). Overview. In S. W. Blackstone (Ed.), *Augmentative communication: An introduction* (pp. 1–28). Rockville, MD: American Speech-Language-Hearing Association.

Venter A., Lord, C., & Schopler, E. (1992). A follow-up study of high-functioning autistic children. *Journal of Child Psychology and Psychiatry, 33,* 489–507.

Wetherby, A. (2006). Understanding and measuring social communication in children with autism spectrum disorders. In T. Charman & W. Stone (Eds.), *Social and communication development in autism spectrum disorders: Early identification, diagnosis, and intervention* (pp. 3–34). New York: Guilford Press.

Wetherby, A. M., Prizant, B. M., & Hutchinson, T. A. (1998). Communicative, social/affective, and symbolic profiles of young children with autism and pervasive developmental disorders. *American Journal of Speech–Language Pathology, 7,* 79–91.

Wetherby, A. M., & Prutting, C. A. (1984). Profiles of communicative and cognitive-social abilities in autistic children. *Journal of Speech and Hearing Research, 27*(3), 364–377.

Yoder, P. J., & McDuffie, A. S. (2006). Treatment of responding to and initiating joint attention. In T. Charman & W. Stone (Eds.), *Social and communication development in autism spectrum disorders: Early identification, diagnosis, and intervention* (pp. 117–142). New York: Guilford Press.

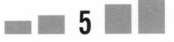

Sensory Processing Disorders in Children with Autism

Nature, Assessment, and Intervention

Eynat Gal
Sharon A. Cermak
Ayelet Ben-Sasson

Children and adolescents with autism often present with sensory processing disorders. In addition to communication and social core deficits, autism is defined by restricted stereotyped behaviors (American Psychiatric Association, 2000). These behaviors include sensory and motor aspects such as unusual sensory interests and stereotyped body movements. Additional sensory–motor features often associated with autism include over- and underresponsivity to sensations, clumsiness, and abnormal postures (O'Neill & Jones, 1997). Firsthand accounts of adults with autism reveal their unusual sensory experiences including sensitivity, distortions in sensory perception, and fascination with the details of sensory input (Grandin, 1995; Grandin & Scariano, 1986; Jones, Quigney, & Huws, 2003; Shore, 2001; Williams, 1998). Several scholars have suggested that sensory processing symptoms underlie the core social and communication deficits in autism (Ornitz, Guthrie, &

Farley, 1978; Talay-Ongan & Wood, 2000). It is important to address sensory processing disorders, as they have been significantly associated with impaired daily living skills (Kay, 2001; Liss, Saulnier, Fein, & Kinsbourne, 2006) and elevated anxiety and depressive symptoms in children with autism (Pfeiffer, Kinnealey, Reed, & Herzberg, 2005). Various intervention methods have been applied to address sensory processing disorders in persons with autism in the form of direct sensory-integrative intervention, caregiver consultation, environmental and task adaptations, and the design of "sensory diets." These interventions aim to improve self-regulation and participation in activities of daily life.

The goal of this chapter is to (1) define sensory processing concepts and theory, (2) describe the nature of sensory processing disorders in children with autism, (3) demonstrate how these disorders may impact the participation of children with autism and their families in activities of daily living, and (4) outline the assessment and intervention methods used by occupational therapists to address sensory processing disorders in children with autism. Although this chapter focuses on types of sensory modulation and sensory processing disorders, motor issues that relate to sensory processing disorders are briefly reviewed. (See Leary & Hill, 1996, and Smith, 2004, for reviews of motor disorders in autism.)

SENSORY PROCESSING CONCEPTS AND THEORY

Sensory processing is a comprehensive term that refers to the way in which the nervous system manages sensory information, including the registration, modulation, integration, and organization of sensory input (Miller & Lane, 2000). Ayres (1985) described the human brain as a "sensory processing machine," as over 80% of the nervous system is involved in processing or organizing sensory input. Children and adults have characteristic ways of processing sensory information. For some people, particular sensory experiences are pleasurable, while these same sensory events are innocuous or noxious to others. Each way of responding to, or experiencing, sensation may have a corresponding pattern of behavior (Huebner & Dunn, 2001). However, for individuals with a sensory processing disorder these differences are extreme and may interfere with daily functioning (Miller, Lane, Cermak, Osten, & Anzalone, 2005)

Classification of Sensory Processing Disorders

Since the 1960s, sensory processing disorders have been defined by occupational therapists using different terms (Ayres, 1965, 1972). Recently, the Interdisciplinary Council for Developmental and Learning Disorders

(ICDL) task force revised the Zero to Three (2005) classification of regulatory sensory processing disorders (Miller et al., 2005). The ICDL classification was designed for young children; however, it is clinically relevant for older children as well. According to the ICDL model there are three types of sensory processing disorders: *sensory modulation, sensory discrimination,* and *sensory-based motor disorders.*

Sensory Modulation

Sensory modulation is one component of sensory processing and is defined as the ability to regulate and manage one's response to sensory input from auditory, visual, tactile, vestibular, and oral modalities in a graded and adaptive manner (Mulligan, 2002). Dunn (1997) defined sensory modulation as the ability to balance habituation and sensitization. Habituation is the ability of the nervous system to recognize a stimulus as familiar and to stop responding to that stimulus, for example the feel of clothing on our skin. Sensitization is the nervous system's ability to identify important or harmful stimuli and respond accordingly, for example responding to a fire alarm. Children with a *sensory modulation disorder* have difficulties regulating and organizing the degree and intensity of responses to sensory input in multiple sensory modalities. They are diagnosed based on their behavioral presentation; however, it is hypothesized that this disorder reflects atypical neurological responses of habituation and sensitization responses (Dunn, 1997). There is research that supports this hypothesis. For example, in an electrodermal response study, children with a sensory modulation disorder either showed reduced physiological response to sensations or showed more distinctive electrodermal responses, and were slower to habituate to sensations than children without a sensory modulation disorder (McIntosh, Miller, Shyu, & Hagerman, 1999).

Sensory modulation disorders consist of three subtypes: *sensory overresponsivity, sensory underresponsivity, and sensory seeking* (Miller et al., 2005). Sensory overresponsivity is defined as exaggerated, rapid-onset, or prolonged reactions to sensory stimulation (Miller et al., 2005). It is hypothesized that children who are overresponsive to sensory input may lack the ability to habituate their response to background stimuli. Children with overresponsivity tend to respond to sensory stimuli with anxiety, fearfulness, avoidance, and/or negative and oppositional behavior.

Sensory underresponsivity is defined as a lack of awareness or slow response to sensory input of typical intensity (Miller et al., 2005). This pattern is also referred to as a low registration pattern, which describes the child's difficulty noticing sensation. It is hypothesized that this behavioral response may reflect overhabituation. The child with under-responsivity may appear self-absorbed, uninterested, lethargic, passive, or slow in reacting to various stimuli.

Sensory seeking is defined as craving of and interest in sensory experiences that are prolonged or intense compared with those that appeal to typical children (Miller et al., 2005). Children with a sensory seeking pattern tend to be active, impulsive, and restless.

These three types of sensory modulation disorders are comparable to the four patterns of sensory modulation disorders defined by Dunn (1997): (1) sensory avoiding, (2) sensory sensitivity, (3) low registration, and (4) sensory seeking. Sensory avoiding and sensitivity are comparable to sensory overresponsivity, low registration is comparable to under-responsivity, and sensory seeking is a subtype in both models.

Sensory Discrimination

Sensory discrimination is the processing of spatial and temporal qualities of touch, movement, or body position, as well as vision and audition, and is important for skill development (Koomar & Bundy, 2002). For example, tactile input coming in through the skin receptors of the body provides information about the size, shape, and texture of objects. If a child were to put his hand in his pocket and feel different objects, he would be able to tell a coin from a key without the use of vision. Children with decreased tactile discrimination, therefore, may rely overly on their visual skills and have difficulties in automatic adjustment when grasping different objects such as cups or eating and writing utensils. Children with decreased proprioceptive discrimination may show difficulty in judging the amount of force or speed needed for a task. Children with poor discrimination also often present with poor awareness of their body and with dyspraxia (Ayres, 1972; Cermak & Larkin, 2002; Koomar & Bundy, 2002; Miller et al., 2005).

Sensory-Based Motor Challenges

Sensory-based motor challenges relate to postural disorders and dyspraxia (impairment in motor planning). Children with sensory-based motor difficulties, specifically somato-dyspraxia, often exhibit poor tactile and proprioceptive processing, clumsiness, poor gross-motor skills (e.g., difficulty in catching a ball, frequent tripping), difficulty with fine-motor and manipulation skills, and poor organization. They may have difficulties with balance, sequencing movements, bilateral coordination, and imitating movements (Miller et al., 2005; Rogers, 1999; Smith &

Bryson, 1994). Such difficulties are especially pronounced when the child learns a new motor skill and requires increased practice compared to typical children in order to automate the new skill.

THE NATURE OF SENSORY PROCESSING DISORDERS IN CHILDREN WITH AUTISM

The prevalence of sensory modulation disorders in school-age children with autism ranges from 30% to 88% across studies (Kientz & Dunn, 1997; Le Couteur et al., 1989; Ornitz, Guthrie, & Farley, 1977; Volkmar, Cohen, & Paul, 1986; Weisblatt, Parr, & Alcantara, 2005). Wide age ranges and differences in measures among studies may have contributed to these variations. Several sensory processing studies in autism (e.g., Ermer & Dunn, 1998; Kientz & Dunn, 1997) used the Sensory Profile (Dunn, 1995), a parent questionnaire assessing sensory processing behaviors during daily activities. Parent report studies demonstrated that school-age children with autism show higher frequencies of extreme sensory processing behaviors compared with their typically developing, age-matched peers (Kientz & Dunn, 1997; Miller, Reisman, McIntosh, & Simon, 2001; Talay-Ongan & Wood, 2000; VerMaas-Lee, 1999) and compared with children with mental retardation (Sagarin, 1998). However, fewer differences were found relative to other clinical populations such as children who have blindness and deafness or receptive aphasia (Wing, 1976). It appears that some aspects of sensory processing are unique to children with autism, while other aspects are common in other clinical populations as well. It is possible that children with autism are unique in their mixed pattern of modulation disorders. Wing (1976) described children with autism as those who typically have odd and contradictory responses to sensory input, including inattention, fascination, and distress. This clinical observation was supported by evidence showing that children with autism present with more than one type of sensory modulation disorder (Liss et al., 2006), specifically over- and underresponsivity (Baranek, David, Poe, Stone, & Watson, 2006; Ornitz et al., 1978). It is possible that this mixed pattern reflects a common underlying mechanism in poor sensory modulation (Dunn, 1997). Poor modulation can be expressed as difficulty maintaining an optimal level of arousal leading to exaggerated responses and fluctuation of response from under- to overresponsivity. Alternatively, underresponsive behaviors may be an attempt to shut down and avoid overwhelming sensations (Lane, 2002), and sensation-seeking responses may be the child's way of increasing arousal (Dunn, 1997).

Overresponse to Sensory Input

School-age children with autism show significantly more sensory over-responsive behaviors than typically developing children (Ermer & Dunn, 1998; Kientz & Dunn, 1997; Miller et al., 2001; Talay-Ongan & Wood, 2001) and other clinical populations such as children with fragile X (Miller et al., 2001) and children with attention-deficit/hyperactivity disorder (ADHD) (Ermer & Dunn, 1998). In a large-scale study of individuals with autism spectrum disorders (n = 248), 80% of parents reported negative sensory reactions by their child (e.g., dislike of certain textures) (Weisblatt et al., 2005). Children with autism and sensory overresponsivity presented 'fight,' 'flight,' and 'fright' reactions toward sensations such as light touch and loud noises. They were also highly distracted by background sensations and showed difficulty performing in overstimulating environments.

Underresponse to Sensory Input

Underresponsivity is considered by some investigators to be the most distinguishing sensory pattern of children with autism (Rogers & Ozonoff, 2005). Children with autism who are underresponsive may appear to be deaf or may show a delayed response to extreme temperature or pain. Some parent-report studies confirm this notion by showing a significantly higher frequency of underresponsivity in school-age children with autism compared with typically developing children (Kientz & Dunn, 1997) and compared with children with milder forms of autism spectrum disorders (pervasive developmental disorders not otherwise specified [PDDNOS]) (Liss et al., 2006; Smith-Myles et al., 2004). However, other studies did not find differences in underresponsivity between children with autism and typically developing children or relative to other clinical populations (Ermer & Dunn, 1998; Miller et al., 2001).

Sensory Seeking

There is contrasting evidence regarding sensory-seeking behaviors in children with autism. In one study, children with autism showed higher frequencies of sensory-seeking behaviors compared with typical children (Kientz & Dunn, 1997) and compared with children with PDDNOS (Liss, 2002), while in another study, they showed lower frequency of sensory seeking behaviors compared with typically developing children and children with ADHD (Ermer & Dunn, 1998). This contrasting evidence may relate to the fact that these studies evaluated the frequency of typical sensory seeking (e.g., seeking physical activities, touching textures), but did not focus on idiosyncratic unusual sensory interests (e.g., flicking fingers, smelling objects). In a study that examined unusual sensory interests in individuals with autism, rates were as high as 90% (Weisblatt et al., 2005), suggesting that the atypical nature of sensory seeking is important to evaluate for understanding sensory seeking in autism.

Sensory Modalities

Response to Auditory Stimuli

Aside from evidence of the unique types of sensory responses of children with autism, there are descriptions of the specific sensory modalities involved. Gillberg and Coleman (1992) argued that abnormal reactions to sound are common in children with autism. These odd behavioral responses to sounds include ignoring some sounds, fascination with other sounds, and display of distress when presented with other sounds. All these responses may occur within the same child. In a study of 248 individuals with autism, more individuals (77%) had noise sensitivity than unusual interest in sounds (9%) (Weisblatt et al., 2005). A recent study reported that children with autism showed superior auditory discrimination abilities relative to chronological age-matched typical peers (O'Riordan & Filippo, 2006). The authors suggested that this may relate to a heightened response to background sounds in children with autism. One must consider the contribution of auditory processing symptoms to the communication deficits of children with autism (Baranek et al., 2006). For example, a child with autism and auditory processing symptoms may respond more effectively when spoken to without background noise or in a certain tone of voice. Verbal and nonverbal communication require processing of both auditory and visual input, hence a child's inability to attend to and integrate auditory and visual input may lead to great disruption in communication and behavior.

Response to Visual Stimuli

In addition to atypical auditory responses, atypical responses to visual stimuli are present in many children with autism. In contrast with the auditory modality, more parents report visual interests than visual sensitivities in their child with autism (Weisblatt et al., 2005). Visual-seeking behaviors include fascination with geometrical figures, close visual examination of objects, and twirling and spinning of circular objects. Unusual visual responses observed in persons with autism include sensitivity to light, especially bright, flashing, or blinking lights, and difficulty finding things due to visual overload (McMullen, 2001). Visual sensitivity may also be manifested in peripheral eye contact or gaze aversion. However, it is difficult to disentangle the sensory, emotional, and social aspects of abnormal eye contact.

Response to Other Sensory Input

Odd responses to proximal sensations, such as touch, movement, taste and smell, pain, and temperature, are also present in children with autism. Again, the response can be fascination, distress, or indifference. Some children with autism seem to explore the world through these proximal senses for much longer time periods than usual, while other children dislike being touched and will pull away even from gentle, affectionate touch. Some children with autism may enjoy or seek deep touch, while others may display this desire in the form of self-injurious behaviors (e.g., head banging, pinching). Some children may be bothered by the feel of certain types of clothing, especially shoes and socks. Baranek and Berkson (1994) found that children with developmental disabilities, including autism, show a higher frequency of tactile over-responsiveness based on a caregiver report and direct examination. Miller and colleagues (2001) found tactile sensitivity to be more characteristic of children with autism than children with fragile X. In the vestibular modality, some children with autism show avoidance of movements that require the feet to leave the ground (e.g., riding an escalator), while others may seek physical activity in the form of stereotyped movements.

Unusual oral (includes taste and smell) responses are highly common in children with autism (Miller et al., 2001; Talay-Ongan & Wood, 2001; Weisblatt et al., 2005). There are children who show sensitivity to smells and negative reaction to faint odors such as perfume worn by others. Other children may frequently smell objects or people. Children may seek oral stimulation by mouthing objects, biting, or eating nonedible materials. Some children restrict their diets and will accept a very small number of food choices, such as only peanut butter and jelly sandwiches, popcorn, and water. Such behavior may represent an insistence on sameness, which is a characteristic of many children with autism. However, it also may result from sensory overresponsiveness to tastes, smells, or textures, leading to a diet limited to "sensory-safe" or preferred foods.

Autism and Sensory-Based Motor Disorders

Autism is associated with a wide range of sensory-based motor disorders that are manifested in fine- and gross-motor impairments and/or atypical movements and postures (Dawson & Watling, 2000; Leary & Hill, 1996; Smith, 2004). Studies have shown that school-age children with autism have impairments in praxis (Smith & Bryson, 1994), gait, posture, and balance (Kohen-Raz, Volkmar, & Cohen, 1992), eye–hand coordination, finger speed (Smith & Bryson, 1998), gesture, and imitation (Rogers, 1999).

SENSORY PROCESSING DISORDERS
AND OCCUPATIONS OF DAILY LIFE

In order to facilitate the occupational performance of children and adolescents with autism, one must consider its interplay with sensory processing. Occupational performance is the participation in meaningful and purposeful activities that produce functional and successful daily living skills and routines (American Occupational Therapy Association, 2002). A school-age child's areas of occupation include performance of activities of daily life, attending school and learning, and participation in play, leisure, and social interactions with family members and peers. Adolescents are expected to be more independent in self-care, home management tasks (e.g., shaving, simple meal preparation), and leisure activities (e.g., going to the cinema with peers) and often engage in prevocational training. In the following section we discuss how different types of sensory processing disorders such as sensory over- or underreactivity, sensory seeking, and dyspraxia may impact the occupational performance and choices of children and adolescents with autism. We also refer to the influence of occupations and their context upon the expression of sensory processing disorders. Sensory processing disorders dynamically interact with other factors such as family context, environmental opportunities, and experience to shape an individual's engagement in occupations throughout the life span (Parham, 2002).

Activities of Daily Life

Activities of daily life, which include self-care, home management, community mobility, health, and safety management (American Occupational Therapy Association, 2002), require the processing of multiple and unpredictable sensations within the home, school, and community environments. Children with sensory overresponsiveness may become highly distressed from certain textures, sounds, tastes, touches, and movements and thus avoid or resist participating in daily activities that consist of these aversive sensations (e.g., brushing teeth, using an escalator). Some children who are overresponsive to sensory input may insist on sameness in daily routines, in the clothes they wear, and in foods they eat in an attempt to increase predictability and control of sensation. The hypervigilance of children who are overresponsive to sensory input can lead to their inability to perform daily tasks in overstimulating environments, as these children may be distracted by background sounds, sights, and smells. Children with underresponsiveness may not process sensations that indicate to them that their shoe is on the wrong foot, that their nose is running, that clothing is entangled or wet, or that they are being called for dinner. These children may not initiate engaging in daily tasks and thus may need reminders to initiate and complete tasks. Children with sensation seeking may require strong input such as loud music or a weighted vest to support their participation in daily activities. Their craving for novel and intense sensation can distract them from completing daily tasks. These children may also benefit from engaging in activities that provide strong sensory input such as raking leaves, mowing the lawn, or vacuuming (although the noise of the vacuum cleaner may be intolerable to children who have auditory sensitivity).

Another aspect of daily activities affected by sensory processing disorders is one's ability to maintain and manage health and to respond to safety hazards. Children with underresponsiveness, who barely feel pain, may not report a severe injury and thus may walk on a broken foot for days, causing further damage. Such children may be prone to various safety challenges such as falls and self-injury. Children who seek sensation are often risk takers and require supervision in safely completing daily tasks. Children with autism who also have a sensory processing disorder may have a restricted and unbalanced food diet, which can cause nutrient deficiencies and contribute to obesity. In addition, the emerging sexuality in teenagers may present an additional challenge to an already confused sensory system. An adolescent may not know how to cope with new body sensations, which may result in anxiety attacks and behavioral expressions (Kinnealey, Oliver, & Wilbarger, 1995). Children may become involved in excessive public masturbation or, alternatively, engage in intensive repetitive movements such as rocking and head banging. Violent behavior toward self or others is another issue that may reflect sensory processing deficits and compromises safety. Violence can be an aggressive response toward unpleasant sensations, a result of underawareness of the amount of force applied, or a craving for intense input.

School and Vocational Activities

Sensory processing disorders can also impact participation in school and vocational activities. The physical and human educational environment may present various sensory–motor challenges for a child with a sensory processing disorder. Children who are overresponsive to sensory input and those who seek sensation often show difficulties in attending to the main stimuli presented by the teacher, and are instead preoccupied by distracting sensations such as cluttered bulletin boards and corridor sounds, or by unusual sensory components of the task. For example, the child with auditory overresponsiveness may have difficulty participating in an inclusive classroom or school cafeteria in which the noise level is high. Similarly, a teacher's high-pitched voice may interfere with the child's ability to listen to the content of what is being said. Seeking behaviors, distractibility, and unawareness of input may impact a child's ability to follow instructions and focus on tasks. Children who are underresponsive to sensory input can become self-absorbed in a task, unaware of the time or the fact that the class has already transitioned to a different task. Children with sensory-based motor disorders may show difficulties in learning to manipulate new objects and utensils. Factors that can impede participation in educational and prevocational training settings include issues related to proximity to other students, sounds, lighting, schedule of breaks, duration of time in seat, and material arrangement. An organized setting with a fixed schedule can increase a child's successful participation in these settings. Later in life, sensory processing challenges may affect vocational skills and choices. For example, a person with autism may not be able to work in environments that present a lot of sensory stimulation, especially noisy environments, and may be so self-absorbed that he or she does not attend to danger signs in the working place.

Leisure Activities

Sensory processing influences how, where, and with whom we spend our leisure time. Leisure, which is the "fun time" for most typical children, may pose a great many demands on children with autism. Many typical leisure settings are highly stimulating (e.g., playground, mall, gym) and thus do not suit children with a sensory processing disorder. Playgrounds require fast response to input, which is difficult for children with underresponsiveness or dyspraxia. Their inability to respond in a timely manner can put them at risk for injury. In addition, learning complex sport activities or engaging in hobbies that require fine-motor skills can be challenging for a child with dyspraxia. Children with overresponsiveness to sensory input may avoid arts and crafts activities, as many of these activities require touching messy materials. They may prefer to engage in sedentary and familiar leisure activities with low motor demands to limit unpredictable stimulation and avoid motor challenges. Children who seek sensation might choose to engage in intense leisure activities such as bike riding, skiing, or viewing fast-paced TV programs.

Friendships and Interactions

Deficits in social interactions are a core feature of autism. Social isolation may not only be a matter of social-communication deficits, but also a by-product of sensory–motor deficits. Human interactions expose all involved people to various sensory stimuli, often unpredictable in nature. A child with sensory overresponsiveness may withdraw from or avoid interactions in order to avoid unpredictable stimuli such as surprising touches and sudden noises. Children who seek sensation may touch or smell their peers in an inappropriate manner, which can lead to ridicule or rejection from peers. Children who are underresponsive may often be slow to respond to their peers' initiations, thus causing lack of communication. Children who have dyspraxia may avoid playing any kind of game that requires motor coordination, which, for many of their peers, may be a preferred activity. Therefore mismatches between the sensory processing of children with autism who also have a sensory processing disorder and their peers' sensory processing may directly impact the friendships and interactions of children with autism. Table 5.1 presents examples for possible implications of various sensory processing disorders such as sensory overresponsivity, sensory underresponsivity, sensory seeking, and sensory-based motor challenges for children's occupations in their everyday lives.

ASSESSMENT OF SENSORY PROCESSING DISORDERS

Given the high incidence of sensory processing disorders in children with autism, assessment of sensory–motor functions is essential. Assessment typically serves as the initial step of the intervention process and should provide sufficient information to guide therapists and families in setting goals, determining the appropriate model for service delivery, and evaluating change. However, assessment is almost always an ongoing process, especially for children with autism, for whom a myriad of internal (e.g., seizures) and external (e.g., moving into a new class) factors influence function (Mailloux, 2001).

TABLE 5.1. Examples of Implications of Sensory Processing Disorders for Occupations of Children with Autism

	Sensory overreactivity	Sensory underreactivity	Sensory seeking	Dyspraxia
Activities of daily life	• Resists nail and hair trimming. • Wears long-sleeved shirts all year round.	• Unaware of mess on hands or face. • Does not adapt clothing to room temperature.	• Twirls shoelaces instead of tying them.	• Difficulty lacing and fastening shoes. • Difficulty in sequencing the steps of dressing.
Health	• Melts down when hears a fire drill. • Eats only soft-textured foods such as yogurts.	• Lack of response to pain, extreme temperature, or injury. • Does not attend to street cues when crossing the street.	• Bangs head, jumps from heights. • Eats nonedible materials. • Runs into the street.	• Prone to falls and accidents. • Difficulty following fire safety procedures.
Learning	• Overwhelmed and distracted by fluorescent lights in classroom.	• Does not follow oral instructions.	• Difficulty staying in seat for extended periods of time and fidgety.	• Difficulty in learning new skills and preference for familiar activities.
Vocational training	• Difficulty working in noisy environments.	• Lack of attention to danger signs at work. • Highly focused on task.	• Perseverates on one sensory aspect of the job ignoring job demands.	• Preference for tasks that require few motor skills, such as computer work, library work.
Leisure	• Anxious at, or avoids going to, a movie or mall.	• Slow response to moving swings or passing bike riders.	• Engages in self-stimulation or unusual sensory interests (water play, wheel spinning). • Seeks intense input through jumping, or loud music.	• Difficulty in learning to ride a bike, swim, or play baseball, resulting in reduced participation with peers.
Friendships/ social interaction	• Overwhelmed by unexpected pushing and yelling of children during recess.	• Bumps into others • Squeezes friend's hand instead of shaking.	• Sniffing or rocking may lead to social rejection.	• Limiting interests to nonmotor activities and enforcing restricted interests on uninterested peers.
Family life	• Distressed by changes in family routines. • Avoids of touch/hugs/kisses from parent.	• Does not notice facial expressions of family members.	• Spinning plates or yelling in a restaurant.	• Demands preplanned family activities. • Limited participation in family sport activities.

The assessment process should include an examination of the child's sensory and motor assets and needs, their impact upon daily occupations, the sensory and motor features of tasks and environments where the child wants to and is expected to perform, and the "fit" of these environments with the child's needs. Such an assessment should answer the following questions: (1) Is the child's response to sensation different in frequency and quality from that of typically performing children, and to what extent? (2) How do these behaviors impact child and family occupations, routines, and well-being? and (3) How do these differences interact with the child's environment and task demands? It is important to evaluate behaviors in different settings and at different times of the day, as sensory behaviors may be more pronounced at certain places and times than at others. For instance, in the school cafeteria a child with overresponsivity may be highly distressed by sensations and respond by not eating, while at home mealtimes may occur in a less stimulating or challenging environment and therefore the child is able to eat.

Information about a child's sensory processing is gained through caregiver report, direct assessment, and clinical observation. Sensory histories and questionnaires provide important insights into various aspects of sensory processing that are not always apparent through direct assessment or observation. Based on parent-completed questionnaires, therapists evaluate where the child is on a scale of over- and underresponsiveness, specifically within various sensory modalities. The onset, duration, and intensity of the behavioral responses are noted as well. Sensory history checklists comprise the majority of standardized, norm-referenced measures of sensory modulation and primarily assess the frequency of sensory behaviors within daily contexts (see Table 5.2 for examples of standardized measures for evaluating sensory processing disorders in school-age children).

There are additional sensory processing questionnaires described in research protocols for children with autism (e.g., Baranek et al., 2006; Liss, 2002) that include the evaluation of unusual sensory responses characteristic of these children. Standardized tests of sensory processing that are directly administered to the child focus on motor planning and sensory-based motor skills rather than sensory modulation. Direct testing may not be feasible for some children with autism due to their communication deficits, short attention span, and difficulties performing in unfamiliar settings. Thus, alternative types of assessment in the child's natural environment may be required.

Although standardized assessments focus primarily on the child's characteristics or skills, in practice, occupational therapists use various observations and apply their knowledge of sensory processing and task

TABLE 5.2. Standardized Measures of Sensory Modulation for School-Age Children

Name of test	Author (year)	Ages	Description	No. of items
Sensory Profile	Dunn (1999)	3–10 years	Caregiver questionnaire: the frequency of sensory daily behaviors are rated from 0 (almost never) to 5 (almost always). Yields composite scores for different types of sensory processing (e.g., low registration, sensation seeking, sensory sensitivity, sensory avoiding) and for different sensory modalities. Composite scores interpreted relative to age norms.	125
Short Sensory Profile	Dunn (1999)	3–10 years	Caregiver questionnaire; assesses sensory processing in seven domains.	38
Adolescent/Adult Sensory Profile	Brown & Dunn (2002)	11 years through older age	Similar to the children' version, but it is a self-report questionnaire.	60
Touch Inventory for Elementary School Age Children (TIE)	Royeen (1986); Royeen & Fortune (1990)	6–10 years	Screening scale to identify children with tactile defensiveness. Administered to child.	26
Sensory Processing Measure (SPM)	School version <u>Miller, Kuhaneck, Henry, & Glennon (2007)</u> Home version <u>Parham & Ecker (2007)</u>	School age	Includes two forms for school and home. The school form looks at child's functioning in the main classroom, art class, music class, physical education class, on the playground, in the cafeteria, and on the school bus. It is completed by school staff. The home form is completed by the parent and assesses the child's sensory functioning in the home environment. Both forms were standardized with the same sample of children.	62 (school) 75 (home)

analysis to evaluate environmental supports and barriers to participation. This is important for understanding the 'impairing' nature of a child's sensory processing deficits and their expression in his or her natural environment. There are participation-based measures such as the School Functional Assessment (Coster, Deeney, Haltiwanger, & Haley, 1998) that are not specifically designed to assess sensory processing disorders, but rather to assess broader areas of functioning (e.g., transitioning between classes, using class materials) that may be affected by sensory processing disorders.

The gross- and fine-motor skills of the child should be examined, including motor planning. These are usually assessed through direct testing of the child rather than questionnaires. The "gold-standard" assessment for sensory discrimination and praxis is The Sensory Integration and Praxis Tests (Ayres, 1989), a set of 17 tests designed to assess aspects of sensory processing and motor planning/praxis. This test is standardized for children ages 4 through 8 years. Other standardized tests that assess motor skills are described in Table 5.3. Many children with motor planning problems also have difficulty in visual-motor integration and handwriting, therefore assessment of these areas is also important.

The repetitive and stereotyped movements of the child should also be assessed. Assessment should examine their presence as well as their function (e.g., increase arousal level, provide intense stimuli, avoid overstimulation) and context. Various studies (e.g., Baranek, Foster, & Berkson, 1997; Gal, Dyck, & Passmore, 2002) suggest that these movements, often called "self-stimulatory movements," may have a sensory base. The assessment of stereotyped movements can provide information about the child's atypical patterns of movement and may contribute to understanding the child's way of processing sensory information.

OCCUPATIONAL THERAPY INTERVENTIONS
FOR SENSORY PROCESSING DISORDERS
IN CHILDREN WITH AUTISM

The main goal of occupational therapy is to enable the child to participate in typical everyday occupations. Interventions involve planning, implementation, and review of outcome (American Association of Occupational Therapy, 2002). There are four primary modes of intervention that address sensory processing disorders in children with autism; these include direct therapeutic intervention, education and consultation within home and school environments, accommodations, and self-

TABLE 5.3. Standardized Measures of Praxis for School-Age Children

Name of test	Author (year)	Ages	Description	No. of items
Sensory Integration and Praxis Tests	Ayres (1989)	4–11 years	Battery of 17 subtests to assess visual perception, visual–motor integration, constructional abilities, praxis, somatosensory perception, and vestibular-proprioceptive processing.	Number of items varies with each subtest
Bruininks–Oseretsky Test of Motor Proficiency—Second edition (BOT-2)	Bruininks & Bruininks (2005)	4–21 years	An individually administered test of fine- and gross-motor skills with eight subtests (fine motor precision, fine motor integration, manual dexterity, bilateral coordination, balance, running speed and agility, upper-limb coordination, and strength). includes composite scores in four areas (Fine Manual Control, Manual Coordination, Strength, and Agility) and a Total Motor Composite.	Eight subtests with 5 to 9 items per subtest (total 53 items). Administration time is 45–60 minutes; a shorter screening version is available.
Movement Assessment Battery for Children (MABC)	Henderson & Sugden (1992)	5–11 years	Two parts, a performance-based assessment and a teacher checklist, both designed to assess everyday motor competence.	
MABC Teacher Checklist			Teacher checklist, completed by teacher, screens children for motor difficulty in the school situation. Items divided into four sections of increasingly complex situations: child stationary–environment stable, child moving–environment stable, child stationary–environment changing, child moving–environment changing.	48 items divided into four sections with 12 items in each section
MABC Test			Four age-related item sets measuring different aspects of motor ability.	8 items with 3 items assessing manual dexterity, 2 items assessing ball skills (throw/catch), and 3 items assessing static and dynamic balance
Dynamic Occupational Therapy Cognitive Assessment for Children (DOTCA-Ch)	Katz, Parush, & Bar-Ilan (2005)	6–12 years	This assessment, designed to examine learning potential and thinking strategies through a dynamic assessment, consists of 22 subtests in 5 cognitive areas: orientation, spatial perception, praxis, visuomotor organization, and thinking operations. Each subtest has a baseline score, a mediation score, and a posttest score.	The praxis area includes three subtests: Imitation, Sequencing, Verbal Directions
Perceived Efficacy and Goal Setting System (PEGS)	Missiuna, Pollock, & Law (2004)	6–9 years	Child's self-reported perception of performance competence at everyday tasks; helps set goals for intervention. Includes a parent and teacher questionnaire on their views of child's competence.	24 pairs of cards for everyday activities

111

employed strategies. All or some of these intervention modes may be applied in the intervention plan for a child with autism, depending on the child's needs, the response to intervention, and the resources available. Intervention should be provided or supervised by an occupational therapist trained in sensory integration to assure quality care and safety.

Direct Therapeutic Intervention

Direct therapeutic sensory intervention is a key component in the process of treatment and takes place in the form of occupational therapy, using a traditional sensory integrative approach on a one-to-one basis in a room with suspended equipment for a variety of movement and sensory experiences (Ayres, 1972). The goal of therapy is not to teach specific skills but to follow the child's lead and artfully select and modify activities according to the child's responses in order to provide appropriate sensory input and elicit adaptive responses. Adaptive responses are goal-directed behaviors that enable an individual to meet with new or changing environmental challenges. The activities designed in this type of intervention afford a variety of opportunities to experience tactile, vestibular, and proprioceptive input in a way that provides the "just right" challenge for the child in order to promote increasingly complex adaptive responses to environmental challenges (Schaaf & Anzalone, 2001). Direct therapeutic intervention is also an opportunity for the therapist to examine which sensations have calming versus arousing effects on the child. This model of intervention requires specialized equipment and typically takes place outside the classroom. Thus, it is important to combine direct therapeutic intervention with other types of intervention methods (Baranek, 2002).

Education and Consultation

Education and consultation is a process that involves *reframing* a student's behavior within a sensory perspective and facilitating problem solving and strategy development (Bundy, 2002). Therapists can reframe teachers', parents', and peers' views of a student's behavior by providing them with an understanding of sensory processing disorders and their possible impact on everyday activities. If caregivers learn to view their child's sensory behaviors of avoidance and inattention (e.g., avoidance of eye contact or hugs) as a sensory response and not as rejection, lack of interest, or low motivation, they may become more tolerant of the child's atypical sensory behaviors. Such consultation can empower caregivers by giving them basic explanations for their child's behaviors that they may have previously viewed as unusual, inexplicable, or confrontational. During facilitation of problem solving, the step following reframing, therapists enable caregivers to identify effective strategies for interacting and working with their child in ways that match their child's sensory needs (Bundy, 2002; Miller et al., 2005). For instance, an overresponsive child may be more likely to look at a parent in a dimmed room without visual distractions or to enjoy play involving firm hugs rather than tickling. In addition, occupational therapists have the knowledge and tools to assist parents and teachers in modifying the human and nonhuman environment, task demands, and routines to optimize the fit between the child and sensations in the home or school environment. For instance, if the mother of a child with overresponsivity to smell refrains from wearing perfume, this may reduce the child's negative response when interacting with her. Consultation often consists of developing a "sensory diet" for a child and supervising caregivers and teachers in carrying it out, a method described hereafter. Consultation does not end in planning strategies for others but requires close evaluation of the effectiveness of program implementation and modification of the program as needed. One of the key factors for the success of interventions is the partnership developed between the consulting therapist and the caregiver or teacher, a relationship that is based on trust, respect, and open communication (Bundy, 2002). It is expected that through consultation caregivers and teachers will gain a sensory perspective on a child's difficult behaviors, improve their parenting and teaching skills, and create environmental changes that will facilitate the child's successful performance.

Sensory-Based Accommodations

Sensory-based accommodations address the child's sensory processing needs throughout the day and within the natural context. These accommodations are commonly implemented through an individualized sensory diet, a carefully planned, practical program of specific sensory activities designed to provide the optimal amount and types of sensation the child needs. The sensory diet is based on the notion that controlled sensory input can affect arousal, alertness, and attention level, and thus affect a child's ability to function (Wilbarger, 1995). An effective sensory diet enables a child to feel calm, alert, and organized and thus enhances occupational performance. It can also help the child with self-regulation, which is the ability to attain, maintain, and change levels of alertness needed for a task or situation (Williams & Shellenberger, 1994). The sensory diet provides the child with opportunities to receive beneficial sensory input at frequent intervals, thereby enabling the child to more fully participate in daily activities. It is important to recognize that preferred input varies from child to child, and sometimes from day to day or hour to hour, depending on the child's arousal level. Many behaviors common in children with autism, such as jumping, repetitive running, head banging, chewing on nonfood objects, masturbating, biting or hitting oneself or others, or hand flapping may be the result of a need for input to the muscles and joints (proprioceptive input). Sensory diet activities often provide proprioceptive, deep touch, pressure, or vestibular input in a more socially or contextually appropriate way, such as wearing a weighted vest (Fertel-Daly, Bedell, & Hinojosa, 2001), having a massage (Escalona, Field, Singer-Strunck, Cullen, & Hartshorn, 2001), or receiving deep pressure using a "therapressure brush" (Wilbarger, 1995). In addition to, or as part of, the sensory diet, the occupational therapist often makes recommendations for accommodations that will afford the child greater opportunities for success throughout the day. A firm hug, wrapping a child in a blanket, or sitting on a vibrating pillow are some examples of such accommodations aimed at assisting children to regulate and organize their behavioral responses and helping them to decrease negative reactions to sensory input. "Heavy work" activities such as jumping on a firm pillow or trampoline, riding bicycles, swimming, stacking chairs, or a supervised exercise program (e.g., running, weightlifting) for older children may provide similar benefits (Escalona et al., 2001). For older students, therapists collaborate with caregivers and with students themselves to identify sensory activities that are age and developmentally appropriate, goal-directed, and functional.

There are also accommodations and strategies designed to meet the needs of children who have sensory-based motor difficulties such as dyspraxia. Children with dyspraxia have difficulty organizing and planning their motor actions and, therefore, often have difficulty varying their play, learning complex motor skills, or transitioning between activities. Familiar routines are very important for children with motor planning difficulties. Use of visual cues may assist the child with completing multistep tasks and with the many transitions expected in a school day. For example, a timer that clearly shows the passing of a prescribed time can help a child to anticipate the end of an activity. Also, pictures of the child's daily activities can be presented to the child prior to a daily routine to assist in reminding the child of the steps involved in routines and to help explain new ones. Children with dyspraxia may benefit from simple step-by-step directions for novel activities using the sensory modality that is the most efficient for them. For example, a child for whom the auditory modality is the most efficient will benefit the most from verbal instructions, while hand-over-hand instructions and touch clues can be more beneficial with the child for whom the kinesthetic modality is preferred.

Children with autism frequently have difficulty with self-care tasks due to problems tolerating or responding to sensory input. It is important to observe the child's reactions in order to determine if some behavioral responses during daily living activities reflect difficulty in sensory modulation or in motor planning or both. Some behaviors may be the result of tactile, taste, or smell oversensitivity. For example, a child with autism may have strong preferences for foods with similar tastes, shapes, or colors. Introducing new foods slowly may help the child to develop tolerance and interest in a greater variety of foods. It also may be helpful to use preferred foods to entice children to try novel foods. Using ice pops or frozen juice ice cubes or applying firm pressure around the mouth prior to eating may be helpful to desensitize the mouth area, thus decreasing the tactile sensitivity in that area and preparing the mouth for better chewing and swallowing. In order to improve self-feeding, the use of a weighted fork or spoon or nonslip surfaces under plates (e.g., dycem mats) may be helpful. The weight gives the child enhanced sensory feedback about where his arm is in relation to his body. Firm pressure to the head, shoulders, legs, and fingers may also provide calming preparation of a child's sensory system before cutting hair and nails, at shower time, or prior to or after putting socks on.

Sensory-Based Self-Employed Strategies

Self-employed strategies are aimed at providing children with tools that are helpful in coping with unpleasant sensory experiences, can be independently employed, and can be accessed in "real time." Self-employed strategies are particularly relevant for older children and adolescents with autism, who are expected to be more independent and may receive few intervention hours. Therefore, it is important to find strategies that a person with autism can implement with minimal supervision. An example of such a program is Sensory Stories, which is designed to help children with sensory overresponsiveness successfully engage in activities within their home, school, and community environment (Marr & Nackley, 2006). Sensory Stories comprise 30 individual stories about daily activities that instruct the child to use calming sensory strategies in order to deal with the unpleasant sensory aspects of a particular situation. When read on a regular basis, Sensory Stories can help the child develop effective routines to manage sensory experiences surrounding typical daily activities. Sensory Stories use a variety of self-employed strategies and may be adapted to a specific child's needs (Marr & Nackley, 2006).

Another self-employed strategy is the Alert Program, which supports children, teachers, parents, and therapists in choosing appropriate strategies to change or maintain states of alertness in the child. In this program, students learn to identify their level of alertness and learn what they can do before or during stressful times to attain a more optimal state of alertness to engage in tasks. Both Sensory Stories and the Alert Program incorporate a cognitive strategy approach to helping the child with self-regulation of sensory input. Because of the cognitive demands, this approach may not suit children with autism who are lower functioning; however there are ways to apply the principles of these strategies to children with lower cognitive abilities, such as creating a picture book with pictures of calming activities that the student can perform independently.

THE INTEGRATION OF SENSORY–MOTOR INTERVENTIONS WITHIN EDUCATIONAL PROGRAMS

Sensory–motor interventions can be applied within broader educational programs for children with autism. Using an inclusive approach, occupational therapists can consult with educators about ways to incorporate sensory-based intervention principles into the child's education plan (Baranek, 2002) to assist in achieving the child's educational goals within specific educational programs. For example, in an intensive Applied Behavior Analysis program, sitting for an extended period of time can challenge children who seek sensation or can result in further reduction of arousal in children who are underresponsive. For these children, incorporating sensory-based physical activity within the child's training schedule may be crucial for achieving an optimal arousal level. Understanding sensory processing preferences can also assist in selecting effective reinforcements for behavioral programs. In the Floor Time program (Greenspan & Wieder, 1998), occupational therapists can guide caregivers in engaging the child by using sensations that the child is more likely to respond to and by designing sensory–motor aspects of the play setting. In TEACCH (Treatment and Education of Autistic and related Communication-handicapped CHildren) programs (Mesibov, 1996), sensory activities can be included in the child's pictorial activity schedule, and environmental accommodations can be integrated to promote the child's independent performance goals in such programs. Finally, occupational therapists can collaborate with educators in designing effective instructional materials (e.g., visual cues), educational settings, sensory activities, and reinforcements to match the child's sensory and motor needs within the educational system.

EFFICACY OF SENSORY–MOTOR INTERVENTIONS FOR CHILDREN WITH AUTISM

Sensory and motor intervention approaches are commonly implemented by occupational therapists treating children with autism (Watling, Deitz, Kanny, & McLaughlin, 1999). However there are no rigorous, large-scale experimental studies that examine the efficacy of sensory and motor interventions for these children (Baranek, 2002; Dawson & Watling, 2000). Case-study, single-system, and small-group research indicates that children with autism who receive sensory-based interventions show gains in their social and communication skills as well as a reduction of stereotyped behaviors (Ayres & Tickle, 1980; Linderman & Stewart, 1999; Reilly, Nelson, & Bundy, 1984; Zissermann, 1992). Other positive outcomes include increased modulation of the child's arousal level, self-regulation, and attention. Edelson, Edelson, Kerr, and Grandin (1999) studied the efficacy of a deep pressure intervention for 12 children with autism, which involved the engagement in a "hug machine." Following this intervention, there was a reduction in behavioral measures of tension and anxiety, as well as in physiological measures of anxiety. Since the outcome of sensory and motor interventions is described in heterogeneous, small-scale, uncontrolled studies, there is a need to close the gap between sensory practice and evidence (Rogers & Ozonoff, 2005). When assuring the quality of a sensory and motor intervention for children with autism, Baranek (2002) recommends close examination of the (1) feasibility within the educational program, (2) cost, (3) maintenance of the outcome across time, and (4) generalizability to other settings.

CONCLUSION

In addition to the core social, communication, and behavioral characteristics of autism, sensory and motor problems can also have a major impact on the occupational performance of children with autism. Sensory–motor difficulties of children with autism can not only create a source of frustration and anxiety, but may further increase their social isolation. This chapter outlined the process of assessment and intervention for sensory processing and motor planning issues. Gaining a sensory perspective on behavior may assist parents and professionals in understanding many of the child's atypical behaviors, in finding ways to modify the human and nonhuman environment to meet sensory and motor needs, and in learning how to implement strategies to promote adaptive behaviors. As occupational therapists, we hope that such interventions will enable the individual with autism to enjoy daily sensations and become a more active and interactive participant in society.

ACKNOWLEDGMENTS

Ayelet Ben-Sasson was supported by The Wallace Research Foundation grant awarded to Dr. Alice Carter at the University of Massachusetts and Dr. Margaret Briggs-Gowan at Yale University.

REFERENCES

American Occupational Therapy Association. (2002). Occupational therapy practice framework: Domain and process. *American Journal of Occupational Therapy, 56,* 609–639.

American Psychiatric Association, (2000). *Diagnostic and statistical manual of mental disorders* (4th ed., text rev.). Washington, DC: Author.

Ayres, A. J. (1965). Patterns of perceptual motor dysfunction in children: A factor analytic study. *Perceptual and Motor Skills, 20,* 335–368.

Ayres, A. J. (1972). *Sensory integration and learning disabilities.* Los Angeles: Western Psychological Services.

Ayres, A. J. (1985). *Developmental dyspraxia and adult onset apraxia.* Torrance, CA: Western Psychological Services.

Ayres, A. J. (1989). *Sensory integration and praxis tests.* Los Angeles: Western Psychological Services.

Ayres, A. J., & Tickle, L. S. (1980). Hyper-responsiveness to touch and vestibular stimuli as a predictor of positive response to sensory integration procedures by autistic children. *American Journal of Occupational Therapy, 34*(6), 375–381.

Baranek, G. T. (2002). Efficacy of sensory and motor interventions in children with autism. *Journal of Autism and Developmental Disorders, 32*(5), 397–422.

Baranek, G. T., & Berkson, G. (1994). Tactile defensiveness in children with developmental disabilities: Responsiveness and habituation. *Journal of Autism and Developmental Disorders, 24*(4), 457–471.

Baranek, G. T., David, F. J., Poe, M. D., Stone, W. L., & Watson, L. R. (2006). Sensory experience questionnaire: Discriminating sensory features in young children with autism, developmental delays, and typical development. *Journal of Child Psychology and Psychiatry, 47*(6), 591–601.

Baranek, G. T., Foster, L. G., & Berkson, G. (1997). Tactile defensiveness and stereotyped behaviours. *American Journal of Occupational Therapy, 51*(2), 91–94.

Brown, C., & Dunn, W. (2002). *Adolescent/Adult Sensory Profile*. San Antonio, TX: Psychological Corporation.

Bruininks, R. H., & Bruininks, B. D. (2005). *Bruininks-Oseretsky Test of Motor Proficiency* (2nd ed.). Circle Pines, MN: American Guidance Service.

Bundy, A. C. (2002). Using sensory integration theory in schools: Sensory integration and consultation. In A. C. Bundy, S. L. Lane, & E. A. Murray (Eds.), *Sensory integration: Theory and practice* (2nd ed., pp. 310–332). Philadelphia: Davis.

Cermak, S. A., & Larkin, D. (2002). Issues in identification and assessment of developmental coordination disorder. In S. A. Cermak & D. Larkin (Eds.), *Developmental coordination disorder* (pp. 86–102). Albany, New York: Delmar Thomson.

Coster, W., Deeney, T., Haltiwanger, J., & Haley, S. (1998). *School Function Assessment*. San Antonio, TX: Psychological Corporation/Therapy Skill Builders.

Dawson, G., & Watling, R. (2000). Interventions to facilitate auditory, visual, and motor integration in autism: A review of the evidence. *Journal of Autism and Developmental Disorders, 30*(5), 415–421.

Dunn, W. (1995). *Sensory Profile*. New York: Psychological Corporation.

Dunn, W. (1997). The impact of sensory processing abilities on the daily lives of young children and their families: A conceptual model. *Infants and Young Children, 9*(4), 23–35.

Dunn, W. (1999). *Sensory Profile*. San Antonio, TX: Psychological Corporation.

Edelson, S. M., Edelson, M., Kerr, D. C., & Grandin, T. (1999). Behavioral and physiological effects of deep pressure on children with autism: A pilot study evaluating the efficacy of Grandin's hug machine. *American Journal of Occupational Therapy, 53*(2), 142–152.

Ermer, J., & Dunn, W. (1998). The Sensory Profile: A discriminant analysis of children with and without disabilities. *American Journal of Occupational Therapy, 52*(4), 283–290.

Escalona, A., Field, T., Singer-Strunck, R., Cullen, C., & Hartshorn, K. (2001). Brief report: Improvement in the behavior of children with autism following massage therapy. *Journal of Autism and Developmental Disorders, 31*, 513–516.

Fertel-Daly, D., Bedell, G., & Hinojosa, J. (2001). Effects of a weighted vest on attention to task and self-stimulatory behaviors in preschoolers with pervasive developmental disorders. *The American Journal of Occupational Therapy, 55*(6), 629–640.

Gal, E., Dyck, M., & Passmore A. (2002). Sensory differences and stereotyped movements in children with autism. *Behaviour Change, 4*, 207–219.

Gillberg, C., & Coleman, M. (1992). *The biology of autistic syndromes*. London: Mac Keith.

Grandin, T. (1995). *Thinking in pictures and other reports from my life with autism*. New York: Vintage Books.

Grandin, T., & Scariano, M. (1986). *Emergence: Labelled autistic*. Novato, CA: Arena.

Greenspan, S. I., & Wieder, S. (1998). *The child with special needs: Encouraging intellectual and emotional growth*. Reading, MA: Addison Wesley.

Henderson, S. E., & Sugden, D. A. (1992). *The Movement Assessment Battery for Children*. San Antonio, TX: Psychological Corporation.

Huebner, R. A., & Dunn, W. (2001). Understanding autism and the sensorimotor findings in autism. In R. A. Huebner (Ed.), *Autism: A sensorimotor approach to management* (pp. 3–40). Gaithersburg, MD: Aspen.

Jones, R. S. P., Quigney, C., & Huws, J. C. (2003). First-hand accounts of sensory perceptual experiences in autism: A qualitative analysis. *Journal of Intellectual and Developmental Disability, 28*(2), 112–121.

Katz, N., Parush, S., & Bar-Ilan, T. (2005). *Dynamic occupational therapy cognitive assessment for children*. Pequannock, NJ: Maddok.

Kay, S. F. (2001). *The relationship between sensory processing and self care for children with autism ages two to four*. Unpublished doctoral dissertation thesis, Nova Southeastern University, Fort Lauderdale, FL.

Kientz, M. A., & Dunn, W. (1997). A comparison of the performance of children with and without autism on the Sensory Profile. *American Journal of Occupational Therapy, 51*(7), 530–537.

Kinnealey, M., Oliver, B., & Wilbarger, P. (1995). A phenomenological study of sensory defensiveness in adults. *American Journal of Occupational Therapy, 49*, 444–451.

Kohen-Raz, R., Volkmar, F. R., & Cohen, D. J. (1992). Postural control in children with autism. *Journal of Autism and Developmental Disabilities, 22*, 419–432.

Koomar, J., & Bundy, A. (2002). Creating intervention from theory. In A. C. Bundy, S. L. Lane, & E. A. Murray (Eds.), *Sensory integration: Theory and practice* (2nd ed., pp. 261–308). Philadelphia: Davis.

Lane, S. J. (2002). Sensory modulation. In A. C. Bundy, S. J. Lane, & E. A. Murray (Eds.), *Sensory integration: Theory and practice* (2nd ed., pp. 101–122). Philadelphia: Davis.

Leary, M. R., & Hill, D. A. (1996). Moving on: Autism and movement disturbance. *Mental Retardation, 34*(1), 39–53.

Le Couteur, A., Rutter, M., Lord, C., Rios, P., Robertson, S., Holdgrafer, M., et al. (1989). Autism diagnostic interview: A standardized investigator-based instrument. *Journal of Autism and Developmental Disorders, 19*, 363–387.

Linderman, T. M., & Stewart, K. B. (1999). Sensory integrative-based occupational therapy and functional outcomes in young children with pervasive developmental disorders: A single subject case study. *American Journal of Occupational Therapy, 53*, 207–213.

Liss, M. N. (2002). *Sensory abnormalities in individuals with autism*. Unpublished dissertation, University of Connecticut, Storrs, CT.

Liss, M. N., Saulnier, C., Fein, D., & Kinsbourne, M. (2006). Sensory and attention abnormalities in autistic spectrum disorders. *Autism, 10*(2), 155–172.

Mailloux, Z. (2001). Sensory integrative principles in intervention with children with autistic disorder. In S. S. Roley, E. I. Blanche, & R. C. Schaff (Eds.), *Understanding the nature of sensory integration with diverse populations* (pp. 365–384). Tucson, AZ: Therapy Skill Builders.

Marr, D., & Nackley, V. L. (2006). Sensory stories. Framingham, MA: Therapro. *www.theraproducts.com/index.php?main_page=product_therapro_info& products_id=321156*

McIntosh, D. N., Miller, L. J., Shyu, V., & Hagerman, R. J. (1999). Sensory modulation disruption, electrodermal responses, and functional behaviours. *Developmental Medicine and Child Neurology, 41,* 608–615.

McMullen, P. (2001). Living with sensory dysfunction in autism. In R. A. Huebner (Ed.), *Autism: A sensorimotor approach to management.* Gaithersburg, MD: Aspen Publishers.

Mesibov, G. B. (1996). Division TEACCH: A collaborative model program for service delivery, training, and research for people with autism and related communication handicaps. In M. C. Roberts (Ed.), *Model programs in child and family mental health* (pp. 215–230). Hillsdale, NJ: Erlbaum.

Miller, H., Kuhaneck, M. S., Henry, D. A., & Glennon, T. J. (2007). Sensory Processing Measure (SPM): Main classroom and school environment forms. Los Angeles: Western Psychological Services.

Miller, L. J., Lane, S., Cermak, S. A., Osten, E., & Anzalone, M. (2005). Regulatory-sensory processing disorders. In S. I. Greenspan & S. Wieder (Eds.), *Diagnostic manual for infancy and early childhood: Mental health, developmental, regulatory-sensory processing and language disorders and learning challenges* (pp. 73–112). Bethesda, MD: Interdisciplinary Council on Developmental and Learning Disorders.

Miller, L. J., Reisman, J. E., McIntosh, D. N., & Simon, J. (2001). An ecological model of sensory modulation: Performance of children with fragile X syndrome, autistic disorder, attention-deficit/hyperactivity disorder, and sensory modulation dysfunction. In S. S. Roley, E. I. Blanche, & R. C. Schaff (Eds.), *Understanding the nature of sensory integration with diverse populations* (pp. 57–88). Tucson, AZ: Therapy Skill Builders.

Mulligan, S. (2002). Advances in sensory integration research. In A. C. Bundy, S. L. Lane, & E. A. Murray (Eds.), *Sensory integration: Theory and practice* (2nd ed., pp. 397–411), Philadelphia: Davis.

O'Neill, M., & Jones, R. S. P. (1997). Sensory-perceptual abnormalities in autism: A case for more research. *Journal of Autism and Developmental Disorders, 27*(3), 283–293.

O'Riordan, M., & Filippo, M. (2006). Discrimination in autism within different sensory modalities. *Journal of Autism and Developmental Disorders, 36*(5), 665–675.

Ornitz, E. M., Guthrie, D., & Farley, A. J. (1977). The early development of autistic children. *Journal of Autism and Childhood Schizophrenia, 7,* 207–209.

Ornitz, E. M., Guthrie, D., & Farley, A. J. (1978). The early symptoms of childhood autism. In G. Sebman (Ed.), *Cognitive defects in the development of mental illness* (pp. 24–42). New York: Brunner/Mazel.

Parham, D. L. (2002). Sensory integration and occupation. In A. C. Bundy, S. L. Lane, & E. A. Murray (Eds.), *Sensory integration: Theory and practice* (2nd ed., pp. 413–434). Philadelphia: Davis.

Parham, D., & Ecker, C. (2007). *Sensory Processing Measure (SPM): Home form.* Los Angeles: Western Psychological Services.

Pfeiffer, M., Kinnealey, M., Reed, C., & Herzberg, G. (2005). Sensory modulation and affective disorders in children with Asperger syndrome. *American Journal of Occupational Therapy, 59,* 335–345.

Reilly, C., Nelson, D. L., & Bundy, A. C. (1984). Sensorimotor versus fine motor activities in eliciting vocalizations in autistic children. *Occupational Therapy Journal of Research, 3,* 199–212.

Rogers, S. J. (1999). An examination of the imitation deficit in autism. In N. Jacqueline & G. Butterworth (Eds.), *Imitation in infancy* (pp. 254–283). New York: Cambridge University Press.

Rogers, S. J., & Ozonoff, S. (2005). Annotation: What do we know about sensory dysfunction in autism? A critical review of the empirical evidence. *Journal of Child Psychology and Psychiatry, 46*(12), 1255–1268.

Royeen, C. B. (1986). The development of a touch scale for measuring tactile defensiveness in children. *American Journal of Occupational Therapy, 40*(6), 414–419.

Royeen, C. B., & Fortune, J. C. (1990). Touch inventory for elementary-school-aged children. *American Journal of Occupational Therapy, 44*(2), 155–159.

Sagarin, J. D. (1998). *Toward a different model of autism: Exploring the sensory experiences of those diagnosed with autism or pervasive developmental disorder.* Unpublished dissertation. Clark University, Worcester, MA.

Schaaf, R., & Anzalone, M. E. (2001). Sensory integration with high-risk infants and young children. In S. S. Roley, E. I. Blanche, & R. C. Schaff (Eds.), *Understanding the nature of sensory integration with diverse populations* (pp. 365–384). Tucson, AZ: Therapy Skill Builders.

Shore, S. (2001). *Beyond the wall: Personal experience with autism and Asperger syndrome.* Shawnee Mission, KS: Autism and Asperger Publishing Company.

Smith, I. M. (2004). Motor problems in children with autistic spectrum disorders. In D. E. Tupper & D. Dewey (Eds.), *Developmental motor disorders: A neuropsychological perspectives* (pp. 152–169). New York: Guilford Press.

Smith, I. M., & Bryson, S. E. (1994). Imitation and action in autism: A critical review. *Psychological Bulletin, 116*(2), 259–273.

Smith, I., & Bryson, S. E. (1998). Gesture imitation in autism: Non-symbolic postures and sequences. *Cognitive Neuropsychology, 15,* 259–273.

Smith-Myles, B., Hagiwara, T., Dunn, W., Rinner, L., Reese, M., Huggins, A., et al. (2004). Sensory issues in children with Asperger syndrome and autism. *Education and Training in Developmental Disabilities, 39*(4), 283–290.

Talay-Ongan, A., & Wood, K. (2000). Unusual sensory sensitivities in autism: A possible crossroads. *International Journal of Disability, Development and Education, 47*(2), 201–212.

VerMaas-Lee, J. R. (1999). *Parent ratings of children with autism on the evaluation of sensory processing (ESP).* Unpublished master's thesis, University of Southern California, Los Angeles.

Volkmar, F. R., Cohen, D., & Paul, R. (1986). An evaluation of DSM-III criteria for infantile autism. *Journal of the American Academy of Child and Adolescent Psychiatry, 25,* 190–197.

Watling, R., Deitz, J., Kanny, E. M., & McLaughlin, J. F. (1999). Current practice of occupational therapy for children with autism. *American Journal of Occupational Therapy, 53,* 498–505.

Weisblatt, E. J., Parr, J. R., & Alcantara, J. I. (2005, May). *Sensory symptoms in autism spectrum disorders.* Paper presented at the 4th International Meeting for Autism Research, Boston, MA.

Wilbarger, P (1995). The sensory diet: Activity programs based on sensory processing theory. *Sensory Integration Special Interest Section Newsletter, 18*(2), 1–4.

Williams, D. (1998). *Autism and sensing: The unlost instinct.* London: Jessica Kingsley.

Williams, M., & Shellenberger, S. (1994). *How does your engine run?: A leader's guide to the Alert Program for Self-Regulation.* Albuquerque, NM: TherapyWorks.

Wing, L. (1976). Diagnosis, clinical description, and prognosis. In L. Wing (Ed.), *Early childhood autism: Clinical, educational and social aspects* (2nd ed.). Oxford, UK: Pergamon Press.

Zero to Three. (2005). *Diagnostic Classification of Mental Health and Developmental Disorders of Infancy and Early Childhood* (rev. ed.). Washington, DC: Zero to Three Press.

Zissermann, L. (1992). The effects of deep pressure on self-stimulating behaviors in a child with autism and other disabilities. *American Journal of Occupational Therapy, 46,* 547–551.

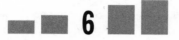

Assistive Technology as an Aid in Reducing Social Impairments in Autism

Ofer Golan
Paul G. LaCava
Simon Baron-Cohen

Social functioning is a core difficulty in children, adolescents, and adults with autism (Frith, 2003). This chapter considers the use of technology to improve social functioning in the autism population. It describes the benefits and possible limitations of assistive technology for helping overcome social impairments in autism. Finally, this chapter discusses the required conditions for tailored interventions targeting social difficulties in individuals with autism.

SOCIAL FUNCTIONING IN AUTISM

Deficits in social functioning are a defining component of autism (American Psychiatric Association, 1994; World Health Organization, 1994).

Impairments in social cognition, interaction, and behavior are evident from early points of development and across the lifespan. These include lack of interest in socializing, difficulties understanding social phenomena, and the absence of typical emotional and social behavior. Individuals with autism typically are limited in their ability to share enjoyment, interests, or achievements with others (e.g., by showing, bringing, or pointing out objects of interest). They also may not look for comfort from others when distressed. They tend to have limited understanding of others' emotional states and may fail to offer comfort to others. Their interaction style lacks social or emotional reciprocity, and they have difficulties using nonverbal cues such as gaze, facial expression, body postures, and gestures to regulate social interaction. Consequently, they often fail to develop age-appropriate peer relationships.

Several theories have attempted to explain the underlying causes for the social deficit in autism. The Theory of Mind (ToM) deficit theory (Baron-Cohen, 1995; Baron-Cohen, Tager-Flusberg, & Cohen, 2000) relates the social impairments in autism to a deficit in the ability to attribute mental states to others ("mindblindness"). Failure to understand others' intentions and to predict their behavior could explain the inability to interact or comprehend the social world, or the feeling that one is like "a Martian in the playground" (Sainsbury, 2000). A similar, though broader view of the social deficit in autism describes it as the result of an empathizing deficit (Baron-Cohen, Wheelwright, Lawson, Griffin, & Hill, 2002; Gillberg, 1992; Wing, 1981). Empathizing includes the drive to identify emotions and mental states in others and to respond to these with an appropriate emotion. The empathizing deficit in autism includes both the understanding of others' intentions, emotions, and beliefs and the ability to respond with an appropriate emotion to another's mental state—in other words, a deficit in both the cognitive and affective aspects of empathy (Baron-Cohen & Belmonte, 2005; Baron-Cohen et al., 2002). The Weak Central Coherence theory of autism (Frith, 2003) suggests that individuals with autism experience a fragmented world due to a cognitive style that focuses on detail at the expense of context and holism. Since the social world is heavily dependent on integration of details (such as facial expression, vocal intonation, gestures, body language, and verbal content) in context, the implications of such a fragmented cognitive style for social functioning are evident. Another theory explaining some aspects of the social deficit in autism is the Executive Dysfunction theory (Ozonoff, 1995; Russell, 1997). This theory argues that autism involves a deficit in executive functions including cognitive flexibility and planning. The social world is usually spontaneous and unstructured, requiring cognitive and behavioral flexibility. In addition, social rules that can be learned have to be implemented flexibly in accordance with the social context. Therefore, an inability to apply social rules flexibly could help explain social functioning difficulties in autism.

SYSTEMIZING STRENGTHS IN AUTISM

In contrast to the difficulties previously described, individuals with autism show good and sometimes even superior skills in "systemizing" (Baron-Cohen, 2003). Systemizing is the drive to analyze or build systems in order to understand and predict the system's behavior and its underlying rules and regularities. Individuals with autism tend to be hyperattentive to detail and to prefer predictable, rule-based environments, features that are intrinsic to systemizing. Clinical descriptions of children with autism denote their obsessive interest in systems from a very early age. Examples include interests in spinning objects (e.g., fans, washing machines), mechanical objects (e.g., trains), and patterns (e.g., on pavement tiles or curtains) (Attwood, 2003; Baron-Cohen & Wheelwright, 1999). Low- and high-cognitive-functioning individuals with autism are superior to individuals from the general population (matched by mental age) and to those with learning difficulties at various tasks that involve searching for details or analyzing and manipulating systems. Example tasks include the Wechsler Block Design subtest (Shah & Frith, 1993); the Embedded Figures Test (Jolliffe & Baron-Cohen, 1997); visual search tasks (O'Riordan, Plaisted, Driver, & Baron-Cohen, 2001); the intuitive physics tests (Baron-Cohen, Wheelwright, Spong, Scahill, & Lawson, 2001; Lawson, Baron-Cohen, & Wheelwright, 2004); and the Systemizing Quotient, a self-report questionnaire for systemizing related behaviors and interests (Baron-Cohen, Richler, Bisarya, Gurunathan, & Wheelwright, 2003). This unique cognitive style may underlie the circumscribed interests often seen in children and adolescents with autism in topics or systems such as trains, geography, and electronics (Attwood, 2003; Baron-Cohen & Wheelwright, 1999).

This affinity for systems and skill in understanding and predicting how systems work could be harnessed to support and enhance coping with areas of difficulty such as social functioning. Skill in systemizing lends itself to the use of predictable, routine, and systems-oriented visual technologies, where rapid social interactions can be minimized and predictable routines and systems can be augmented. Next we review such existing technologies.

TECHNOLOGY TO SUPPORT SOCIAL SKILLS TRAINING

What Is Assistive Technology?

Assistive technology (AT) is a broad term describing a range of equipment and products that are used to enhance or improve how a person functions. AT can help increase social interaction, independence, and functioning in natural settings and improve daily living and communication skills. It can be used to teach social interaction skills by modeling appropriate social behavior and to teach social rules and emotional understanding. A spectrum of devices ranging from low- to high-tech applications, AT can be as simple as a homemade visual schedule or as complex as a virtual reality system. AT can be purchased commercially and used as is or customized to fit the individual's needs. All levels of AT may be appropriate for use with individuals with autism to teach social conventions and rules, emotion recognition, emotional expression, and prosocial behaviors such as sharing or turn taking, making eye-contact, and conversation skills. Sometimes, combinations of high and low AT levels are used. For example, a visual support system can be created that uses computer-generated pictures that are then laminated and inserted into a binder. The following sections describe the different AT levels, providing examples of each. Although AT devices can be used in a multitude of ways to address skill deficits in areas such as communication, mobility, and adaptive functioning, the focus of this chapter is on using AT to (1) teach social skills, (2) encourage social interaction, and (3) foster social support.

Low-Tech AT

Low-tech AT devices are usually products that are relatively inexpensive and do not rely on electricity or battery power to operate. These devices may require some degree of modification and creation by the user or caregivers. Visual supports can be considered low-tech AT and include the use of any visual tools such as schedules, pictures, icons, or drawings. Visual supports assist individuals by improving their understanding of expectations and social interactions, along with improving their ability to tolerate transitions and make choices (Savner & Myles, 1999). Types of visual supports include social-communication devices, schedules, social scripts, and social stories. Visual supports can be created using basic materials such as markers, paper, binders, and icon or symbols as well as mid- and high-tech resources such as cameras (traditional, instant, or digital), computers, and software (e.g., *Boardmaker, Makaton, Picture This, Writing with Symbols 2000*).

Visual supports allow the user to learn any number of social skills by visually structuring social-communication interactions and by presenting visual cues to the user in a systematic way. This can include using visual cues to teach social rules, emotion recognition and expression, turn taking, and reading others' body language, or as self-monitoring nonverbal signals when communicating. For example, materials previously described can be used to make a topic ring or wallet (Stokes, 2001), which can be used by an individual to initiate conversations with others. Each card or page on the ring or in the wallet can have a picture or symbol (with or without text) to help the individual initiate conversations and interactions with others. The topic ring or wallet can help prompt an individual to talk about topics of interest or provide reminders about ways to engage in a variety of conversations and interactions with others (Stokes, 2001).

Back-and-forth worksheets are another example of the use of low-tech visual supports to assist with social-communication and engagement activities. Sharing daily activities with families and friends is a typical event for many children. In schools, teachers can help students with autism complete back-and-forth or school-to-home communication worksheets to help students share what they did during the school day with their families. Back-and-forth worksheets can be created in a low-tech manner by having students complete worksheets with pictures or icons/symbols. Visuals can be created using computers and icon or symbol programs.

Manual communication boards can be created in a low-tech manner by using picture symbols (from products such as *Boardmaker* or *Makaton*) on clipboards or in three-ring binders, notebooks, or manila folders. Manual communication boards are low-tech, relatively inexpensive, and portable. Symbols are placed onto the board and the user can either point, point and verbalize, or just use the board as a prompt to verbalize. Communication boards are personalized to meet the unique needs of the user.

The Picture Exchange Communication System (PECS; Bondy & Frost, 1994) is a well-known and widely used system for those with communication difficulties. PECS has a foundation in applied behavioral analysis and can be used with a number of visual materials. The core of this system is an exchange of pictures, symbols, icons, or actual photographs between the individual with autism and a communication partner. The use of a visual cue to represent a word, concept, or idea helps the user to communicate when speech–language difficulties are present. Representing words with visual symbols helps to simplify and structure social communication for those with autism.

Social Stories are short narratives created to enhance the socialization of individuals with autism (Gray, 2004). They can be created using a number of low-tech materials (pens, paper, visual symbols) or with high-tech materials such as computers and software. Social Stories have become a very popular method for teaching social skills to individuals with autism. Research has revealed initial support for this promising method, although more rigorous studies need to be designed and implemented (Reynhout & Carter, 2006; Rust & Smith, 2006; Sansosti, Powell-Smith, & Kincaid, 2004). Similarly, comic strip conversations (Gray, 1994) use drawings to engage in conversations that foster communication, understanding, and social interaction in individuals with autism. As with several of the previously mentioned resources, comic strip conversations can be created with a number of different low-tech resources, including dry-erase boards, paper products, or small chalkboards, or through high-tech means such as computers and programs that allow for drawing.

Social scripts are a way to teach and support social interaction skills (Ganz, Cook, & Earles-Vollrath, 2006; Myles & Simpson, 2003). These scripts provide structure to rapid-paced social interactions, help those with autism practice skills prior to interaction, and provide a routine for real-life conversations. Scripts can be created using generic paper products or with computers. The systematic presentation of social information in scripts allows individuals with autism to master acceptable forms of social interaction. Finally, tailoring the scripts to meet the needs of the individual with autism is paramount.

Mid-Tech AT

Mid-tech AT is generally more complex than low-tech, costs more, and is usually battery operated or runs on electricity. There is a wide spectrum of augmentative and alternative communication (AAC) devices that can be used as AT to support and teach social skills. Voice output communication aid (VOCA) refers to a number of different portable, battery-powered devices that assist in expressive communication by producing recorded speech. Visual symbols represent words or phrases and when the user presses the symbol, the voice output for the corresponding word or phrase is heard. Devices can range from one simple switch, offering a few choices to complex boards of 128 choices with multiple levels. For example, the *Wrist Talker (http://enablingdevices.com/ home.aspx)* can record up to 10 seconds of a greeting or other voice output and can be worn around the wrist like a watch. Such greeting phrase recordings can also be used as segments of social scripts to be repeated by the user in appropriate situations.

Talking photo albums or picture frames can assist individuals with autism to arrange information (both social and nonsocial) in a systematic way by associating visual with verbal information. Talking photo albums or picture frames can be purchased at any number of AT resource sites (e.g., *shop.augcominc.com/*), as well as off the shelf at department or other stores. Generally, these photo albums and picture frames allow the user to insert pictures, icons, or other graphics and text and to record short phrases or sentences. The voice output can then be played back when the photo or button is touched.

Videotaped recordings of television shows or movie segments can be used to teach and model appropriate social skills. Myles and Southwick (2005) recommend using videotapes of popular TV shows to highlight appropriate use of social skills and social interaction. For example, using videotapes of programs such as *Saved by the Bell* or *Third Rock from the Sun* can provide social skills instruction through modeling of behaviors, including both socially appropriate behaviors and social errors.

High-Tech AT

High-tech AT is typically the most expensive and usually involves microcomputer components, computer systems, and software. The use of computer software for individuals with autism has several advantages in that the computerized environment is predictable, consistent, and free from the social demands that individuals with autism may find stressful. Users can work at their own pace and level of understanding. Social lessons can be repeated until mastery is achieved. In addition, interest and motivation can be maintained through individually selected computerized rewards (Bishop, 2003; Moore, McGrath, & Thorpe, 2000; Parsons & Mitchell, 2002).

Software is commercially available to teach various social skills such as manners, perspective taking, emotion recognition and expression, and conversation skills. For example, The Birthday Party and My Community by Social Skills Builder *(www.socialskillbuilder.com)* teach social understanding and behavioral social skills in different settings through interactive video sequences. Other educational software focuses on understanding emotions and recognizing them through facial expressions, vocal intonation, and context. Among these programs are Mind Reading (Baron-Cohen, Golan, Wheelwright, & Hill, 2004; *www.jkp.com/mindreading*), Gaining Face *(http://ccoder.com/GainingFace/)*, The Emotion Trainer (Silver & Oakes, 2001; *www.emotiontrainer.co.uk*), and Fun with Feelings *(www.ultimatelearning.net)*.

Musselwhite and Burkhart (2001) have done extensive work in the area of social or participation scripts and AT. Various high-tech devices such as computers, software, and VOCAs can create sequenced social scripts to use in the natural environment. For example, scripts can be used to prompt and support conversations of those with autism with their peers, families, and others.

Video modeling is another popular method to teach daily living and social skills (Ayres & Langone, 2005; Hitchcock, Dowrick, & Prater, 2003, Mechling, 2005). Video modeling can be used as a stand-alone method or integrated within an activity schedule or Social Story (Charlop & Milstein, 1989; Hagiwara & Myles, 1999; Kimball, Kinney, Taylor, & Stromer, 2004). Peers, actors, other individuals, and the individual with autism can be videotaped role-playing the appropriate social skill. Afterwards, the video can be played back during social skill groups, direct instruction, or prior to social interactions. The peer or self-modeling of the targeted social skills can be reviewed multiple times. This type of technology is optimal for teaching social skills in individual, small-group, or whole-classroom settings because it is motivating, acceptable, and modern.

VOCAs run the gamut from mid-tech, moderately priced devices to expensive high-tech products. *Speaking Dynamically Pro (www.mayer-johnson.com/)* is a speech output program that is available for Windows and Macintosh platforms. It uses the *Boardmaker* symbols and has many features including abbreviation and word expansion features. *Dynavox* is another brand line that produces several models of fast, flexible, computerized speech output products. Users of these products have flexibility because they can link pages, record various voices, and choose symbols.

Clicker 5 is multimedia software that is very flexible and easy to use *(www.cricksoft.com/)*. It allows the user to create text and graphic output that can be augmented with voice output as well. Typed text can be augmented with pictures, symbols, videos and audio files, and other graphics. Social scripts, journal entries, social processing, and Social Stories can be created using *Clicker 5* and then printed to take with the user and used on the computer. Users can record their own voices for the output or use included voice options.

Some of the ATs reviewed were developed specifically for individuals with autism. Others have been useful for individuals with autism as well as for those with other disabilities or with typically developing individuals. The effectiveness of many of these technologies is supported by clinical evidence, parent report, and user feedback. However, not many of them have been evaluated in scientifically controlled studies. The following section describes a piece of software evaluated and used for teaching children, adolescents, and adults with autism to recognize emotions in faces and voices.

HIGH-TECH AT: *MIND READING: THE INTERACTIVE GUIDE TO EMOTIONS*

Mind Reading (Baron-Cohen et al., 2004; *www.jkp.com/mindreading*) is an example of a high-tech AT method for improving emotion recognition. It is an interactive guide to emotions and mental states that is a teaching tool tailored for emotion recognition by learners on the autism spectrum. Using visual, auditory, and contextual information, *Mind Reading* aims to assist individuals with autism to improve their emotion and mental state recognition skills. This software was created to use with children and adults at various levels of functioning, from young children with cognitive impairment to high-functioning adults who struggle with emotion recognition. Vocal and animated *helpers* or characters give instructions on every screen. Figure 6.1 provides sample screen shots from the software.

Mind Reading is based on the Theory of Mind and Empathizing models described in the beginning of this chapter. It is aimed at improving understanding of others' mental states to reduce the uncertainty individuals with autism may experience in the social domain and improve their social integration skills. In order to harness the systemizing skills of many individuals with autism, information in *Mind Reading* was organized systematically with a taxonomy of emotions that includes 412 emotions and mental states grouped into 24 emotion groups and six developmental levels from age 4 years to adulthood. Each emotion group is introduced and demonstrated by a short video clip giving some clues for later analysis of the emotions in this group. Each emotion is defined and demonstrated in six silent films of faces, six voice recordings, and six written examples of situations that evoke this emotion. This is, therefore, a rich and systematically organized set of educational materials. The face videos and voice recordings use male and female actors of various ages and ethnicities to facilitate generalization. Faces and voices are presented separately for each emotion, with silent face films and faceless voice recordings. This is provided to encourage analysis of the emotion in each modality as well as to facilitate the learning process by not overburdening the user perceptually and cognitively. All face video clips and voice recordings have been validated by a panel of 10 independent judges. This emotion database can be accessed using three applications: *The Emotions Library, The Learning Center,* and *The Games Zone.*

The Emotions Library: An emotion page

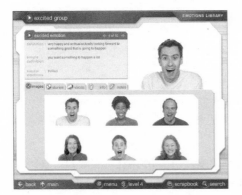

6 out of the 24 emotion groups

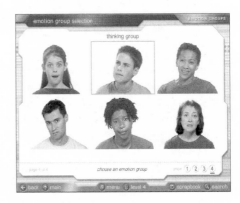

The Learning Center: A quiz question

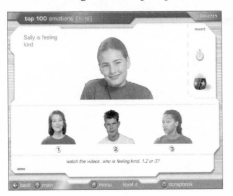

The Games Zone: "Hidden Face"

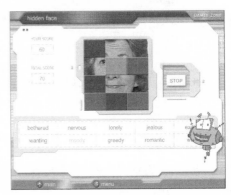

FIGURE 6.1. Screenshots from *Mind Reading: The Interactive Guide to Emotions* (Baron-Cohen, Golan, Wheelwright, & Hill, 2004).

1. *The Emotions Library* allows users to browse freely through the various emotions and emotion groups. Users can watch a short video introducing each emotion group in a social context. They can then learn more about particular emotions in the group by browsing the emotion pages (see Figure 6.1). An emotion page includes the emotion's definition, a simple definition for children, and media tabs with the six facial expression video clips, six vocal expression audio clips, and six written examples of situations that evoke the emotion. Users can add their own notes in a notes tab and compare different emotional expressions in the face and voice, using a scrapbook.

2. *The Learning Center* uses lessons and quizzes to teach about emotions in a more structured and directive way. In addition to teaching about the 24 emotion groups, it also includes lessons and quizzes about the most commonly used emotions and has a "build your own lesson/quiz" option. As emotional expressions may not be particularly rewarding to users with autism, the Learning Center includes various reward collections that users can "win" in order to motivate them to complete the lessons and quizzes. The reward collections, selected for their potential appeal to users with autism, are arranged systematically (e.g., pictures and information about space elements, clips of birds arranged by families, and different types of trains to collect).

3. *The Games Zone* is comprised of five educational games, allowing users to enjoy a game while studying about emotions. Examples include a memory game requiring matching cards with identical emotional faces, a game requiring matching thought and feeling bubbles to characters in a series of real-life situations, and a game requiring recognition of an emotion by gradually revealing different parts of a face.

The effectiveness of *Mind Reading* was evaluated in three separate studies. Two studies evaluated the software with high-functioning adults with autism (Golan & Baron-Cohen, 2006a) and with school-age children with autism (Golan, 2006; Golan & Baron-Cohen, 2006b) in the United Kingdom. Following 20 hours of using *Mind Reading* over a period of 10–15 weeks, software users significantly improved in their ability to recognize emotions from facial and vocal expressions, compared to control children with autism not using the software. This included improvement on recognition of quite complex emotions and mental states such as *insincere* or *intimate* for adults and *jealous* or *embarrassed* for children. For the adult users, this improvement was limited to material included in the software or to closely related stimuli. This limitation is reflective of the generalization difficulties often characteristic of individuals with autism. The children, however, demonstrated better generalization, since they also improved on recognition of facial and vocal expressions not included in the software. In addition, adult users with autism reported an increased interest in emotions and facial expressions following the use of the software as well as improved use of eye contact with others. Parents of children using the software reported an improvement in their child's ability to talk about emotional and mental states.

A third evaluation study of *Mind Reading* conducted in the United States with school-age children (LaCava, Golan, Baron-Cohen, & Myles, in press) replicated the findings of the U.K. studies, supporting the software's cross-cultural validity. Future evaluation studies should focus on more cognitively and language-impaired users with autism, as well as on the use of *Mind Reading* in combination with other ATs and with human mediators to further improve generalization of skills learned.

FUTURE POSSIBILITIES OF AT

Over the last decade, the World Wide Web and Internet have become household words. Using the Internet to facilitate and learn social skills is now possible. Currently, there is limited research supporting its effectiveness for improving social skills in individuals with autism. However, the previously discussed strengths and impairments of the autism population make the Internet a good match as a teaching tool. The use of e-mail, instant messaging, chat rooms, list servers, media groups, and other means of communication allows individuals with autism to communicate in a secure and controlled social atmosphere. Therefore, the increasing number of websites, online forums, and communities set up by and for individuals with autism and their families provides not only information and support but also increased opportunities for social interaction. Access to the Internet via home computers as well as via mobile communication interfaces, such as cellular phones and hand-held computers, offers new opportunities for social interaction for individuals with autism. Bishop (2003) conducted research that examined the use of the Internet to help individuals with autism better understand emotions and communicate with peers. By using mobile phones with Internet capabilities, participants with autism were able to translate unknown words, access interpretations, and obtain suggestions for responses in real time. el-Kaliouby and Robinson (2005) described a portable piece of AT that uses samples of facial expressions and vocal intonation to highlight the emotional or mental state of the speaker's feedback to the user (el-Kaliouby & Robinson, 2005). Future research should evaluate the effectiveness of AT systems in supporting the social understanding and behavior of individuals with autism.

Interesting attempts to support socializing in children with autism have come from the field of robotics. Children with autism may find robots more predictable and less intimidating than humans. Through child–robot interaction, social skills such as joint attention, turn taking, sharing, and greeting can be practiced. Through the interaction with a robot, children can engage in three-way interactions (child–robot–adult/ another child). Robots can be designed to have magnified facial features in order to increase attention to these features—an important aspect of socioemotional communication (Michaud & Théberge-Turmel, 2002). Robins, Dautenhahn, Boekhorst, and Billard (2005) studied the interaction of four children with autism with a humanoid robot over a period of 3 months. They reported an improvement in the children's imitation, turn taking, and role-switching abilities, as well as improved communicative competence (Robins et al., 2005). Though further research is needed, these preliminary results suggest that robots could serve as effective social mediators, bridging the gap between the human social world and individuals with autism.

Virtual Environments (VE; also called virtual reality) are another domain with immense potential for individuals with autism and related social difficulties. VE are artificial, computer-generated, three-dimensional simulations in single- or multi-user forms. In either format, the user can operate in realistic scenarios to practice social skills, conversations, and social problem solving. Moore and colleagues investigated the use of VE with children and adolescents with autism and found that over 90% of their participants used the VE to recognize basic emotions (Moore, Cheng, McGrath, & Powell, 2005). Other studies have also shown the potential for using VE to teach social skills to individuals with autism (Parsons et al., 2000; Parsons & Mitchell, 2002; Parsons, Mitchell, & Leonard, 2005).

How effective VE, the Internet, and future high-tech devices are in assisting those with autism remains to be seen. Although many products exist for individuals with Asperger syndrome or high-functioning autism, attention is needed to develop AT to teach social skills to individuals with more cognitive and language impairments. More research in AT is merited, especially in the area of helping this population generalize skills to natural environments.

POSSIBLE LIMITATIONS OF AT

As described in this chapter, there are a wide range of benefits to using AT to teach and support social skills in the autism population. There are some limitations to consider as well. Individuals with autism may have characteristics and behaviors that limit the use of some AT. For example, if an individual with autism has a history of destructive behaviors, it may be inadvisable to purchase an expensive machine that could easily be destroyed. In such cases, it is necessary to first teach the individual replacement behaviors. Also, some individuals may have motor deficits that make certain devices too difficult to use. Finally, some individuals may need to be taught the language necessary to operate certain high-tech devices.

Certainly time, talent, budgetary constraints, and other resources are needed to find and purchase the appropriate AT for individuals with autism. If these components are not given adequate consideration, the devices may not meet user expectations. In some instances, more creativity by stakeholders is needed, as money may not be available to purchase the optimal and most expensive technologies.

Individuals with autism have problems with skill generalization and this issue needs consideration when using AT with this population. Many studies have shown that AT has helped individuals with autism make gains in clinics or research settings, but skills have not been shown to generalize across time or to other settings (Bolte et al., 2002; Hadwin, Baron-Cohen, Howlin, & Hill, 1996; Swettenham, 1996, 2000). The tendency to focus on small details at the expense of being able to see the larger picture (Frith, 2003), abstraction difficulties, and insistence on sameness may make generalization a challenge for individuals with autism. AT systems may be able to teach principles through examples, but their flexibility and adaptability for the world of individuals with autism may be limited. To address this potential generalization problem, the involvement of human mediators (teachers, parents, siblings, or peers) should be a central consideration. Human mediators can assist in associating the knowledge acquired through AT with examples from the user's experience, and in providing flexible context-related interpretations to learned social rules (e.g., even though it is important to share, one should not share the ball with the opponents' team in a football game). On the other hand, it is important to allow the individual with autism to use the AT product as independently as possible, that is, fading caretaker prompts as soon as possible and helping the individual use AT in natural settings. The attitudes of caretakers and other stakeholders also play a role in AT success. For example, if those involved have a fear of technology or prior negative experiences with AT, this can affect the successful use of AT with an individual who has autism. Therefore, it is important for all stakeholders to support the use of AT across settings.

Training is another possible limitation of AT use. There must be initial and follow-up training of the caregivers who will help the individual with autism use the AT. As technology advances every year, diligently staying abreast of new information and training is also a necessary consideration.

Finally, possible limitations related to the use of AT devices also include portability, durability, ease of use, need for technological support, and understanding of speech output voices. If a device is not easy to use, carry, and service then the AT may be abandoned or used only occasionally, thus limiting its potential. Addressing these limitations will help individuals with autism use AT effectively to increase their social skills and interaction.

CONCLUSION

The affinity children, adolescents, and adults with autism have for technology, due in part to their relative ease in using clear rule-based systems, makes AT ideal for supporting them in various areas of functioning, particularly social functioning. AT can be used to teach a variety of social skills including emotional understanding, social scripts, and prosocial behaviors. The rapid progress of technological solutions may offer human-like support to individuals with autism while retaining the qualities of a technological system. In the meantime, due to the flexible, context-dependent nature of social phenomena, along with the inherent generalization difficulties in autism, the use of AT should go hand in hand with human interactive support to assist in the transference of the skills learned using AT to everyday life.

ACKNOWLEDGMENTS

Ofer Golan was supported by the National Alliance for Autism Research, the Corob Charitable Trust, the Wingate Foundation, and B'nai B'rith Leo Baeck scholarships. Paul LaCava was supported by the Organization of Autism Research. Simon Baron-Cohen was supported by the Shirley Foundation, the Medical Research Council, and the Three Guineas Trust.

REFERENCES

American Psychiatric Association. (1994). *Diagnostic and statistical manual of mental disorders* (4th ed.) Washington, DC: Author.

Attwood, T. (2003). Understanding and managing circumscribed interests. In M. R. Prior (Ed.), *Learning and behavior problems in Asperger syndrome* (pp. 126–147). New York: Guilford Press.

Ayres, K. M., & Langone, J. (2005). Intervention and instruction with video for students with autism: A review of the literature. *Education and Training in Developmental Disabilities, 40,* 183–196.

Baron-Cohen, S. (1995). *Mindblindness: An essay on autism and theory of mind.* Boston: MIT Press/Bradford Books.

Baron-Cohen, S. (2003). *The essential difference: Men, women and the extreme male brain.* London: Penguin.

Baron-Cohen, S., & Belmonte, M. K. (2005). Autism: A window onto the development of the social and the analytic brain. *Annual Review of Neuroscience, 28,* 109–126.

Baron-Cohen, S., Golan, O., Wheelwright, S., & Hill, J. J. (2004). *Mind Reading: The interactive guide to emotions.* London: Jessica Kingsley.

Baron-Cohen, S., Richler, J., Bisarya, D., Gurunathan, N., & Wheelwright, S.

(2003). The Systemising Quotient (SQ): An investigation of adults with Asperger syndrome or high functioning autism and normal sex differences. *Philosophical Transactions of the Royal Society, Series B, 358*, 361–374.

Baron-Cohen, S., Tager-Flusberg, H., & Cohen, D. J. (2000). *Understanding other minds: Perspectives from developmental cognitive neuroscience* (2nd ed.). Oxford, UK: Oxford University Press.

Baron-Cohen, S., & Wheelwright, S. (1999). "Obsessions" in children with autism or Asperger syndrome: Content analysis in terms of core domains of cognition. *British Journal of Psychiatry, 175*, 484–490.

Baron-Cohen, S., Wheelwright, S., Lawson, J., Griffin, R., & Hill, J. J. (2002). The exact mind: Empathizing and systemizing in autism spectrum conditions. In U. Goswami (Ed.), *Handbook of childhood cognitive development* (pp. 491–508). Malden, MA: Blackwell Publishers.

Baron-Cohen, S., Wheelwright, S., Spong, A., Scahill, V. L., & Lawson, J. (2001). Are intuitive physics and intuitive psychology independent? A test with children with Asperger syndrome. *Journal of Developmental and Learning Disorders, 5*, 47–78.

Bishop, J. (2003). The Internet for educating individuals with social impairments. *Journal of Computer Assisted Learning, 19*(4), 546–556.

Bolte, S., Feineis-Matthews, S., Leber, S., Dierks, T., Hubl, D., & Poustka, F. (2002). The development and evaluation of a computer-based program to test and to teach the recognition of facial affect. *International Journal of Circumpolar Health, 61*(Suppl. 2), 61–68.

Bondy, A., & Frost, L. (1994). The picture exchange communication system. *Focus on Autistic Behavior, 9*, 1–19.

Charlop, M. H., & Milstein, J. P. (1989). Teaching autistic children conversational speech using video modeling. *Journal of Applied Behavior Analysis, 22*, 275–285.

Frith, U. (2003). *Autism: Explaining the enigma* (2nd ed.). New York: Blackwell Publishers.

Ganz, J. B., Cook, K. T., & Earles-Vollrath, T. L. (2006). *How to write and implement social scripts*. Austin, TX: PRO-ED.

Gillberg, C. L. (1992). Autism and autistic-like conditions: Subclasses among disorders of empathy. *Journal of Child Psychology and Psychiatry, 33*(5), 813–842.

Golan, O. (2006). *Systemising emotions: Teaching emotion recognition to people with autism using interactive multimedia*. Unpublished PhD, University of Cambridge, Cambridge, UK.

Golan, O., & Baron-Cohen, S. (2006a). Systemizing empathy: Teaching adults with Asperger syndrome and high-functioning autism to recognize complex emotions using interactive multimedia. *Development and Psychopathology, 18*(2), 591–617.

Golan, O., & Baron-Cohen, S. (2006b). *Teaching children with Asperger syndrome and high-functioning autism to recognize emotions using interactive multimedia*. Manuscript in preparation.

Gray, C. A. (1994). *Comic strip conversations: Colorful, illustrated interactions with students with autism and related disorders*. Jenison, MI: Jenison Public Schools.

Gray, C. A. (2004). *Social Stories, 10.0*. Jenson MI: Jenison Public Schools.

Hadwin, J., Baron-Cohen, S., Howlin, P., & Hill, K. (1996). Can we teach children with autism to understand emotions, belief, or pretence? *Development and Psychopathology, 8*(2), 345–365.

Hagiwara, T., & Myles, B. S. (1999). A multimedia social story intervention: Teaching skills to children with autism. *Focus on Autism and Other Developmental Disabilities, 14,* 82–95.

Hitchcock, C. H., Dowrick, P., & Prater, M. A. (2003). Video self-modeling intervention in school-based settings: A review. *Remedial and Special Education, 24,* 36–45, 56.

Jolliffe, T., & Baron-Cohen, S. (1997). Are people with autism and Asperger syndrome faster than normal on the Embedded Figures Test? *Journal of Child Psychology and Psychiatry and Allied Disciplines, 38*(5), 527–534.

el Kaliouby, R., & Robinson, P. (2005). The emotional hearing aid: An assistive tool for children with Asperger syndrome. *Universal Access in the Information Society, 4*(2), 121–134.

Kimball, J. W., Kinney, E. M., Taylor, B. A., & Stromer, R. (2004). Video-enhanced activity schedules for children with autism: A promising package for teaching social skills. *Education and Treatment of Children, 27,* 280–298.

LaCava, P. G., Golan, O., Baron-Cohen, S., & Myles, B. S. (in press). Using assistive technology to teach emotion recognition to students with Asperger syndrome: A pilot study. *Remedial and Special Education.*

Lawson, J., Baron-Cohen, S., & Wheelwright, S. (2004). Empathising and systemising in adults with and without Asperger syndrome. *Journal of Autism and Developmental Disorders, 34*(3), 301–310.

Mechling, L. (2005). The effect of instructor-created video programs to teach students with disabilities: A literature review. *Journal of Special Education Technology, 20,* 25–36.

Michaud, F., & Théberge-Turmel, C. (2002). Mobile robotic toys and autism. In K. Dautenhahn, A. Bond, L. Cañamero, & B. Edmonds (Eds.), *Socially intelligent agents: Creating relationships with computers and robots* (pp. 125–132). New York: Springer.

Moore, D., Cheng, Y., McGrath, P., & Powell, N. J. (2005). Collaborative virtual environment technology for people with autism. *Focus on Autism and Other Developmental Disabilities, 20,* 231–243.

Moore, D., McGrath, P., & Thorpe, J. (2000). Computer-aided learning for people with autism: A framework for research and development. *Innovations in Education and Training International, 37,* 218–228.

Musselwhite, C. R., & Burkhart, L. J. (2001). *Can we chat?: Co-planned sequenced social scripts*. Eldersburg, MD: Special Communications.

Myles, B. S., & Simpson, R. L. (2003). *Asperger syndrome: A guide for educators and parents* (2nd ed.). Austin, TX: PRO-ED.

Myles, B. S., & Southwick, J. (2005). *Asperger syndrome and difficult moments: Practical solutions for tantrums, rage, and meltdowns*. Shawnee Mission, KS: Autism Asperger Publishing.

O'Riordan, M. A., Plaisted, K. C., Driver, J., & Baron-Cohen, S. (2001). Superior visual search in autism. *Journal of Experimental Psychology: Human Perception and Performance, 27*(3), 719–730.

Ozonoff, S. (1995). Executive functions in autism. In E. Schopler & B. Mesibov (Eds.), *Learning and cognition in autism* (pp. 199–219). New York: Plenum Press.

Parsons, S., Beardon, L., Neale, H. R., Reynard, G., Eastgate, R., Wilson, J. R., et al. (2000b, September). *Development of social skills amongst adults with Asperger's syndrome using virtual environments: The AS interactive project.* Proceedings of the 3rd International Conference on Disability, Virtual Reality, and Associated Technologies, Alghero, Italy.

Parsons, S., & Mitchell, P. (2002). The potential of virtual reality in social skills training for people with autistic spectrum disorders. *Journal of Intellectual Disability Research, 46,* 430–443.

Parsons, S., Mitchell, P., & Leonard, A. (2005). Do adolescents with autistic spectrum disorders adhere to social conventions in virtual environments? *Autism, 9,* 95–117.

Reynhout, G., & Carter, M. (2006). Social stories for children with disabilities. *Journal of Autism and Developmental Disabilities, 36,* 445–469.

Robins, B., Dautenhahn, K., Boekhorst, R., & Billard, A. (2005). Robotic assistants in therapy and education of children with autism: Can a small humanoid robot help encourage social interaction skills? *Universal Access in the Information Society, 4*(2), 105–120.

Russell, J. (1997). *Autism as an executive disorder.* Oxford, UK: Oxford University Press.

Rust, J., & Smith, A. (2006). How should the effectiveness of social stories to modify the behaviour of children on the autistic spectrum be tested? *Autism, 10,* 125–138.

Sainsbury, C. (2000). *Martian in the playground: Understanding the schoolchild with Asperger's syndrome.* London: Lucky Duck Publishing.

Sansosti, F. J., Powell-Smith, K. A., & Kincaid, D. (2004). A research synthesis of social story interventions for children with autism spectrum disorders. *Focus on Autism and Other Developmental Disabilities, 19,* 194–204.

Savner, J. L., & Myles, B. S. (1999). *Visual supports in the classroom for students with autism and related pervasive developmental disorders.* Shawnee Mission, KS: Autism Asperger Publishing.

Shah, A., & Frith, U. (1993). Why do autistic individuals show superior performance on the block design task? *Journal of Child Psychology and Psychiatry and Allied Disciplines, 34*(8), 1351–1364.

Silver, M., & Oakes, P. (2001). Evaluation of a new computer intervention to teach people with autism or Asperger syndrome to recognize and predict emotions in others. *Autism, 5,* 299–316.

Stokes, S. (2001). *Autism: Interventions and strategies for success.* (Report by Cooperative Educational Service Agency #7, Department of Special Education) WI: Retrieved August 15, 2006, from *http://www.cesa7.K12.wi.us/SPED/autism/AUTISM.pdf.*

Swettenham, J. (1996). Can children with autism be taught to understand false belief using computers? *Journal of Child Psychology and Psychiatry, 37,* 157–165.

Swettenham, J. (2000). Teaching theory of mind to individuals with autism. In S. Baron-Cohen, H. Tager-Flusberg, & D. J. Cohen (Eds.), *Understanding other minds: Perspectives from developmental cognitive neuroscience* (2nd ed., pp. 442–456). Oxford, UK: Oxford University Press.

Wing, L. (1981). Asperger's syndrome: A clinical account. *Psychological Medicine, 11*(1), 115–129.

World Health Organization. (1994). *International classification of diseases* (10th ed.). Geneva, Switzerland: Author.

FAMILY AND CAREGIVERS OF THE INDIVIDUAL WITH AUTISM

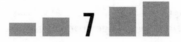

Advocating for Services

Legal Issues Confronting Parents and Guardians

Wayne Steedman

An understanding of the laws impacting children with autism is integral
to their care, treatment, and assimilation. This chapter explores how
statutes, regulations, and court decisions impact children with autism
and those involved with their care and treatment. The statutes that are
the focus of this chapter include the Individuals with Disabilities Education Improvement Act of 2004[1] (IDEA), Section 504 of the Rehabilitation Act of 1973,[2] and the No Child Left Behind Act[3] (NCLB). Additionally, relevant court cases are discussed. Finally, long-term planning
and residential options are addressed.

UNDERSTANDING HOW THE LAW WORKS

Our legislative system has parallel federal and state tracks. Federal laws
are passed by Congress and signed by the president. State laws are
passed by state legislatures and signed by the governor. In accordance
with the supremacy clause of the United States Constitution,[4] state laws

may not in any way interfere with or diminish the rights or protections established by federal laws. A state may enact a law that expands rights and protections beyond those that the federal law provides. For example, the IDEA requires states to provide special education to eligible students between the ages of 3 and 21 years, inclusive. However, some states have expanded the age range from birth through 25 years of age. This is acceptable; however, if a state attempted to change the age range to above 3 or below 21 years, the state law would be declared invalid and in violation of the supremacy clause.

Our judicial system is similarly bifurcated. The federal courts hear a variety of cases including those in which a federal law is at issue, claims involving two or more states, treaties, Constitutional claims, and more. The state courts hear cases pertaining to their own state laws. If a state law parallels a federal law, an aggrieved party may choose to sue in either state or federal court. This is true in special education cases, as there is the federal law, the IDEA, and there are state laws that parallel the IDEA.

In special education cases, the aggrieved party, usually the parents, must first "exhaust" administrative remedies. In other words, before parties can file a complaint in a court, they must first have their case decided by an administrative officer, specifically an administrative law judge or a hearing officer.[5] The administrative officer's decision can be appealed to a state or federal trial court. That judicial decision can then be appealed to the appellate court above the trial court. Ultimately, the case could be appealed to the U.S. Supreme Court. It is important to understand that some judicial decisions are "binding," meaning that they must be followed by other "lower" courts within the jurisdiction of that court, and some decisions, though not binding, are "persuasive." Administrative rulings and trial court decisions are not binding, but may be persuasive. Administrative decisions tend to be less persuasive than trial court decisions. Appellate court decisions are binding but may be reversed by a higher court or, potentially, by Congress.

THE IDEA

History

The IDEA was first enacted in 1975 as the Education for All Handicapped Children Act[6] (EAHCA) and has been amended multiple times since. The act was officially renamed the IDEA in the 1990 amendments.[7] When enacting the EAHCA, Congress found that more than 1 million children with disabilities had been barred from attending school and more than half of the children with disabilities attending school were not receiving appropriate educational services.[8] Although Congress had enacted previous legislation to provide children with disabilities access to public schools,[9] it became clear following two landmark court cases that more was needed. The first case, *Pennsylvania Association for Retarded Children v. Commonwealth of Pennsylvania (PARC)*,[10] was brought on behalf of retarded children challenging the constitutionality of a Pennsylvania law that excluded children with mental retardation from education and training. The case resulted in a consent decree, which ensured children with mental retardation access to public education and training. The second case, *Mills v. Board of Education*,[11] also involved the exclusion of children with disabilities from public schools in the District of Columbia. The judge ruled that a child with a disability who was eligible for public education could not be excluded from public school. The *PARC* and *Mills* cases convinced Congress that comprehensive federal legislation was needed to guarantee that disabled children were provided access to an appropriate education.

Purpose

The IDEA represents an ambitious federal effort to promote the education of children with disabilities.[12] The primary purpose of the act is "to ensure that all children with disabilities have available to them a free appropriate public education [FAPE] that emphasizes special education and related services designed to meet their unique needs and prepare them for further education, employment, and independent living."[13] The act goes on to note the need to protect the rights of children with disabilities and their parents, provide assistance to the states and local educational agencies, ensure that parents and educators have available to them the tools needed to improve educational results for children with disabilities, and ensure the effectiveness of efforts made to educate children with disabilities.[14] Although the IDEA has been successful in opening the school doors to children with disabilities, Congress recently found that its implementation "has been impeded by low expectations and an insufficient focus on applying replicable research on proven methods of teaching and learning for children with disabilities."[15] The newly amended IDEA seeks to redress these shortcomings by placing greater emphasis on the use of scientifically based instructional practices and raising the standard for what constitutes a FAPE.

Special Education

Special education is defined as "specially designed instruction, at no cost to the parents, to meet the unique needs of a child with a disability."[16] It may be provided in a classroom, home, hospital, institution, or other setting. Specially designed instruction means adapting, as appropriate, the content, methodology, or delivery of instruction to address the unique needs of the child.[17] The law requires schools to provide the related services a child may need to benefit from special education.[18] Related services include, but are not limited to, speech and language therapy, occupational therapy, school nurse services, psychological services, transportation, or recreation. This list is not exhaustive. A related service can be any developmental, corrective, or supportive service a child with a disability needs to benefit from special education. It is important to note that the law does not permit schools to refuse a service because it is too expensive. In *Cedar Rapids Community School District v. Garrett F.*,[19] the Supreme Court held that the IDEA "does not employ cost" in its definition of related services.[20]

Each child with a disability must have an *individualized education program* (IEP).[21] The IEP must be designed to address the educational needs of the child that result from the child's disability.[22] It is developed by a team of individuals that includes the parents, who are considered equal participants in its development.[23] The importance of the IEP cannot be overstated. It identifies the child's level of academic achievement and functional performance as of the time of its development. It also identifies measurable academic and functional goals[24] that are to be accomplished in 1 year.[25] If the annual goals are the heart of the IEP, what gives it "legs" is the statement of special education instruction, related services, and program modifications or supports for school personnel that will be provided to the child. In essence, the IEP is the document that both describes and ensures the educational program the child will receive for the next year. It has been described as the primary vehicle by which a FAPE is provided.[26]

What constitutes a FAPE has been the subject of much debate and litigation. In *Board of Education v. Rowley,* the Supreme Court interpreted a FAPE to require school districts to provide a disabled child "personalized instruction with sufficient support services to permit the child to benefit educationally from that instruction."[27] The court explicitly noted that the act does not require school districts to provide the "best" education or to "maximize each child's potential commensurate with the opportunity provided other children."[28] *Rowley* established the standard by which a FAPE is measured and set the bar low. However, it is noteworthy that *Rowley* was decided in 1982 and the IDEA has been amended several times since. Most recently, the IDEA was amended in 2004 and the amendments took effect July 1, 2005. The new amendments create some requirements for schools that should prove helpful to parents of all children with disabilities and particularly for children with autism.

Least Restrictive Environment

Least restrictive environment (LRE) refers to the extent to which a child with disabilities is educated with nondisabled peers. The less time a child with disabilities spends with nondisabled peers in school, the more restrictive the educational environment is considered. There is a preference in the law that children with disabilities be educated in the least restrictive environment. The IDEA mandates that removal of children with disabilities from regular classes occur only when the nature or severity of the child's disability is such that the child can not be sufficiently educated in regular classes with the use of supplementary aids and services.[29]

The term "mainstreaming" was used for many years to describe the practice of reintegrating children into the regular class who had been placed in self-contained, or segregated, special education classrooms. The more commonly used term today is "inclusion," which, though similar to mainstreaming, is different. Inclusion refers to the practice of providing special education and related services to children in the regular classroom in lieu of placing them in separate classes or programs. There are many benefits to inclusion. Children with disabilities, especially children with autism, benefit from the presence of appropriate peer models. Additionally, children with disabilities are made to feel a part of mainstream society. Nondisabled children can be taught to better understand individuals with disabilities and respect their similarities as well as their differences. (See Chapter 10 for more information on nondisabled peer models.)

However, inclusion also has its shortcomings. An unintended consequence of inclusion is that the special education services the child receives are often a diluted version of what the child would receive in a self-contained special education class. Inclusion requires special education teachers to be assigned to multiple classrooms, thereby reducing their time within each classroom. Many school systems have resorted to hiring paraprofessionals (individuals without a teaching certification) to provide special education instruction. Paraprofessionals may provide special education instruction to a child, but only under the direct supervision of a special education teacher.[30] Unfortunately, many schools violate this provision of the law and students may receive a large part of their instruction from paraprofessionals while the special education teacher is in another classroom.

Inclusion also requires a high degree of coordination and collaboration between the special education teacher, the regular education teacher, and other individuals involved in the child's education. Given the demands placed on teachers' time, the requisite level of coordination is frequently lacking. Although the special education teacher is generally responsible for implementation of the child's IEP, in an inclusion model it is not unusual for the regular education teacher to be partially, or even equally, responsible for the goals and objectives outlined in the IEP. This requires that the general education teachers have more training, advanced skills, and a greater flexibility in their teaching style and approach, a combination not often seen. Finally, the need for school-to-home communication, while particularly important for all children with disabilities, is even more acute in the inclusion program. Children with disabilities as a whole require more parental support for their education than their nondisabled counterparts. Because multiple teachers typically participate in the delivery of instruction in an inclusion model, parents need clear, timely, and complete information about their child's progress, problems, and class assignments if they are to provide effective support. Failure to receive this degree of communication is a common complaint from parents of children with autism in inclusion programs.

Research-Based Instructional Practices

A major change in the 2004 amendments to the IDEA emphasizes the use of research-based instructional practices. As noted earlier in this chapter, Congress blamed the failure of the IDEA to achieve better results in part on a failure to adequately employ scientifically proven teaching methods.[31] The IDEA now requires that the IEP include "a statement of the special education and related services and supplementary aids and services, based on peer-reviewed research to the extent practicable, to be provided to the child."[32] This new requirement forces schools to utilize methods of instruction and practices that have been proven to be effective through replicable research when it exists.

Schools may resist identifying educational methodology in the IEP, claiming that if a methodology is specified in the IEP the school is limited to the use of only that methodology even if it is not effective. This argument has always been specious, as schools may not only hold an IEP meeting at any time to change an IEP that is not working, they are required to do so. Thus, even if a research-based method is included in a child's IEP, the IEP can be changed if is ineffective. Schools may claim that they utilize an "eclectic approach," creating the impression that they employ a variety of methodologies. However, research has shown that an eclectic approach is generally not effective for children with autism.[33]

School officials further claim that the law provides them the exclusive authority to make decisions concerning educational methodology. This claim finds its roots in the *Rowley* decision. There the Supreme Court noted that the "primary responsibility for choosing the educational method most suitable to the child's needs was left by the act to state and local educational agencies *in cooperation with the parents*."[34] Schools sometimes forget that parents were to be included in the decision-making equation albeit in a somewhat diminished role. The multiple amendments to the IDEA since the *Rowley* decision have strengthened the role of parents in the IEP process.[35] The Congressional committee reports from the 1997 amendments identify one of the purposes of the act as expansion of opportunities for partnerships between parents and public school officials.[36] Parents are expected to be "equal participants" with school officials in developing and revising their child's IEP.[37] The requirement that schools utilize research-based educational intervention places parents in a stronger position to ensure that schools identify those methodologies in their child's IEP. This is particularly beneficial to parents of children with autism. Extensive research exists on effective teaching methods for children with autism.[38] Nevertheless, many schools have been slow to implement proven interventions, choosing instead to continue the use of methods that have no scientific support or empirical evidence of success. Schools frequently use interventions they know rather than what the child needs. This violates the IDEA's requirement that the school design the IEP to meet the child's unique educational needs.[39] Armed with a clear mandate from IDEA 2004, parents can now insist that schools utilize research-based teaching methods and hold the school accountable.

IDEA 2004: A New Definition of FAPE

As noted previously in this chapter, the Supreme Court set the bar low for what constitutes a FAPE in its seminal decision *Board of Education v. Rowley*. The court explicitly rejected any contention that the IDEA (at that time the EAHCA) required school districts to maximize a child's potential or provide the best educational program for a child with disabilities.[40] Rather, it held that the primary goal of the act was to give children with disabilities access to public education and provide them with "some educational benefit."[41] However, in IDEA 2004, Congress raised the bar. In the act's "Findings," Congress noted that almost 30 years of research and experience have demonstrated that the education of children with disabilities can be made more effective by having high expectations and educating them in the regular classroom so they can "meet developmental goals and, to the *maximum extent possible,* the challenging expectations that have been established for all children" as well as "be prepared to lead productive and independent adult lives, to the *maximum extent possible.*"[42] Additionally, Congress found that the education of children with disabilities can be made more effective if professionals who work with disabled children receive "high quality, intensive" training so that they have the skills and knowledge necessary to "improve the academic achievement and functional performance of children with disabilities, including the use of scientifically based instructional practices, to the *maximum extent possible.*"[43] Congress further noted that "[i]mproving educational results for children with disabilities is an essential element of our national policy of ensuring equality of opportunity, full participation, independent living, and economic self-sufficiency for individuals with disabilities."[44] Note also that Congress added preparing children with disabilities for "further education" as one of the purposes of the act.[45]

These Congressional findings, intermixed with the added purpose of the act and the requirement of research-based teaching methods in the child's educational program, establish a higher standard than simply access to public education with *some* benefit. Thus, in accord with the IDEA's new requirements, a FAPE is one in which a child receives special education and related services that use scientifically based instructional practices to ensure that the disabled child is given the opportunity to meet educational expectations that have been established for all children as well as to improve his or her academic achievement and functional performance to the maximum extent possible. This is important in order to prepare the child for further education, employment, and independent living. This definition incorporates the essential elements of IDEA 2004 and provides school districts and parents of children with disabilities a framework from which to conceptualize a child's educational program.

SECTION 504 OF THE REHABILITATION ACT OF 1973

The Rehabilitation Act of 1973 is a civil rights act designed to prohibit discrimination against individuals with disabilities in federally funded facilities. Section 504 of the act provides that:

No otherwise qualified individual with a disability in the United States . . . shall, solely by reason of his or her disability, be excluded from the participation in, be denied the benefits of, or be subjected to discrimination under any program or activity receiving Federal financial assistance or under any program or activity conducted by any Executive agency or by the United States Postal Service.[46]

The Act defines an individual with a disability as any person who (i) has a physical or mental impairment which substantially limits one or more of such person's major life activities, (ii) has a record of such an impairment, or (iii) is regarded as having such an impairment.[47]

Section 504 covers a much broader array of individuals with disabilities than the IDEA. Whereas the IDEA pertains only to the education of children, Section 504 covers children and adults. Section 504 does not limit the types of disabilities covered. Anyone who qualifies for services under the IDEA is also covered by Section 504. However, the reverse is not true. For example, a child with diabetes would likely be covered under Section 504 but not by the IDEA because diabetes is not one of the disabilities identified under it. Of course the child with diabetes would only be covered under Section 504 if the disability substantially limited a major life activity. Major life activities include, but are not limited to, breathing, speaking, walking, hearing, eating, seeing, learning, working, and caring for oneself.

Section 504 imposes certain requirements on public schools though not as extensively as the IDEA. Public schools are required to provide a free appropriate public education for all qualified individuals with a disability regardless of the nature or severity of the disability.[48] However, Section 504 defines an *appropriate* education as one that is designed to meet the individual needs of the child with a disability "as adequately as the needs of" a nondisabled child.[49] Compare this with the IDEA's requirement that a child with a disability benefit from the educational program. Section 504 has no corresponding requirement. Theoretically, a school could comply with Section 504's requirements without providing any educational benefit to the child, unless that child also has an IEP.

Section 504, like the IDEA, requires that children with disabilities receive their education in the "least restrictive environment."[50] As with the IDEA, children with disabilities are not to be removed from the regular classroom unless an appropriate education can not be provided in the regular environment with the use of supplementary aids and services.

Although Section 504 provides many protections to children with disabilities in public schools, they are far fewer than the safeguards available under the IDEA. For example, as noted previously in this chapter, the IDEA mandates that an eligible child with a disability receive an IEP, which is a comprehensive description of the educational program the child will receive. An IEP is not required under Section 504.[51] Many schools develop what they may call a *504 Plan* or an *Accommodations Plan*, but even this is not mandated by Section 504.

Another example is how discipline is addressed by the two statutes. A publicly funded school may not suspend or expel a child who is covered under Section 504 or IDEA for more than 10 days without first holding a meeting to determine whether the behavior for which the child is being disciplined is a manifestation of the child's disability.[52] Under either statute, if the child's behavior is determined not to be a manifestation, the child may be disciplined in the same manner as the school would discipline a child without a disability, so the child could be expelled. Under the IDEA, however, the school district must continue to provide the child a FAPE. Under Section 504, continuation of a FAPE is not required.

Section 504 and Children with Autism

Most children with autism are covered by the IDEA. Children with autism almost always require direct and intensive special education and related services, something found in an IEP but rarely found in a 504 plan. Autism is also one of the IDEA's identified disabilities. Nevertheless, parents of children with autism should not ignore Section 504 because it emphasizes equal protection in areas not covered by the IDEA, specifically extracurricular activities. Section 504's emphasis on equal treatment requires public schools to provide nonacademic and extracurricular services and activities in a manner that ensures equal opportunity for participation. Thus, a child with autism could not be excluded from participating in a school club, play, dance, field trip, or other activity simply by virtue of his or her disability. Further, the school must make reasonable accommodations to ensure the student has access to the activity. The IDEA requires publicly funded schools to provide physical education but does not address athletics. Under Section 504 children with autism can not be prohibited from trying out for the school basketball team, for example, although they, like other children, are not guaranteed to make it.

The story of Jason McElwain is worth mentioning. Jason is a 17-year-old young man with autism attending Greece Athens High School, located just outside of Rochester, New York. Jason was the manager of the school's basketball team, which means he was not a player. Nevertheless, his coach allowed him to suit up for the last game of the season, held on February 15, 2006. Once the coach decided his team had a comfortable lead, he put Jason in. Jason proceeded to score 20 points in 4 minutes—a remarkable achievement for anyone. His teammates carried him off the court on their shoulders. His story has made national news and serves as a reminder to all not to underestimate the potential of individuals with autism. Given his remarkable scoring ability, one wonders, though, why he was not a player on the team.

Section 504 can also be used to protect the rights of individuals who advocate for children with disabilities. In *Settlegode v. Portland Public Schools,*[53] a teacher who taught adapted physical education to disabled children, many of whom had autism spectrum disorders, was fired for having advocated for better services and treatment for her students. Pamela Settlegode had sent numerous letters to her supervisors complaining of inadequate materials and equipment for the children she served, as well as difficulty finding a place to teach. She was frequently forced to teach her adapted physical education classes in the hallway because the regular physical education classes had first use of the gymnasium. Her supervisors admonished her to stop writing letters. When she did not, her teaching contract was terminated. Ms. Settlegode sued, alleging retaliation for a protected activity under Section 504 and several other statutes and thus won a $1 million judgment against the school district and her supervisors. Though the IDEA will provide more services and safeguards for children with autism spectrum disorders, Section 504 can also be a valuable tool for protecting children's rights.

THE NCLB

The NCLB was signed into law by President Bush on January 8, 2002. It represents the most recent amendments and reauthorization of the Elementary and Secondary Education Act of 1965 (ESEA). When President Lyndon Johnson signed the ESEA in 1965 he stated, "No law I have signed or will ever sign means more to the future of America." Yet, more than 40 years later, only approximately one-third of fourth graders in public schools are able to read at grade level.[54] Although NCLB is designed to address the education of all children and is not specific to the needs of children with disabilities, it places requirements on publicly funded schools that have implications for children with disabilities.

The purpose of NCLB "is to ensure that all children have a fair, equal, and significant opportunity to obtain a high-quality education and reach, at a minimum, proficiency on challenging State academic achievement standards and state academic assessments."[55] Twelve steps are identified to achieve this purpose, most notably "closing the achievement gap between high- and low-performing children"[56] and "affording parents substantial and meaningful opportunities to participate in the education of their children."[57]

In the IDEA, Congress noted the need to coordinate the act with NCLB.[58] NCLB identifies children with disabilities as one of several disaggregated groups of children whose progress must be tracked by the state. At the heart of NCLB is accountability. Every publicly funded school is required to meet *adequate yearly progress* (AYP) standards. AYP is defined by each state, but must ensure that all students are proficient in reading, math, and science by 2014.[59] School districts are required to report how all students perform on statewide assessments, including specific groups of students identified as low-income students, students with disabilities, limited English proficiency students, and minority students. Consistent failure to attain AYP for students in general or in any of the disaggregate groups could result in increasingly severe sanctions against the school.[60]

The primary means of ensuring achievement of AYP is by hiring highly qualified teachers trained in the use of "effective methods and instructional strategies that are based on scientifically based research."[61] NCLB requires schools to inform parents whether their child is being taught by a teacher who is highly qualified and to report on the school's progress in achieving AYP.

NCLB recognizes parent involvement as an important component of a successful schoolwide program.[62] Schools, in collaboration with parents, are required to develop written policies that encourage parent involvement.[63] Such policies must include the following: (1) opportunities for parents to participate in the planning, review, and improvement of school programs; (2) the education of school personnel to value parent contributions and learn how to work with them as equal partners; and (3) the development of a school–parent contract that outlines how parents, school personnel, and students share responsibility for improved student achievement. A key component of NCLB's parental involvement requirements is communication between teachers and parents that includes conferences, frequent progress reports, and "reasonable access to staff, opportunities to volunteer and participate in their child's class and observations of classroom activities."[64]

Although NCLB provides no individual cause of action, parents of children with autism can, nevertheless, use it to further their child's education. Not infrequently parents complain that schools set the bar too low for their child's functional and academic development. Schools have adhered to the *Rowley* standard of "some educational benefit" and most likely, will continue to do so until the courts recognize IDEA 2004's higher standard. In the meantime, NCLB's requirement that all children, including children with disabilities, achieve AYP forces schools to raise their expectations. This may help close the achievement gap between high- and low-performing children through intensive and individualized educational programs delivered by highly trained school staff. NCLB's parental-involvement requirements better position parents to hold schools accountable.

LONG-TERM PLANNING FOR CHILDREN WITH AUTISM

Long-term planning for more severely impaired children with autism is unique and complicated and requires the expertise of individuals experienced in such planning. What is prudent for a child without disabilities could be a costly mistake for a child with autism. For example, buying stocks or bonds in the child's name or identifying the child as a beneficiary in a will or life insurance policy could result in the child with disabilities losing important government benefits.

Once more severely impaired children "age out" of special education,[65] they will likely continue to need individual care and services. Funding for those services must be carefully planned. Additionally, parents must plan for the likelihood that their child will outlive them. Long-term planning is crucial for the child with autism, yet too few parents have developed a plan. According to a survey conducted by Metlife in 2005, less than a third of parents of children with special needs have a will or have done any financial planning for their children's future.[66] Most children with autism will be eligible for Supplemental Security Income (SSI) and Medicaid if their parents plan appropriately.

SSI and Medicaid are available to individuals with very limited income and minimal assets. The income limitations vary from state to state and are tied to the federal poverty level. An individual's liquid assets can not exceed $2000.[67] Liquid assets include bank accounts, stocks, and bonds, among other holdings. Assets such as an individual's clothing, furniture, the home they live in, and one automobile used for their transportation usually are not counted.

Medicaid is a joint federal- and state-funded health insurance program that is administered by each state. Although the federal government sets broad guidelines, each state establishes its own rules for eligibility and coverage. Medicaid pays for some or all medical care including prescriptions, dental, and vision care for eligible persons. An individual must be characterized as low income and have no private health insurance to meet federal Medicaid eligibility requirements.

SSI is a federal supplement income program designed to help elderly (65 or older), blind, or disabled individuals with low income. It provides cash to meet basic needs of shelter, clothing, and food. The amount SSI provides has traditionally been below the federally identified poverty level. Thus families must often supplement SSI payments to ensure that the disabled individual has some degree of comfort. Funding such supplementary assistance without running afoul of government restrictions must be carefully planned. Establishing a savings account or investing in other liquid assets in the child's name is a mistake if the combined assets exceed $2,000. Keep in mind that interest or dividends, if deposited or reinvested in the child's account, could eventually exceed the federal limit if not monitored carefully.

Special-Needs Trust

Perhaps the best and safest way to provide supplementary assistance to a child and, ultimately, adult with autism, while protecting his or her right to government benefits is through a special needs trust (SNT). An SNT is a legal entity that permits donors to give assets to a trustee for the benefit of the disabled individual. The assets are owned by the trust and managed by the trustee. The beneficiary, the child or adult with autism, has no control over the assets of the trust. An SNT is governed by state law and, therefore, should be drafted by an attorney with experience in and knowledge of state law as it pertains to such instruments.

There are many advantages to an SNT. Parents or guardians can be the trustee or another relative, or a friend, attorney, accountant, or even an institution (e.g., a bank) can serve as the trustee. The trust can and should identify a line of successors should the initial trustee become unable to manage the trust. Perhaps the greatest advantage of the trust is that assets such as cash, stocks, bonds, personal property, or real estate can be placed in the trust without impacting the disabled individual's right to government benefits. As manager of the trust, the trustee has authority to invest, sell, and use the trust's assets to the benefit of the disabled individual. Parents and other individuals can designate the SNT as a beneficiary in their will. Note that the trust, not the disabled individual, is the designated beneficiary. They can also designate the SNT as a beneficiary in a life insurance policy. Parents and other individuals can also make contributions to the SNT that may be tax deductible. Thus, the SNT is an important planning tool for parents of children with autism. The following section describes several types of SNTs.

Revocable versus Irrevocable Trusts

As the name implies, an irrevocable SNT is one that, once created, can not be changed. Any assets in the trust must remain in the trust to be used only for the disabled individual. A revocable SNT can be changed. Although on its face the revocable SNT appears better, there are certain advantages to the irrevocable SNT that may make it the preferred choice for parents.

Most states consider a revocable SNT to be a part of the parents' estate. Therefore, when the parents die, all assets in the SNT are potentially subject to estate taxes, payment of debts, and even lawsuits. The potential exists that all of the assets in the SNT could be frozen during a lengthy legal proceeding or used to satisfy outstanding claims. On the other hand, an irrevocable SNT, if set up properly, is separate from the parents' estate and protected from any claims made against the estate. However, because it is untouchable once it is set up, extreme care and planning must go into establishing an irrevocable SNT.

Testamentary versus Living Trusts

A testamentary SNT is a trust established for the benefit of the disabled individual as a part of the parents'/guardians' last will and testament. It is established upon the death of the parents. A living SNT[68] is a trust established while the parents are still living. The primary disadvantage to the testamentary SNT is that it is subject to probate, which could take months or even years. In the meantime the disabled individual could be without any assistance beyond that provided by SSI and Medicaid. The living SNT is a better choice. The trust can be set up for the child at any age. The parents, if they are the trustees, can establish a checking account to develop a record of payments from the trust on behalf of the child. Later, if someone other than the parents becomes the trustee, the checking account can serve as a record of acceptable expenditures from the trust.

A further advantage of the living SNT is that it offers additional financial protection to not only the disabled individual but the parents as well. Generally, people are all living longer. More and more people will spend the last 5 or more years of their lives in nursing homes or other types of assisted living. Such services are expensive and can use up large portions if not all of the parents' assets. However, any assets that have been placed in the SNT cannot be used for such care or factored into what portion of the parents' assets will have to be exhausted before other benefits become available.

RESIDENTIAL PLACEMENTS

For the purposes of this chapter, residential placement is defined as a 24-hour care facility located outside of the parents' or guardians' home. It could be a residential treatment center (RTC), a group home, or a medical facility. Placement may be necessitated by a variety of factors and can range from a few days to years. Residential placements can be very expensive, exceeding $100,000 per year in some facilities. Therefore, funding for a residential placement can be a challenge.

For children who are eligible for special education, funding through the school system is a possibility. The IDEA requires school districts to place children in the least restrictive educational setting in which the child can receive an appropriate education.[69] Schools are required to consider a continuum of educational placements including "hospitals and institutions." In order for a child to receive a residential placement, the school district must have determined that the child could not receive an appropriate education in a less restrictive environment even with the use of supplementary aids and services. The placement must be necessitated for educational reasons, not because of health, medical, or familial problems, although they can be contributing factors. Education, especially under IDEA 2004's broader definition, encompasses more than academics. A child's IEP must include functional goals in addition to academic goals. Judicial decisions have favored an expansive definition of education to include social and emotional needs.[70] The IDEA's mission includes preparing disabled children for further education, employment, and independent living. For children 16 and older, the IEP must include postsecondary transition goals and services related to training, employment, and independent living.[71] If a residential placement is the only means by which a disabled child may have an opportunity to achieve such goals, the school must fund the placement regardless of the costs.[72]

If the child needs a residential placement for reasons unrelated to his or her education, Medicaid may be the only other viable funding source. Private health insurance rarely covers residential placements except for very short-term stays. As noted previously in this chapter, Medicaid is a government-funded health insurance program for individuals with low income and few assets. Because parents' income and assets are considered, many disabled children are not eligible for Medicaid. Some states have adopted a Medicaid waiver program for children with autism, which excludes the parents' income and assets when determining whether the child meets the financial needs requirements. However, if the child has an income exceeding the state's income limitation or has assets in his or her name in excess of $2000, the child will not qualify. The need for long-term planning at an early age cannot be overemphasized.

CONCLUSION

This chapter has only broadly discussed important legal issues confronting parents and guardians of children with autism. It is important that parents recognize that there are many laws, regulations, and programs that provide a means of obtaining needed services for their children. In many cases parents will be able to effectively navigate on their own. However, knowledgeable legal expertise is a must in establishing a special needs trust as well as for dealing with certain other legal issues relating to education and residential placements. Some organizations parents can turn to for help include the Autism Society of America (ASA; *www.autism-society.org*), the Council of Parents, Advocates and Attorneys (COPAA; *www.copaa.com*), and Wrightslaw *(www.wrightslaw.com)*.

NOTES

1. Public Law 108-446; 20 U.S.C. § 1400 *et seq.*
2. 29 U.S.C. § 706(7)(B).
3. Public Law 107-110; 20 U.S.C. § 6301 *et seq.*
4. U.S. Constitution, Art. VI, § 2.
5. 20 U.S.C. §1415(b)(6).
6. Public Law 94-142.
7. Public Law 101-476.
8. 20 U.S.C. § 1400(c) (1976).
9. See Elementary and Secondary Education Act of 1965 as amended by Public Law 89-750 (1966); Education of the Handicapped Act of 1970, Public Law 91-230.
10. 334 F. Supp. 1257 (E.D.Pa. 1971), 343 F. Supp. 279 (E.D. Pa. 1972).
11. 348 F. Supp. 866 (D.D.C. 1972).
12. See *Board of Education v. Rowley,* 458 U.S. 176 (1982).
13. 20 U.S.C. § 1400(d). Note that "further education" is new in IDEA 2004.
14. *Id.*
15. 20 U.S.C. § 1400(c)(4) (2004).
16. 20 U.S.C. § 1401(a)(29).
17. 34 C.F.R. §300.26(b)(3).
18. 20 U.S.C. § 1401(a)(26).
19. 526 U.S. 66 (1999).

20. *Id.* at 77.
21. 20 U.S.C. § 1414(d).
22. 20 U.S.C. §1414(d)(1).
23. *Id.*
24. Prior to the 2004 Amendments, the IDEA required short-term objectives or benchmarks that related to the annual goals. The new IDEA requires only annual goals, except that the IEPs of children who will take alternate assessments must include short-term objectives or benchmarks.
25. IDEA 2004 offers up to 15 states an opportunity to participate in a pilot program designed to evaluate the efficacy of 3-year IEPs. However, the provision continues the requirement that the IEP include measurable *annual* goals. See §1414(d)(5).
26. See *Honig v. Doe,* 484 U.S. 305, 310 (1988).
27. 458 U.S. 176, 189 (1982).
28. *Id* at 198.
29. 20 U.S.C. § 1412(a)(5).
30. 20 U.S.C. § 6319.
31. See note 18.
32. 20 U.S.C. §1414(d)(1)(A)(i)(IV).
33. Howard, J. S., Sparkman, C. R., Cohen, H. G., Green, G., Stanislaw, H. (2005). A comparison of intensive behavioral analytic and eclectic treatments for young children with autism. *Research in Developmental Disabilities 26,* 359–383.
34. *Rowley* at 207 [emphasis added].
35. 20 U.S.C. §1400(c)(4)(B).
36. H. Rep. 105-95 at 82 (1997); S. Rep. No. 105-17 at 4-5(1997).
37. 34 C.F.R. §300, App. A, question 5.
38. See generally National Research Council. (2001). *Educating Children with Autism.* Washington, DC: National Academies Press.
39. 20 U.S.C. §1414(d)(1).
40. See note 31 and related text.
41. 458 U.S. 176, 200.
42. 20 U.S.C. §1400(c)(5)(A) [emphasis added].
43. §1400(c)(5)(E) [emphasis added].
44. 20 U.S.C. § 1400(c)(1) (2004).
45. §1400(d).
46. 29 U.S.C. § 794(a).
47. 29 U.S.C. § 705(20).
48. 34 C.F.R. § 104.33(a).
49. 34 C.F.R. § 104.33(b)(1)(i).
50. 34 C.F.R. § 104.34.
51. Section 504 states that an IEP is one means of meeting its requirement for an appropriate education, but it is not required.
52. See 20 U.S.C. § 1415(k). An exception to this rule is that a child may be immediately placed in an alternative educational setting for up to 45 days if, on school property or at a school function, the child possesses a weapon, possesses or uses illegal drugs, or inflicts serious bodily injury upon a person.
53. Case No. 02-35269 (9th Cir. 2004).

54. See Wright, P. W. D., Wright, P. D., & Heath, S. W. (2004). *Wrightslaw: No Child Left Behind*. Hartfield, VA: Harbor House Law Press.
55. 20 U.S.C. § 6301.
56. 20 U.S.C. § 6301(3).
57. 20 U.S.C. § 6301(12).
58. 20 U.S.C. § 1400(c)(5)(C).
59. 20 U.S.C. § 6311.
60. Sanctions range from identification of the school or school district as "in need of improvement" for failure to meet AYP for 2 consecutive years to a state takeover of the school for failure to meet AYP for 5 consecutive years. 20 U.S.C. § 6316(b).
61. 20 U.S.C. § 6314(b)(1).
62. 20 U.S.C. § 6314(b)(1)(F).
63. 20 U.S.C. § 6318(b).
64. 20 U.S.C. § 6318(d).
65. The IDEA requires states to provide special education to eligible children through age 21, but some states have extended the age cut-off .
66. See Reeves, S. (2005). Financial planning for kids with special needs. Retrieved March 2005, from *www.forbes.com*.
67. Understanding SSI. (2005). Retrieved from *www.socialsecurity.com*.
68. Also sometimes referred to as an "Intervivos Special Needs Trust."
69. 20 U.S.C. § 1412(a)(5).
70. See *County of San Diego v. California Special Education Hearing Office*, 93 F.3d 1458 (9th Cir. 1996).
71. 20 U.S.C. § 1414(d)(1)(A)(VIII).
72. *Cedar Rapids Community Sch. Dist. v. Garret F.*, 526 U.S. 66 (1999). School districts are not required to pay for the most expensive program if another less expensive program can meet the child's needs. *Florence County Sch. Dist. No. IV v. Carter*, 510 U.S. 7 (1993).

8

Family Resources during the School-Age Years

April W. Block
Stephen R. Block

Caregivers may face inconsistencies between the services professionals recommend for their school-age child with autism and the simultaneous inability to gain access to or afford those important therapeutic and supportive services. Such a paradox is the subject of this chapter, with the goal of providing insights and suggestions to professionals in order to better help families navigate systems to obtain necessary service supports. The chapter reviews some of the barriers that prevent families from obtaining needed services and then describes some of the models and strategies that can be used to gain access to these services. While some of the principles and strategies may benefit families outside of the United States, the focus of the chapter is U.S.-based.

Caregivers who have school-age children with autism generally experience extraordinary barriers in their attempt to obtain the appropriate scope of services that might benefit their sons and daughters. Accessing appropriate and effective services is difficult for families of children with a variety of mental disorders, even those families with substantial financial resources (U.S. Public Health Service, 2000). Availability of services for a specific child usually is interrelated with costs for a particular type of service, as well as general costs to an agency deemed responsible for offering a range of autism services, such as a public school. For example, anecdotal reports and existing research (Block & Hartsig, 2002) indicate that once a child has received a diagnosis of autism, families often do extensive searches on autism (typically now on the Internet) to find out what they can do to best help their child. In their searches, they may find a model they believe will be the best and advocate for those specific services to be delivered through agencies such as their public schools. Schools typically are responsible for implementing the Individuals with Disabilities Education Act (IDEA). While school districts may want to accommodate the needs of the child, most state and local educational agencies simply cannot afford to do so. The struggle to choose an intervention model, the commitment by various entities that any given model they identify is the most effective approach for a child, and the associated costs create a great deal of tension between families and the public schools.

In the United States, according to the basic tenets of the IDEA, children of school age are entitled to receive a free and appropriate public education. Children with a diagnosis of autism are not excluded from this statutory right. The IDEA emphasizes the importance of a child's access to special education and related services and is designed to meet the unique learning needs of children and to prepare them for eventual independence and employment.

Furthermore, the principles contained in the IDEA are intended to support (1) the child's readiness for education by ensuring access to an appropriate evaluation, (2) placement in the least restricted learning environment, (3) parent and student participation in decision making, (4) development of an individualized education plan (IEP) designed to meet the unique needs of the child, (5) implementation of the IEP, and (6) procedural safeguards to ensure that the parents' and child's rights are protected, and that the child receives what he or she is entitled to under the law.

Despite the clarity of the federal mandate to provide educationally related supports and services, many school districts throughout the nation are incapable of complying with the IDEA because they claim to have insufficient financial resources, particularly for specific treatments requested by the parents. Consequently, it is not difficult to demonstrate that school districts throughout the nation are out of compliance with their statutory obligations; one only has to examine the hundreds of due process cases that caregivers have filed against school districts for violations of the special education law. Among these legal cases, Mandlawitz

(2002) identified approximately 150 cases with issues centering on education and services for children with autism. The most common theme in these cases was caregivers seeking reimbursement or continuing payments for applied behavioral analysis or discrete-trial teaching programs conducted in the home, over and above the more typical therapies such as speech/language, occupational therapy, sensory integration, or physical therapy.

Most complaints and lawsuits stem from disagreements during a child's transition from 0–3 services into a school district preschool program. Not surprisingly, the key issues are differences of opinion between the caregivers and school districts over the intensity of treatment needed. The caregivers seek to hold on to extensive in-home therapeutic services, while the school districts promote less expensive in-school services.

Barriers to obtaining specific types of autism services are not exclusive to the United States. They also extend into Canada. In 2004, the Canadian Supreme Court overturned two earlier rulings and found that the provinces were not obligated to cover costly forms of autism treatment. The Court did not accept the view that a denial of payment for Lovaas therapy services was discriminatory (Campbell, 2004).

While the IDEA seems to be clear that cost cannot be a consideration when it comes to providing a free and appropriate public education, the U.S. Supreme Court has actually provided school districts a backdoor way out of providing optimal services for children. In the case of *Board of Education of the Hendrick Hudson Central School District v. Rowley* (458 U.S. 176, 1982), the U.S. Supreme Court recognized that every child has unique learning needs and therefore did not establish a benchmark for the meaning of "appropriate" education. Consequently, school districts have used the absence of a prescribed standard to mean that educational programs only need to be adequate, thus equating "adequate" with appropriate. Using this form of logic, school districts have often prevailed in cases in which families demanded specific forms of high cost treatment. Given the *Rowley* outcome, judges and administrative hearing officers frequently defer to the school or school district to establish their idea of adequate educational methods. Despite the legal mandates in the IDEA, the courts frequently appear sympathetic to school districts' financial limitations arguments. Money is often a major obstacle that sparks adversity and tension between families and schools districts. While school districts may want to accommodate the needs of the child, most state and local educational agencies simply cannot afford to do so.

Treatment costs can often exceed $25,000 per year (Freudenheim, 2004). Assuming that autism services are available in one's community, families may take on significant debt to cover the cost of services, including draining retirement savings and taking on second mortgages (Freud-enheim, 2004). With debt, the risk to families, beyond the obvious risk of bankruptcy, is the psychological strain that this adds to their already stressful situation. There is ample anecdotal evidence of how far families will go to obtain services for their children with autism, such as selling valued possessions, mortgaging homes, borrowing from credit cards, or working extra jobs. Some families can endure the compound stress of caregiving and financial hardship, while others break up over it (Bolman, 2004).

Because of the high personal and financial costs for autism services, families may also look to the government for assistance. For almost four decades, federal Medicaid law has undergone significant revisions to become the primary funder of long-term care services for individuals with disabilities. The law permits the U.S. Secretary of Health and Human Services to grant waivers of various statutory provisions that normally govern the operation of a state's Medicaid program. In the 1980s, with the addition of the §1915(c) waiver authority, states were able to launch home- and community-based services (HCBS) waiver programs to assist individuals with developmental disabilities to avoid institutionalization and to remain in the community.

Each state determines which type of Medicaid waiver program it will participate in, sets a cap on the number of people it will serve, and establishes the dollar limits for each service. Faced with skyrocketing medical costs throughout the nation, the trend is for states to search for ways to contain, if not cut, their matching share of participation in the Medicaid program (Ruble, Heflinger, Renfrew, & Saunders, 2005). Consequently, one of the major barriers experienced by families of children with autism is the eligibility determination process specified by the state agency responsible for reviewing applications for developmental disability services. Bureaucratic procedures can make the application or appeals process a difficult one to follow. Complicated rules and regulations can deter efforts to apply for services or make it difficult to comprehend and navigate the system.

Another possible avenue for covering the cost of autism services is through private insurance companies and health maintenance organizations (HMOs). However, many health insurance companies do not cover needed autism services. Anecdotal reports about insurance claim rejections have led to a widespread belief that insurance companies will automatically reject claims for the treatment of children with autism. Many families struggle with insurance carriers who would prefer not to cover the expenses for autism services, which can easily run into the tens of thousands of dollars per year for each child receiving services. On this point, the *New York Times* (Freudenheim, 2004) reported that insurance companies use a variety of excuses to avoid covering the claims filed by the families who have children with autism. Excuses included claims that treatment approaches have not been proven effective and that there is a paucity of scientific evidence that one treatment modality is better than another. Other excuses used by insurance companies included challenging the qualifications of the therapists or denying payments due to dual diagnosis issues (e.g., if the child has autism, sometimes considered a medical diagnosis, along with a mood disorder). (See Chapter 1 for more information regarding dual or comorbid diagnoses in children with autism.) According to Campbell (2004), even in 17 states where autism coverage is required by law, insurers often delay or avoid payment in individual cases by questioning the qualifications of the therapist or even a physician's affirmation that treatment is medically necessary.

STRATEGIES FOR OBTAINING SERVICES

At a time when families need support and assistance to help their child with autism, the state's human services agency may refuse services, the school system may balk at covering the services that the caregivers prefer, and the insurance carrier may flatly refuse to pay for services. In such times, families need help from professionals, both to understand what resources are available and to find ways to access financial support to pay for the extensive services children with autism can require. This section provides an overview of strategies for professionals and families in developing a collaborative game plan for accessing the appropriate services specific to the unique needs of each child.

Develop Parent–Professional Relationships

Over the years, caregivers who have children with special needs may interact with a variety of medical, human service, and educational professionals. These professionals may range in approach from those who assume the role of all-knowing expert, not viewing the family's role as integral to the treatment program, to those who are "family-friendly" and operate with a different set of values concerning the role of the family. The family-oriented practitioner recognizes the importance of family involvement in all phases of treatment, services, and supports (Block & Block, 2002). The family and their professionals must work together to assist the growth and development of the school-age child with autism. This type of parent–professional relationship has been characterized as being an association between a family and one or more professionals who function collaboratively, in that the family and professionals use agreed upon roles in pursuit of a joint interest and common goal (Dunst & Paget, 1991). Working as a coherent team is especially important because of the lack of agreement among professionals over the appropriate choice of treatment modalities when working with children with autism (Sperry, Whaley, Shaw, & Brame, 1999). As a result of disagreements among researchers and practitioners on the value of different treatment approaches, the parents and professionals must share confidence in each other in order to communicate and to make mutually agreeable decisions to develop and implement a plan of support and services. When it comes to making decisions about their child with autism, caregivers need encouragement from professionals to be active participants in all aspects of obtaining appropriate services for their child, and the effective professional will recognize the need to be inclusive. If the family does not receive the type of response that promotes a parent–professional partnership, they should seek services and supports elsewhere.

Become Empowered through Knowledge of the IDEA

One major strategy that has proven successful for caregivers and supportive professionals includes reading sections of the IDEA. The attained information can be powerful, with caregivers as well as professionals learning how to use knowledge of the law in pragmatic ways to obtain needed services for the child with autism. While professionals, in general, and school personnel, in particular, are assumed to know the law, in fact many do not. Professionals and families who know what the law states are often surprised to see how much their particular school official may not know. Unfortunately, in our experience, many have never read through the statutes and requirements, relying on information provided by their particular administration, which may or may not be an accurate source of information about the law.

One way to attempt to ensure that everyone involved is familiar with the regulations related to the child's condition is to cite relevant portions of the law in meetings with school officials. Families and their professional partners who understand their rights can often gain immeasurable benefits for their school-age child. Also, school officials who become more familiar with the law can avoid providing the type of incorrect information that could lead the knowledgeable parent to file a grievance.

The application of one's knowledge of the law is likely to be tested during IEP meetings. Although some may claim that school staff might intentionally write a deficient IEP in order to eliminate or reduce costly expenditures, the greater likelihood is that an inadequate IEP is the result of team members' unfamiliarity with the law. In those situations, parents can be quite influential if they are able to discuss with confidence and accuracy what their child is entitled to under the law. To ensure that parents are involved in decisions concerning their child with autism, the 1997 reauthorization of the IDEA stipulated that parents must be included in any group that makes decisions on the educational placement of the child. The foundational message in this provision is that the parent is a fundamental *team* participant and cannot be left out of the meeting. For that reason, the school must attempt to schedule the IEP meeting with proper notification, allowing the caregivers to arrange to participate. If parents are unable to attend at the scheduled time, the school must be flexible and accommodate the parent. Both parents and school personnel should reach a mutual agreement as to when and where the meeting will be held. If an IEP meeting is not going well, parents and supportive professionals can ask questions about the mediation process that must meet the requirements of the IDEA and be made available to the family. Parents can inform the school's officials that they would prefer to resolve the differences of opinion during the IEP meeting than partake in an expensive and time-consuming process.

Maintain Good Record Keeping

By the time a child with special needs enters the school system, the family will have already amassed mounds of documents, reports, and therapeutic recommendations. Once he or she is enrolled in school, the paperwork not only will continue, but it may take on even greater importance to ensure that the child is receiving a free and appropriate education. By keeping all of their child's information in order and accessible when needed, caregivers can be more effective as their child's advocate and arranger of services.

The Autism/PDD Support Network *(www.autism-pdd.net/about-us.html)* recommends that caregivers develop a record-keeping system that includes notes about the child's development, medical records and reports, types of inoculations and dates of shots, therapist evaluations and assessment reports, and school records such as IEPs and individualized family service plans (IFSPs).

Become Educated about Resources and Their Service Parameters

Families and professionals should be aware that each state has its own governmental department responsible for the provision of developmental disability services. The types of funded services that are offered throughout the states are as varied as the names of the state departments

responsible for the administration of developmental disabilities programs (see Table 8.1).

It is also essential to know timelines for service provision, because
this differs across states as well. Even if a child qualifies for government-
funded developmental disability services, this does not mean that services will be available when the family is ready to access them. Waiting
lists may exist, such as in Colorado, where wait time can span from a
few months to more than a few years. The demand for autism services
throughout the nation far outweighs resources allocated for services
(Jacobson & Mulick, 2000). Consequently, families face a remarkable
challenge in depending on overburdened, publicly funded systems with
limited resources when the prevalence of autism is escalating.

In addition, parents should know, if they plan to move from one
state to another, that eligibility for developmental disability services in
one state does not guarantee eligibility for services in another. Although
there is a federal definition of developmental disability, most states have
adopted their own definitions that are tied to eligibility determination.
For example, some states do not recognize the diagnosis of Asperger disorder as a developmental disability for purposes of qualifying for state-
funded services, even if the person with high-functioning autism or
Asperger disorder has fairly low adaptive behavior skills.

Eligibility is usually determined by two factors. One is the age of the
child when the condition was diagnosed. A second factor is the number
of functional life skill areas in which there are substantial limitations. To
illustrate the differences, we compare the legal definitions of South
Dakota, Washington, and North Carolina. The following **bolded words**
are intended to help the reader make comparisons and are not part of
the original texts. While there are a great many similarities in the definitions used across the country, they are not all alike.

In South Dakota, a developmental disability is defined in a state
statute as any severe, chronic disability of a person that is (1) attribut-
able to a mental or physical impairment or combination of mental and
physical impairments; (2) manifested before the person attains **age 22**;
(3) likely to continue indefinitely; (4) resulting in substantial functional
limitations in **three or more of the following areas of major life activity:**
language, learning, mobility, self-direction, capacity for independent living, and economic self-sufficiency; and (5) reflects the person's need for
an array of generic services, met through a system of individualized planning and supports over an extended time, including those of lifelong
duration (*www.state.sd.us/dhs/dd/Division/faqs.htm*).

Compare South Dakota's definition with the following eligibility
requirements from the state of Washington: Evidence of an eligible condition under "mental retardation" requires a diagnosis of mental retar-

TABLE 8.1. Departments Responsible for the Administration of Developmental Disabilities Programs in the 50 U.S. States

- Agency for Persons with Disabilities (FL)
- Bureau for Behavioral Health and Health Facilities (WV)
- Department of Aging and Disability Services (TX)
- Department of Community Health (MI)
- Department of Developmental Services (CA)
- Department of Disabilities and Special Needs (SC)
- Department of Disabilities, Aging and Independent Living (VT)
- Department of Economic Security (AZ)
- Department of Health (WY)
- Department of Health and Family Services (WI)
- Department of Health and Hospitals (LA)
- Department of Health and Social Services (AK, DE)
- Department of Health and Welfare (ID)
- Department of Human Services (CO, DC, HI, IL, IA, MN, NJ, ND, OK, OR, UT)
- Department of Mental Health (MS, MO)
- Department of Mental Health and Developmental Disabilities (TN)
- Division of Mental Health, Developmental Disabilities and Addictive Services (GA)
- Department of Mental Health, Retardation and Hospitals (RI)
- Department of Mental Health, Retardation, and Substance Abuse Services (VA)
- Department of Mental Health and Mental Retardation (AL, KY)
- Division of Mental Health, Developmental Disabilities and Substance Abuse Services (NC)
- Department of Mental Retardation (CT, MA)
- Department/Office of Mental Retardation/Developmental Disabilities (NY, OH)
- Department of Public Health and Human Services (MT)
- Department of Public Welfare (PA)
- Department of Social and Health Services (WA)
- Family and Social Services Administration (IN)
- Social and Rehabilitation Services (KS)
- Department of Health (NM)
- Department of Health and Human Services (ME, NE, NV, NH, AR)
- Developmental Disabilities Administration (MD)

dation by a licensed psychologist or a finding of mental retardation by a certified school psychologist or a diagnosis of Down syndrome by a licensed physician.

1. This diagnosis is based on documentation of a lifelong condition originating **before age 18.**
2. The condition results in significantly below average intellectual and adaptive skills functioning that will not improve with treatment, instruction, or skill acquisition.

centers throughout the country. Respite is one service often offered through family resource centers.

Increasing respite service options for families who have school-age children with autism was the focus of a project developed by Openden and colleagues (2006). They reported successful outcomes using a "babysitter"/respite provider list composed of university undergraduate students who expressed an interest in working with children with special needs. Most of the student providers were majoring in psychology, sociology, or education and met certain criteria including a high GPA. University students did not receive any organized preparation or training. The list of prospective respite providers was disseminated to the families. They had the responsibility of screening, interviewing, and selecting those students they wanted to serve as their respite providers. The caregivers also had the responsibility of training these respite providers on how to care for and work with their child with autism, such as prompting communication or using behavioral intervention strategies. Families paid for the services either directly or with the financial support of local human service agencies. The researchers indicated that their project was successful, based on feedback from the parents who utilized the university students as respite providers. Also, the researchers suggested that their approach to developing respite providers from the base of university students could be replicated by colleges and universities throughout the country (Openden et al., 2006).

Access Advocacy Support

The Administration on Developmental Disabilities (ADD) is a federal government agency within the U.S. Department of Human Services. One of the responsibilities of ADD is to oversee the implementation of the Developmental Disabilities Assistance and Bill of Rights Act of 2000. This law provides funding for three sources of advocacy efforts in each state: protection and advocacy (P&A) agencies, state councils, and university centers for excellence in developmental disabilities education, research, and service (UCEDDs).

Each state has a P&A agency, which offers information and referral services for legal, administrative, and other remedies to resolve problems for individuals with developmental disabilities. While the focus of the P&A agency in each state may be different, the P&A agency mission nationwide is to enhance the quality of life for people with developmental disabilities by investigating incidents of abuse, neglect, and discrimination based on disability. The state P&A agency also can gain access to all client records without permission when there is probable cause to suspect that abuse or neglect is involved. Families can seek support from their state's P&A agency if their child is not receiving services which they are entitled to under the law.

State councils (sometimes referred to as developmental disability planning councils) are composed of individuals appointed by a state's governor. They include individuals with developmental disabilities, caregivers and family members of people with developmental disabilities, representatives of state agencies, and interested community members. Families who have children with special needs can attend council meetings and seek to participate in efforts to promote services in their own state. According to ADD,

> State Councils pursue systems change (e.g., the way human service agencies do business so that individuals with developmental disabilities and their families have better or expanded services), advocacy (e.g., educating policy makers about unmet needs of individuals with developmental disabilities), and capacity building (e.g., working with state service agencies to provide training and benefits to direct care workers) to promote independence, self-determination, productivity, integration and inclusion of people with developmental disabilities in all facets of community life. *(www.acf.hhs.gov/programs/add/states/ddcs.html)*

Some may still refer to the third type of advocacy agency (UCEDDs) by their former title, university-affiliated programs (UAPs). Every state has a UCEDD that manages a range of responsibilities to meet a goal of increasing independence, productivity, and community integration of individuals with developmental disabilities. This is accomplished through a variety of services including interdisciplinary training, technical assistance, research and information dissemination activities, and support for community service activities. Families might discover that their state's UCEDD is involved in autism research or service delivery. Moreover, caregivers should contact the UCEDD to access recommendations for parent training programs to promote knowledge about autism and provide the skill development necessary to navigate the systems of services and funding.

Additional advocacy groups include the Parent Training and Information Centers (PTICs), which are devoted to helping families with children who have disabilities. Each state has at least one PTIC that receives funding from the U.S. Department of Education. The goal of the PTIC is to help families obtain appropriate education and services for their children with disabilities. PTICs also provide training programs to help caregivers and professionals work more effectively with each other, and to resolve problems between families and the various service systems that they must work with. They are also a resource for information and provider referrals.

Chapters of the Arc of the United States (formerly known as the Association for Retarded Citizens) can be found throughout the country. The Arc describes itself as a grassroots organization with 140,000 members who are affiliated through approximately 1,000 state and local chapters across the nation. These local and statewide nonprofit organizations provide advocacy to ensure that children and adults with developmental disabilities have access to the programs and services in their community. They are supported in many different ways including membership dues, individual and corporate contributions, foundation or government grants, and, for some chapters, thrift stores. Some focus their primary activities on resolving issues between individuals, families, and service providers. Others focus on improving access to services by influencing public policy, guided by the national organization's advocacy with Congress and the executive and judicial branches of government.

Several other organizations are devoted to providing information for families who have children with autism. The most notable is the 40-year-old Autism Society of America, and its affiliated chapters throughout the United States. Chapter activity may vary from state to state, but generally, one is likely to find support groups, information, referral services, and educational programs.

Access Additional Resources

There are many informative websites dedicated to helping families who have children with autism. The following websites can assist families in becoming informed about autism and the latest research news.

1. Current Alerting Service for Autism *(www.onlinecasa.org/)* provides abstracts of journal articles in order to keep readers abreast of the latest research findings.
2. National Alliance for Autism Research (NAAR) *(www.naar.org/about/about.htm)* funds global biomedical research to discover causes, prevention, effective treatments, and a cure for autism and to educate the public on the critical role research plays in achieving these goals.
3. National Institute of Child Health and Human Development (NICHD) *(www.nichd.nih.gov/autism/)* is part of the National Institutes of Health. This is one of several institutes doing research into various aspects of autism including its causes, prevalence, and treatments.

4. The Arc *(www.thearc.org)* is the site of the national organization described earlier, with local affiliates devoted to improving supports and services to persons with mental retardation and related developmental disabilities.

5. National Institute of Mental Health (NIMH) *(www.nimh.nih. gov/healthinformation/autismmenu.cfm)* is part of the National Institutes of Health. The focus of NIMH is working to improve mental health through biomedical research on mind, brain, and behavior.

6. Autism PDD Support Network *(www.autism-pdd.net/about-us.html)* is an information and resource site for coping with autism. This site provides an online support community forum to express personal views and ask for information and assistance. This site also offers a comprehensive list of resources by state and can be accessed at *(www.autism-pdd.net/resources-by-state.html#bystate)*.

7. Exploring Autism *(www.exploringautism.org/)* is a collaborative effort of 22 universities and medical centers exploring research into the genetics of autism.

8. Autism Society of America (ASA) *(www.autism-society.org/)* is a 40-year-old organization that is dedicated to increasing public awareness about autism and the day-to-day issues faced by individuals with autism, their families, and the professionals with whom they interact. The society has 200 chapters sharing a common mission of providing information and education, supporting research, and advocating for programs and services.

9. Autistic Society *(www.autisticsociety.org/autism-content-6.html)* was formed in 2003 with a mission to unite caregivers, families, friends, people with autism, and professionals by creating a strong, supportive community worldwide. The society shares firsthand knowledge, information, news, and research about autism.

10. MAAP Services for Autism and Asperger Syndrome *(www. maapservices.org/index.html)* is a nonprofit organization dedicated to providing information and advice to families of individuals with autistic disorder, Asperger disorder, and pervasive developmental disorder not otherwise specified (PDDNOS).

11. National Dissemination Center for Children with Disabilities (NICHCY) *(www.nichcy.org/)* describes itself as the nation's central source of information on disabilities in infants, toddlers, children, and youth, in addition to the IDEA, No Child Left Behind (as it relates to children with disabilities), and research-based information on effective educational practices.

12. Parent Training and Information Centers (PITC) and Community Parent Resource Centers *(www.taalliance.org/Centers/index.htm)* are found in every state and serve families of children and young adults from birth to age 22 with any disability. They help families obtain appropriate education and services for their children and offer a variety of support services such as training and information referral. The website noted here helps parents find the PITC in their own state.

CONCLUSION

Families of children with autism are confronted with many issues from the time they learn of the diagnosis of autism. Caregivers experience inconsistencies in recommendations of treatment modalities as they discover that eligibility criteria differ for government-funded services and supports from state to state, with some states having long waiting lists for funding. Despite these barriers to services and supports, families can prevail and find the resources that they need to assist their child in making developmental gains. The information contained in this chapter provides the edge that families need in obtaining information and accessing services in their local community. With these identified resources, caregivers will have some tools to navigate what may feel like unfriendly terrain. The key to helping caregivers access resources for their child with autism is to encourage them to be open to support from others in order to surmount stress by (1) creating a network with other families of children with autism; (2) discussing some of the child's differences with relatives and other children in the household; (3) developing partnerships with medical and educational professionals; (4) developing a plan for the child's daily and long-term care; and (5) not taking "No" for an answer.

REFERENCES

Block, A. W., & Block, S. R. (2002). Strengthening social work approaches through advancing knowledge of early childhood intervention. *Child and Adolescent Social Work Journal, 19,* 192–208.

Block, A., & Hartsig, J. (2002). What families wish service providers knew. In R. Gabriels & D. Hill (Eds.), *Autism: From research to practice.* London: Jessica Kingsley.

Block, S. R., & Block, A. W. (2003). Respite care, child. In J. J. Ponzetti et al. (Eds.), *International encyclopedia of marriage and family relationships* (2nd ed.). New York: Macmillan.

Bolman, W. M. (2004, July 13–15). *The autistic family life cycle: Family stress and divorce.* Paper presented at the 37th National Conference of the Autism Society of America, Providence, RI.

Campbell, C. (2004, November 20) World briefing Americas: Canada court rules province need not finance autism treatment. *New York Times,* p. 6.

Dunst, C. J., & Paget, K. D. (1991). Parent–professional partnerships and family empowerment. In M. Fine (Ed.), *Collaborative involvement with parents of exceptional children* (pp. 25–44). Brandon, VT: Clinical Psychology Publishing.

Freudenheim, M. (2004, December 21). Most resist big payments, challenging therapists and disorder's nature. *New York Times,* p. 1.

Jacobson, J., & Mulick, J. (2000). System and cost research issues in treatments for people with autistic disorders. *Journal of Autism and Developmental Disorders, 30*(6), 585–593.

Long, S. K., & Coughling, T. A. (2004, Winter). Access to care for disabled children under Medicaid. *Health Care Financing Review, 26,* 89–103.

Mandlawitz, M. R. (2002). The impact of the legal system on educational programming for young children with autism spectrum disorder. *Journal of Autism and Developmental Disorders, 32,* 495–508.

Nebraska Special Education Advisory Council. (2001). *Autism Spectrum Disorders (ASD): Nebraska State Plan,* Lincoln, NE.

Openden, D., Symon, J. B., Koegel, L. K., & Koegel, R. L. (2006). Developing a student respite provider system for children with autism. *Journal of Positive Behavior Interventions, 8,* 119–123.

Rizzolo, M. C., Hemp, R., Braddock, D., & Pomeranz-Essley, A. (2004). *The state of the states in developmental disabilities.* Washington, DC: American Association on Mental Retardation.

Ruble, L. A., Heflinger, C. A., Renfrew, J. W., & Saunders, R. C. (2005). Access and service use by children with autism spectrum disorders in Medicaid managed care. *Journal of Autism and Developmental Disorders, 35,* 3–13.

Schulz, R., & Beach, S. R. (1999). Caregiving as a risk factor for mortality: The caregiver health effects study. *Journal of the American Medical Association, 282,* 2215–2219.

Smith, G. J. (2001). *Status report: Litigation concerning Medicaid services for persons with developmental disabilities.* Alexandria, VA: National Association of State Directors of Developmental Disabilities Services.

Sperry, L. A., Whaley, K. T., Shaw, E., & Brame, K. (1999). Services for young children with autism spectrum disorders: Voices of caregivers and providers. *Infants and Young Children, 11,* 17–33.

U.S. Public Health Service. (2000). *Report of the Surgeon General's Conference on Children's Mental Health: A national action agenda.* Washington, DC: U.S. Department of Health and Human Services.

9

Family Vacations and Leisure Time

Considerations and Accommodations

Sharon Lerner-Baron

Leisure time has been valued as an important part of life since ancient Greek civilization (Fain, 1986). Vacations and leisure time can offset the common stressors of daily life, such as work, raising a family, dealing with friends and relatives, marital problems, sibling concerns, and school hassles. For parents of children who have autism, the challenges of daily life can be magnified. For example, caring for a child with a chronic disability such as autism can involve considerable expenditures of time and effort beyond the typical responsibilities of parenting, and impose financial strain, marital strain, and caregiver depression (Quittner, DiGirolamo, Michel, & Eigen, 1992; Quittner, Opipari, Regoli, Jacobsen, & Eigen, 1992; Thompson et al., 1994). Therefore, the amount of stress in families of a child with autism can be extraordinary and, all too often, these families feel alone and overwhelmed.

People often feel the need to take a vacation and relax with their families. Families with a child who has autism also have a great need for a vacation but may assume that a vacation will create even more stress. Unfortunately, these are the very families who most need a week to escape from everyday hassles such as therapy appointments, carpools, and school meetings and to relax and have fun together. Although it makes intuitive sense that vacations or leisure time might be beneficial for children with autism and their families, the discussion of this topic is almost nonexistent in the autism and general disability literature. Therefore, this chapter offers practical tips and ideas derived from clinical practice for use by clinicians to assist parents in making preparations necessary to help ensure more successful vacation and leisure experiences. The emphasis is on how to prevent challenges that may disrupt a variety of vacation or leisure experiences. The last section of the chapter highlights suggestions for after-school and summer programs.

FAMILY VACATIONS

Many people have a story to tell about childhood vacations—the whirlwind trip they took to the West Coast as a child, the chaotic, yet fun trips to a favorite relative's house, or the fantastic time they had looking for shells on the beach. We may have a mixed bag of recollections from various family vacations during our childhood and young adult lives that evoke both positive and, sometimes, unpleasant emotions, reminding us of old stories and family memories.

Even though stress can be created during the time when families are preparing for the vacations, people often look forward to taking a trip. Families who have children with autism also want vacation time but may experience a host of anxieties related to vacationing. They may hesitate because of their concerns that their child may not travel well or may miss too much therapy, that relatives may be insensitive, or that the vacation may be too much work. Indeed, vacationing does require more preparation, arrangements, and adjustments than a family with typical children may encounter; however, it can be very rewarding. In addition to having an opportunity to enjoy a new location or spend time with relatives and friends, the time away can allow family members to experience joy and relaxation and to become reenergized. Another advantage is that typical siblings can have the chance to see their brother or sister who has autism in a different light! Imagine the feeling of delight that family members may experience seeing the child with autism trying new things of interest in a different environment. Parents, siblings, and the child who has autism face numerous challenges and may miss out on many experiences that families who do not have a child with special needs may take for granted; however, vacations do not have to be one of those missed opportunities.

Vacation Planning

The first step in any vacation is planning. For families of children with autism, this requires extra work and special considerations, but they are well worth the time. It is important to remind parents that they engage in planning on a regular basis, and that vacations are no different. Additionally, it may be helpful to put vacations into perspective. For example, encourage parents to think back to their own childhood vacations—rushing to the airport, arguing with a parent about how much to pack, or not wanting to leave friends. Help normalize the experience by reminding parents that families with typically developing children also find it stressful to plan vacations.

Planning Tips

Because additional planning is required for a family traveling with a child with special needs, it is necessary to emphasize the importance of starting the process a few weeks in advance of the trip. These suggestions may appear to be common sense; however, when parents are so involved in their everyday activities and are coping with the daily issues of raising a child with special needs, it is easy to overlook the obvious.

• If the child does not wear an identification bracelet, advise parents to order one at least 6 weeks prior to the trip. This is important in case the child wanders away and gets lost. Medical ID jewelry can be ordered from various stores online or by telephone. Two companies that work with families of children with special needs are American Medical ID (1-800-363-5985) and N-Style ID (1-775-833-1271). The child's name, phone number, and any medical conditions or allergies should be noted on the ID bracelet. Additionally, parents' home phone numbers and cell phone numbers should be included for emergencies. The diagnosis of autism should be placed somewhere on the bracelet, so that if the child does get separated from the parents, the person reading the bracelet may have a better understanding of how to interact with the child.
• Two weeks prior to the trip, parents should begin introducing the child to wearing the ID bracelet. If the child is opposed to wearing the bracelet due to tactile sensitivity, propose that an engraved tag be attached to a shoelace. Another suggestion is to have parents laminate a pocket-sized card that includes child identification information and the

name of the hotel where the family is staying during the vacation. The child can carry the card in his or her pocket during the trip.

• Remind parents to refill their child's prescription medications and cancel all therapy and medical appointments to avoid missed appointment charges. Local Autism Society of America (ASA) chapters may have autism information brochures or business-size cards with autism facts. Parents can give these cards to strangers who make rude or intrusive comments about their child's behavior. Even if they are not read, this can give the parent a feeling of being in control and taking action.

• Parents should contact the local ASA chapter in the area where the family will be traveling to find grocery stores that carry necessary special-diet food items, restaurants that accommodate special dietary restrictions, and sitters in the area qualified to provide respite care for a child with autism or to assist if the parent needs an extra hand at a museum, park, or beach. This is especially helpful for single parents traveling alone with a child.

• Parents may raise the possibility of purchasing a cell phone for a teen with autism. Most teens carry cell phones, and this may help foster acceptance in inclusive settings, as well as providing teens with autism with the security of knowing that they can contact the parent if they get lost. Even though it may take some time to teach the teen how to access preprogrammed phone numbers, it is worth the sense of security it gives parents to know that they have the option to call their child. Parents need to make sure the phone is charged, turned on, and placed in the child's pocket. There should be a plan to practice using the phone prior to the trip.

• Parents may want to call the hotel ahead of time to request rooms with a handicapped-accessible bathroom (for larger bathrooms) and a refrigerator, if it is required for medication or food.

• Parents should request a letter from their child's pediatrician to explain the child's diagnosis if needed to assure that accommodations are made available at theme parks, restaurants, and airports.

• Parents may want to carry a bag of incentives such as preferred snacks or toys for challenging moments. These items can be used as reinforcements to prevent "meltdowns" and other difficult moments.

Sibling Issues

Brothers and sisters are usually the people we spend most of our time with growing up. Having a sibling with a disability impacts the whole family. The National Dissemination Center for Children with Disabilities (Kupper, 2003) points out that many brothers and sisters describe the experience of having a sibling with a disability as a positive one. Additionally, they report that typical siblings feel that this has helped them to accept other people's differences. On the other hand, Powell and Gallagher (1993) state that some siblings may experience feelings of fear, anger, loneliness, jealousy, embarrassment, and/or resentment about their sibling with autism. Harris (1994) points out that all families encounter sibling frustrations, and that it is important to distinguish whether the challenges are normal family frustrations or unique to having a sibling with autism.

A family trip with a sibling who has autism may introduce special challenges for typical siblings that need to be addressed. If the child with autism requires extensive supervision, parents may not realize that they are giving less attention to the typical sibling. During vacations, this issue may become more pronounced for typical siblings for various reasons. For example, siblings may rationalize the lack of parental attention at home as therapy or school time; but when on vacation, it may seem more unfair to them if the sibling with autism continues to receive most of the attention, as this is also their vacation. Another concern arises when siblings are asked to be caretakers. It may be helpful to explain to parents that there is a possibility for resentment toward both the parents and the child with autism when siblings are placed in this adult role. Additionally, self-stimulating or repetitive behaviors, outbursts, or refusal to follow directions may be more embarrassing to the siblings when on vacation, because the family is away from their neighborhood, where community members may be more aware of and accepting of the issues related to the child with autism.

Planning Tips

The following are suggested ways for parents to address sibling issues prior to going on vacation. Such preparation may help decrease family tension and promote positive, successful vacation experiences.

• Schedule a family therapy meeting to discuss the vacation, highlighting potential problems as well as anticipating positive experiences. For example, if siblings have worries about hand flapping or yelling while they are waiting in line for luggage at the airport, the solution might be to assign one parent to take a walk with the sibling with autism or to give him or her a fidget toy (e.g., squish ball) to hold while waiting for the other parent to retrieve the luggage. The family can also write out expected behaviors for each member of the family. All members should participate in creating this list, so that there is shared ownership. Encourage parents to take this list on the trip so that if a question or problem occurs while traveling, they can refer back to it.

• Prior to the trip, remind parents that they or another adult, *not* the sibling, should be the one responsible for ensuring the safety of the child with autism.

• Encourage parents to schedule special time alone with the typical siblings while on vacation. For example, one parent can take the typical siblings out to dinner or to a movie while the sibling with autism is with a sitter or the other parent. Another option is to allow the typical sibling to choose the next day's activities from a list of choices.

Airplane Travel

Airplane travel requires unique considerations for children and teens with autism due to the range of social, communication, and behavior characteristics particular to this diagnosis including a tendency to be very concrete, perseverate on odd topics, not understand what is said to them, or have sensory sensitivities (American Psychiatric Association, 1994; Rogers & Ozonoff, 2005). For example, a child with autism was on a very long flight and had to use the bathroom. When he saw the long line to use the restroom, he ran up to the first-class section and proceeded to open the door to the lavatory. The flight attendant informed him that he was not allowed to use the first-class facilities and directed him back to the long line in coach. The child screamed at the flight attendant saying that he had to go to the bathroom. At that point, the parent intervened and attempted to discreetly explain that, since the child had autism, it was hard for him to understand why he could not use an unoccupied restroom. Most people also have a hard time with this concept, but they are able to censor their response to be more socially acceptable. The flight attendant insisted this was the rule, and an uncomfortable confrontation ensued in the middle of the aisle. Meanwhile, the child with autism was embarrassed, physically uncomfortable, and agitated. This unfortunate situation could have been avoided if the parent knew ahead of time that she could have requested a notation be made in the computer regarding accommodations for a person who has a disability. Another option would have been to give the flight attendant a small business-like card with facts regarding autism when she initiated the confrontation with the parent.

Preflight Planning Tips

In order to prepare for the flight, parents should consider whether or not this is the first time flying on an airplane for the child with autism. If he or she has never flown before, this section describes strategies that can be shared with the family to help alleviate potential challenges at the airport.

- Recommend that parents read a developmentally appropriate book about airplanes to their child with autism. Helping the child become familiar with airplanes may decrease anxiety and ambiguity as well as introduce a potential new area of interest.
- Suggest that the family plan a visit to the airport prior to the actual vacation at least 1 week before the trip. It may be helpful for parents to call the airport prior to the visit and obtain a contact name that they can reference if they encounter difficulties when allowing the child to observe security routines.
- Help parents identify their goals for this airport visit and formulate ideas to achieve these goals. For example, if the child perseverates about signs and the parents are concerned the child will repeatedly make comments about this topic, it may be advantageous to educate the child as to what may or may not be said in the presence of security personnel. Let the child observe the security process (e.g., the lines and security guards). Encourage the child to look out from the viewing areas and watch the planes. Make this "field trip" functional, but also fun! If the family chooses to have lunch the day of the "field trip" to the airport, caution them that the child may expect to eat at the airport the day of the actual trip and to be prepared to deal with this issue prior to the day of departure.
- When booking the flight, have parents inquire where the seats are located. This is an important consideration for children who may have sensory challenges and experience discomfort if, for example, they are too close to the bathrooms and are bothered by flushing noises or by the constant motion of people lining up to use the bathroom. Mention to parents that they might want to consider requesting the bulkhead area of the plane if they think their child may require a bit more space. This area will also eliminate the problem associated with children who have a difficult time refraining from kicking the seat in front of them.
- If the child is on a special diet, have parents contact the airline a couple of days in advance. The airlines can tell parents what meals are

available. This information will help the parent know whether or not to bring extra food for the flight.

• Recommend that parents inform the airlines when making flight reservations that they will be traveling with a child who has autism in case special assistance is required during the flight. The reservation clerk can note this information in the computer. When assistance is requested for people with special needs, airlines may allow relatives or friends without tickets to obtain special passes to go through security to assist the parent.

• Prepare the child with autism for the flight by helping parents write a social story about airports and airplane travel. Two helpful references for writing a social story are *The New Social Story Book: Illustrated Edition* (Gray, 2006) and *Writing Social Stories with Carol Gray* (Gray, 2000). Specific topics to consider when writing a social story about air travel include having limited personal space, how to react when babies cry, when it is permissible to use electronic devices, or what to do while sitting on a plane. The following is an example of a general story about going to the airport. Parents can individualize this story for their child with autism. Remind parents to read the social story a few times a day with their child prior to taking the trip.

Going to the Airport

Sometimes people fly on an airplane when they go on a vacation. I will go to a place called an airport to fly on an airplane. Airports can be interesting and fun.

Airplanes are usually parked on a runway outside of the airport, so I probably won't see the plane when I first go into the airport.

When we go to an airport, we sometimes take suitcases or backpacks that hold our things like clothes, shoes, toothbrush, and hairbrush.

When I arrive at the airport, my mom or dad may give our suitcases and backpacks to a person at the airport who makes sure that the suitcases and backpacks also fly to (city traveling to) so I will have my things when we get there. It is okay to give my suitcase to the person who takes suitcases and backpacks at the airport—this is that person's job. The suitcase is usually too big to fit next to me on the plane.

My mom and dad may also give this person a ticket so we can ride on the plane. We may have to wait in line to do this. When I am standing in line, I will try to wait quietly. If I have any questions, I can ask my mom or dad.

Before we get to the plane, we will probably walk through a part of the airport called security. It is a good idea to stay close to my mom and dad so they can show me what to do. When Mom or Dad tells me to go in line, I will try to listen to what they ask me to do.

If I have a small suitcase or backpack, I will be told to put it on a moving machine called a conveyor belt. I also may be asked to take off my shoes and coat and put them on the moving machine. It is okay because I will get my things back soon.

It is a good idea to do what the airport person tells me to do. The airport people behind the conveyor belt have a special kind of screen that they use to see what kind of things I am bringing on the trip. I will walk forward when they ask me to. One person goes through the line at a time and then I can get my backpack or small suitcase back. This is a safe thing to do.

Next, we will probably walk to the part of the airport where the planes are waiting outside. We will wait in a place called a terminal until we are allowed to go on the plane. In the terminal, there are seats where we can wait. It may be fun to look at all the things around us in the terminal while we wait. Sometimes, if there is time, we may get something to eat while we wait. While we are waiting it is a good idea to ask Mom or Dad for something to do.

When it is time to go on the plane, my mom or dad will tell me to stand up and get in line. I will try to listen to their directions and go where they tell me to go. It is a good idea to stay next to Mom and Dad while we stand in line to get on the plane.

Soon we will be sitting on the plane and ready to go on our vacation!

In-Flight Tips

- Many airports allow people with special needs to preboard. Parents should evaluate if this will be a helpful accommodation, as sometimes sitting on a plane while people board can be more bothersome than waiting in a larger terminal area.
- A backpack filled with favorite toys, earphones and music, earplugs or noise-blocking headphones, fidget toys, or electronic devices will help make the flight more enjoyable for everyone. A portable DVD and CD player can alleviate the boredom during a long flight.
- For single parents traveling with a child who has autism, it may be helpful to have a friend or a family member who is not traveling accompany the parent to the airport to provide assistance with the child.

Theme Parks

Children, teens, and adults tend to be delighted by the magic and thrills of the rides, shows, parades, and displays put forth by amusement parks. The popularity of these locations as vacation spots is one reason why parents of children with autism may consider the option of visiting a theme park. When helping families evaluate the appropriateness of visiting amusement parks, provide assistance in defining their goals for the trip. If the goal is to have fun, seek entertainment, experience new things, enjoy family members in a different environment, or build happy memories, then amusement parks are a good option. The key is to prepare and plan for the experience to ensure that it is meaningful for all family members by making accommodations and allowances for flexible plans. For example, if the child is hypersensitive to noise, providing earplugs or a head set to muffle unpleasant noises might allow the child to partake in enjoyable activities without the aversive component. Too often, parents avoid theme parks because of concerns that they may be too overwhelming for their special needs child. This is done at the expense of exposing the child to a novel situation that could potentially elicit positive risk taking. With careful planning, the child's fears can be alleviated. Once the parents decide that a theme park will be their vacation destination, the following considerations can be reviewed together as a family.

Planning Tips

Introduction of external structure (e.g., visual cues and organization) has been found to help increase engagement and on-task behaviors, and to decrease the presence of behavior problems in children with autism (Hume, 2005; MacDuff, Krantz, & McClannahan, 1993). Thus, clinicians may want to help families find ways to structure the theme park vacation by researching the theme park before the visit. Bookstores carry numerous references about popular theme parks. Online resources are also valuable. Disneyland, Disneyworld, SeaWorld, Universal Studios, and Legoland are some examples of parks that offer online information about rides and shows and provide maps of the park. This information might also be shared with the child with autism to prepare him or her emotionally for the trip, thus decreasing ambiguity about the vacation.

- Prior to arriving at the theme park, suggest that parents call and inquire whether any of the rides or other attractions will be closed for the day. Preparation for potential disruptions in expectations may be easier to explain to the child with autism prior to visiting the park. Social stories or a list of alternative rides can be provided to the child.

• Encourage parents to write a social story to prepare their child with autism for things such as crowds, noise, and costumed characters, or special holiday decorations and music.

• Children with autism should wear bright-colored shirts so that it is easier to visually track them in a crowd if they start to wander. Also, parents should make sure that the children are wearing their ID bracelet.

• Parents should bring cell phones or walkie-talkies in case the family needs to separate or a child gets lost.

• If the child is not comfortable when wet, a plastic cover-up can be worn so that he or she can try water rides.

• Some children with autism are hypersensitive to temperature and light. Suggest bringing sunglasses, sunscreen, and hats in warm weather—and extra coats, scarves, and gloves in the winter.

Theme Park Passes

Long lines are common at theme parks. Typical children may not like to or understand how to wait, but it is a reality that they can learn to cope with in order to experience the thrill of riding the roller coaster or whirling on the teacup ride. Instant gratification is not a necessary component for them to enjoy the adventure. Typical children possess the ability to comprehend that just because they can hear the music associated with the ride, it does not mean immediate boarding. In contrast, children and teens with autism may not understand the wait time and may begin to express this confusion in a socially unacceptable manner. To avoid unnecessary outbursts and awkward moments while waiting in long lines, it is advantageous to request a *special assistance pass*. These passes offer alternate, shorter lines for people who have disabilities, as well as early entry to shows to avoid a crowd of people rushing in all at once. At Disneyworld, children with special assistance passes do not have to wait in long lines to greet characters. Also, the pass allows the child with autism and an accompanying adult to view parades from a special roped-off section. Typically, there isn't a lot of room to move around when people begin lining up for a parade; therefore this roped-off area is ideal for a child who may be sensitive to being in close proximity to many people. Parents can prepare for a parade experience by lining up early and by having a backpack with fidget toys and snacks and a social story about waiting to keep the child engaged and to prevent potential problem behaviors.

It is advisable that parents contact the park prior to the visit to investigate the procedure for obtaining special assistance passes. The following section includes a few popular tourist attractions that offer special assistance passes. This is not an endorsement of any particular park, but rather it is provided to facilitate planning a trip for a child with autism. The material presented was provided by park employees and accurate at the time this chapter was written. It would be prudent to check for possible policy changes before visiting these parks.

Parents should be sensitive about how they request a pass. Although they may not think that their child is aware of the information being conveyed to park employees, these discussions may impact the child. Therefore, respectful explanations in a discreet tone of voice are important to avoid embarrassing a child in order to obtain a pass. Another challenge is the comments and stares from others while using a special assistance pass. It is helpful to talk with typical siblings about these possible reactions, so that they can be prepared to shrug them off as ignorance and enjoy their time at the theme park.

Special Assistance Passes

Disneyworld in Florida will provide a special assistance pass based on the child's individual needs. Parents can visit the guest relations office in the park. Disneyworld will give a pass that is valid for the entire stay at any of their five theme parks. Disneyland in California distributes special assistance passes at City Hall, located inside the park. This pass will allow for a shorter wait, but parents should be informed that this pass does not guarantee being able to go directly to the front of the line.

California Adventures in California makes decisions on a case-by-case basis, according to the representative contacted via telephone. The pass may be obtained at Guest Relations.

The FastPass system is available at Disneyworld, Disneyland, and California Adventures. This option is free and is available to all Park visitors. FastPass allows all guests, with and without disabilities, to reserve a specific time frame to return to a ride and enter a line with a shorter wait time than the regular line. Upon entry to the park, parents might want to familiarize themselves with the rides that offer the FastPass system. Each member of the family requires a FastPass ticket. Guests insert their theme park ticket into a FastPass machine located in close proximity to the ride. They receive a ticket with a time range to return for admission to the FastPass line (Knight & Knight, 2006).

Legoland in California offers a ride exit pass at their guest services. Parents are instructed to ask the ride attendant to write down on a special card an exact time to return to board the ride.

SeaWorld provides passes at Guest Services. These passes are for front-line privileges at rides, but not for shows. Additionally, there is a provision for a free companion ticket for a person to assist the guest who has autism.

Universal Studios offers a Guest Assistance Pass that can be purchased at Guest Relations. These are front-line passes. Families traveling with a child with autism can obtain this pass for free. The pass allows the child with autism and up to three people in the party to go through the special area.

Other Planning Tips

• Restaurants at theme parks usually have long lines. Some places take reservations, which should be made upon entry to the park to obtain a reasonable time slot. Try to plan meals when it is not a popular eating time in order to avoid crowds.

• Parents should always bring plenty of snacks for picky eaters and children with dietary restrictions. Tantrums can be exacerbated by hunger or thirst, which some children with autism may be unable to identify or verbally express to parents.

• Some parks offer family bathrooms and it would be helpful to inquire upon entering the park where the family bathrooms are located. These bathrooms are especially helpful for single parents visiting a park with a child of the opposite gender. If traveling with an older child or teen of the opposite gender, one restroom option is to locate a first aid station and use that facility. Another is to bring a companion to assist with these types of issues.

• If the child is having a difficult time and is overwhelmed, have a prearranged quiet spot to visit to calm down. Bring sensory toys to help the child to settle down.

• Bring a camera and assign the child with autism the task of taking pictures. This activity will keep the child busy, and perhaps help him or her feel important. Parents should be encouraged not to worry if the child's picture taking is accurate but rather to make sure that there is another person taking pictures with a different camera.

• Keep the child engaged in the activity of checking off rides as they are completed. Then, have the child circle the next ride on the list as a way to transition without conflict.

• If the child is accustomed to a special system for communication, parents should remember to bring this device or picture system with them to the park.

- Be aware of how sensory issues may affect the child and attempt to modify the environment. For example, if the child doesn't like loud noises but is excited about participating in a ride, bring earplugs. Write a social story or use a rules card that explains why it is not safe to let go of the safety bar to cover one's ears. Review the rules verbally and visually. Explain rules in a way that will help the child understand the expectations for safe behavior.

- Have the child sit on the inside of the ride away from open doors. If the parent notices that the child looks a little nervous but still wants to ride, explain what to do if scared, and that he or she should not stand up or try to get out while the ride is still moving. Remind the child, using visuals aids, to keep hands and legs inside. Some children prefer to observe the ride first to prepare for the unknown. Consider whether or not this will be helpful. For some children, it can prepare them so that they will easily board the ride; however, for others, it may lead to anxiety and perseveration.

Visiting Friends and Relatives

Holidays are a special time to relax, spend time with family and friends, cook elaborate meals, and open gifts. Holidays can be joyous times of the year. However, there are also a lot of unspoken expectations, hassles, and stresses that can accompany the holiday seasons. Families who have a child with autism may experience additional concerns. For example, if children are surrounded by many relatives, new toys, or unfamiliar activities, they may become overstimulated and display behavior that other family members may not understand. Additionally, it may be painful for parents to watch as nieces and nephews delight in opening presents with great anticipation, while their child sits in a separate area fixated on parts of a toy. The following planning tips may assist parents to anticipate and address potential stress caused by well-meaning relatives of children with autism.

Planning Tips

- When the destination is a relative's home, evaluate whether or not sending a letter containing information about autism and the specific strengths and needs of the child with autism might be helpful. This letter can be written by the parents from the parents' or child's perspective. The purpose is to create an atmosphere of acceptance and under-

Vacations and Leisure Time   197

standing, and to decrease the anxiety caused by a lack of understanding that may interfere with the trip.

• Some children with autism do not respond to gifts with the same excitement as typical children. For relatives who are unfamiliar with the child who has autism, this can be confusing and perceived as unappreciative. If the child does not enjoy opening gifts or responds with indifference, this can be highlighted in the aforementioned letter to the relatives. Explain that because the child may not respond in the same manner as the typical child, that does not mean he or she does not like the gift. It might be suggested that a relative wrap up the child's favorite toy to give the child, who might be more excited by unwrapping a gift of a familiar toy or movie than a new, unfamiliar one.

• If the child with autism has an interest in a specific topic, parents can ask relatives to have books or items available to facilitate conversations or interaction with the child.

• If the child is on a restricted diet, bring food or ask for a list of grocery stores that carry items that meet the dietary needs of the child.

• Prepare the child in advance for the trip by showing pictures of relatives and make a book with these pictures to bring on the trip. This will help familiarize the child with the people who may expect to be recognized and will make it easier to identify the person if the child forgets. It also demonstrates to relatives that the parents have put thought into having the child engage with the family.

• If the child is uncomfortable in the relative's home, parents can develop a list of places to visit for a few hours, so the family can take a break. Siblings can be given the choice of not going and may appreciate the special time staying with relatives and friends.

RECREATION AND LEISURE ACTIVITIES

Recreation and leisure activities promote physical health and provide opportunities for individuals with disabilities to build relationships with others (Schleien & Ray, 1988). Involvement in these activities allows children the opportunity to have fun and relax, which can offset the more regimented agenda that may accompany various therapies. Unfortunately, recreational activities are not always available for children with autism. It is not uncommon to discover that television, computers, electronic devices, or other solitary nonphysical activities are the preferred recreational choices for children with autism. Although these activities may be preferred by the child, they should not encompass an entire afternoon or evening, because of the isolated, sedentary nature of these activities.

There are many obstacles that may prevent children with autism from enjoying leisure activities. Parents may fear that their child may not be accepted, will be teased, or may require unusual accommodations. It is imperative that professionals who work with families of these children respect these concerns and explore avenues to overcome barriers that may be preventing the child with autism from being included in recreational activities. Parents can contact local parks and recreation services, Jewish Community Centers, church groups, and local Autism Society chapters to ascertain what resources are available in the community. Professionals can assist parents in making informed choices, contact programs to include the child with autism, and educate parents about the Americans with Disabilities Act and their child's right to participate in community activities. Professionals should offer options that are inclusive or segregated, depending upon the family's wishes. It is important not to judge the type of activity the family selects, since only the family can choose the type of recreation that is best for their child.

Children and teenagers who are included in recreational activities have increased self-esteem, opportunities for friendships, and increased physical fitness, learn leisure skills, and usually have a better quality of life (Hall, 2005). Additionally, Devine and King (2006) report that a benefit of inclusive recreation is that it challenges stereotypes about people with disabilities. Therefore, typical peers become more at ease with differences and more accepting of individuals with disabilities (Hall, 2005).

After-School and Summer Recreation Activities

Parents may not be aware of recreation options available for their child with autism outside of the school day. It is important to first determine the types of activities of interest to the child. Swimming, gymnastics, music, or drama classes are just a few examples that parents can explore for their child with autism. After deciding on an activity, question the parents about whether or not they want to enroll their child in an inclusive setting. If they choose not to include their child with typical peers, they may want to contact Special Olympics, the local Autism Society chapter, the special education advisory committee in their school district, or the parks and recreation department to ask for a list of programs that cater specifically to children who have special needs. There also may be special camps that have a high ratio of staff to children and serve only children who have a diagnosis of autism. Another option that is offered in some states is family camp. Parents can search on the Internet or contact local Autism Society chapters to research family camps that the child with autism and the family members can attend together. Each camp is unique, so parents should contact the director of the family camp to explore whether or not the activities, therapy alternatives, and philosophy will fit with the needs of the family.

If parents are looking for a program that includes both typical children or teens and those diagnosed with autism, they can contact parks and recreational centers, Boys' and Girls' Clubs, the YMCA, Jewish Community Centers, church programs, and local Autism Society chapters. It is important to have parents inform programs that their child has autism prior to enrollment so that personalized adaptations, modifications, and flexibility can be provided. Encourage parents to find out if the program (1) has a mission statement that promotes inclusion, (2) provides training for staff, (3) promotes people-first language, (4) works together with the family to help the child be successful, (5) is open to providing disability awareness for typically developing children, (6) groups children with peers who are the same chronological age, and (7) provides disability-specific accommodations and modifications.

It may be helpful to illustrate how to modify activities, so that parents have an idea of how the child can be included. The following are a few examples of how programs can make accommodations to serve children of differing abilities:

Recreation Accommodations

- *Sports games.* Have the child pick teams, keep score, buddy up with a peer to be the goalie, or stand on first base.
- *Swimming.* Provide visual aids for safety instructions and make sure that directions are simple, to the point, organized, and sequenced.
- *Art projects.* Provide sticks to dip in the glue (if the child has sensory issues) or have the projects cut out ahead of time for the child with motor coordination difficulties.
- *Board games.* Modify games that may have confusing rules. Visual and tactile boundaries can be created if the children are playing a game that requires them to stay in certain areas without crossing a line.
- *Gymnastics.* Physically guide the child with autism through the activity at first. Provide prompting and encouragement and modify the movements if necessary.
- *Drama classes.* Modify so that the nonverbal child with autism can also participate. Have the child with autism help with scenery, makeup, or costumes. Suggest that the staff write a nonspeaking part for the child.

- *Teens in leadership roles.* Explore the option of teaching the teen to become a counselor in training. If the teen needs aide support to be successful, train the aide to facilitate, rather than hover, over the teen. This is an excellent opportunity to prepare for job training and to allow campers to understand that teens with disabilities are valued members of the community and can be placed in leadership roles. Another benefit is that it builds self-esteem in the teen with autism.

SUMMARY

Traveling with a child who has autism introduces a number of concerns that may discourage some parents from taking a much-needed break. Traveling and vacationing together as a family can be a very positive experience, provided that plans are made in advance. Children with autism deserve the opportunity to participate in leisure activities with their families. Implementing preplanning and accommodation strategies can allow families of children with autism to experience the joys and adventures of travel and leisure time.

REFERENCES

American Psychiatric Association. (1994). *Diagnostic and statistical manual of mental disorders* (4th ed.). Washington, DC: Author.

Devine, M. A., & King, B. (2006, May). The inclusion landscape: Park professionals can break down common inclusion barriers with practical considerations. *Parks and Recreation Magazine,* 22–25.

Fain, G. (1986). Leisure: A moral imperative. *Mental Retardation, 24*(5), 261–263.

Gray, C. (2000). *Writing Social Stories™ with Carol Gray* (VHS). Arlington, TX: Future Horizons.

Gray, C. (2006). *The New Social Story™ book: Illustrated Edition.* Arlington, TX: Future Horizons.

Hall, E. (2005, Spring). Living well in 2005! The benefits of leisure for people with disabilities. *Access Today.* Retrieved July 27, 2006, from *www.ncc.online.org/monographs/18livingwell.shtml.*

Harris, S. (1994). *Siblings of children with autism: A guide for families.* Bethesda, MD: Woodbine House.

Hume, K., Loftin, R., & Odom, S. (2005, May). *Effects of an individual work system on the independent academic work skills in children with autism.* Paper presented at the 4th International Meeting for Autism Research (IMFAR), Boston, MA.

Knight, M., & Knight, T. (2006). *Disneyland and Southern California with kids* (8th ed.). Fodor's Travel Publications.

Kupper, L. (Ed.). (2003). *Parenting a child with special needs* (3rd ed.). (News Digest 20). Washington, DC: National Dissemination Center for Children with Disabilities.

MacDuff, G. S., Krantz, P. J., & McClannahan, L. E. (1993). Teaching children with autism to use photographic activity schedules: Maintenance and generalization of complex response chains. *Journal of Applied Behavior Analysis, 26*(1), 89–97.

Powell, T. H., & Gallagher, P. A. (1993). *Brothers and sisters: A special part of exceptional families* (2nd ed.). Baltimore: Brookes.

Quittner, A. L., DiGirolamo, A. M., Michel, M., & Eigen, H. (1992). Parental response to CF: A contextual analysis of the diagnostic phase. *Journal of Pediatric Psychology, 71,* 683–704.

Quittner, A. L., Opipari, L. C., Regoli, M. J., Jacobsen, J., & Eigen, H. (1992). The impact of caregiving and role strain on family life: Comparisons between mothers of children with CF and matched controls. *Rehabilitation Psychology, 37,* 289–304.

Rogers, S. J., & Ozonoff, S. (2005). Annotation: What do we know about sensory dysfunction in autism? A critical review of the empirical evidence. *Journal of Child Psychology and Psychiatry, 46,* 1255–1268.

Schleien, S., & Ray, M. T. (1988). *Community recreation and persons with disabilities: Strategies for integration.* Baltimore: Brookes.

Thompson, R. J., Gil, K. M., Gustafson, K. E., George, L. K., Keith, B. R., Spock, A., et al. (1994). Stability and change in the psychological adjustment of mothers of children and adolescents with cystic fibrosis and sickle cell disease. *Journal of Pediatric Psychology, 17,* 171–188.

COMMUNITY ASPECTS OF INTERVENTION

10

Building a Foundation for Successful School Transitions and Educational Placement

Ramona Noland
Nancy Cason
Alan Lincoln

Educating a student with autism presents perhaps the most unique and difficult set of challenges facing educational professionals and families today. Schools are required to provide students with autism, who demonstrate a tremendous range of needs and abilities, a "free and appropriate education" in a "least restrictive" setting. These services often vary widely among both districts and states. Educational transition times, such as changes in grade-level placements, can involve changes in educational service delivery plans, educational settings, and teachers. All this can be challenging, particularly as students with autism have unique impairments in social communication and cognitive skills that hinder their ability to be easily mainstreamed into typical educational settings. The decisions surrounding the development and implementation of educational programs for this subgroup of the autism population can also be challenging for caregivers and educators. This chapter identifies possible conflicts that may arise between caregivers and educators around school-related transitions and provides suggestions to address these issues. Suggested school program components and examples of model school programs are included to assist professionals in having a positive impact on school placements and school transitions for students with autism. Finally, the importance of including caregivers in educational planning and service delivery and peers as social role models for individuals with autism is discussed.

FACTORS INFLUENCING SCHOOL TRANSITION CHALLENGES

Given the myriad of decisions that must be made over the course of a student's education, there are bound to be times of conflict between educators and caregivers. This section reviews potential difficulties involved in the process of making school-related transitions, including differences in educator expectations, education plan focus, and coordination of care practices.

Educator Expectation Differences

When educating students with autism, educational philosophies tend to differ, sometimes greatly, among educators. These differences often depend upon typical grade or age-level expectations. Grade- or age-dependent school expectations are not easily translated into what is educationally necessary for students with autism, who tend to have isolated and very unique strengths and needs specific to the core features of this diagnosis in the areas of social-communication skills and restrictive, repetitive, stereotyped behaviors and interests (American Psychiatric Association, 2000). Educational services and accompanying educator philosophies can be divided into the following five grade-based service levels:

1. Early childhood (ages birth to 3)
2. Preschool (ages 3–5)
3. Elementary school (ages 5–10; grades K–5)
4. Middle and junior high school (ages 10–13; grades 6–9)
5. High school (ages 13–21; grades 10–12).

Differences in educators' philosophies and expectations regarding these grade levels can make these times of major transition difficult for students with autism and their families (Stormont, Beckner, Mitchell, & Richter, 2005). In clinical settings, caregivers often express fears of "the next level" of education for their child, including concerns about what will be expected of their child or concerns that their family belief systems may not mesh well with the overarching philosophy of new educators. Improved understanding of the factors that influence differing educator philosophies at each grade level of education can help caregivers better understand the reasons behind the differing approaches to educating the student at different grade levels. Such increased understanding might encourage more productive discussions and problem solving between caregivers and educators during transition times. The educational focus changes in terms of four main factors, depending upon the student's age or grade level. These include the (1) family, (2) educational setting, (3) expectations for independent functioning of the student, and (4) student's socialization skills.

Many students with autism are initially identified as needing educational intervention when they are very young. Early Childhood (EC) services are highly focused on meeting the needs of the family and are delivered to students and their families in the "natural environment," which is most often in the home or in a child care setting (Mandlawitz, 2006). At this time, educators may want to have student and family needs identified as early as possible so as to provide services that are as intensive as possible, with developmental skill acquisition being a paramount focus. EC services can occur from a student's birth through just prior to his or her third birthday and are provided through Part C of the Individuals with Disabilities Education Act (IDEA). This federal law is now in its fifth incarnation following reauthorization by the federal legislature in 2004 (Public Law 108-446). (See Chapter 7 for more information about the IDEA.)

The transition at 3 years of age from EC services to preschool services provided through Part B of the IDEA may well be the most challenging transition for caregivers. During this transition, the educational setting shifts from the home to the school environment. As part of this shift, caregivers may experience a loss of control regarding their child's daily life. They must now negotiate with educators around issues such as transportation and their child's reaction to the new educational environment. There are increased demands for social interaction placed on the student with autism, given the many educators and students in the preschool educational environment. Additionally, academic skill acquisition goals expand to include preacademics and appropriate classroom social behavior.

The transition to elementary school can be another challenge for students with autism and their caregivers. This is due in part because educational experiences during the previous educational environments may have been more accepting of the student's differing developmental needs and abilities. However, students with autism entering the elementary school years must adjust to more formal instruction that involves increased expectations of behavioral attending and mastery of specific academic skills by predetermined deadlines (Schulting, Malone, & Dodge, 2005). The social demands first placed on students during the preschool years increase exponentially during elementary school as students begin to develop more sophisticated social skills and friendships. Thus, interventions related to socialization may become both more important for the student with autism as well as more difficult to implement. For example, the communication and social needs of a student with autism who has few if any words may require intervention in a segregated setting with a trained peer and an adult supervisor. Arranging this type of intervention could take a significant investment of time and energy. Given the focus on academic skill acquisition during the elementary years, the student's need to develop social skills beyond those specifically needed for the classroom setting can go unaddressed.

The middle, junior, and high school years are important educational transition times for students as the educational focus begins to incorporate more functional academics (e.g., how to purchase items, how to read a menu, reading and understanding traffic signs and signals), vocational skills, and life skills training. A cooperative relationship between home and school is necessary to ensure that both home and school settings provide consistent learning environments to promote skill generalization in students with autism. Unfortunately, direct caregiver involvement at school or work is often less of a priority as the student enters these grade levels, because independent functioning is generally emphasized for students at this age. Socialization among peers becomes heavily linked to school organizations or events and, even though the need remains, socialization is not always an educational focus. The IDEA mandates providing services to students until their successful graduation or the age of majority. This is intended to improve the educational opportunities and educational results of students with disabilities, eventually preparing them for employment, independent living, and economic self-sufficiency (Wells, Sandefur, & Hogan, 2003). For many students with autism, these additional years of educational training between ages 18 and 21 can assist with exploration of possible employment roles and provide time needed to learn job skills and routines and to further practice and develop social skills within various community settings.

Differences in Education Plan Focus

Another factor influencing potential transition difficulties are the types of service plans used to guide educational service provision. These education plans differ as the student transitions between the five service levels and include (1) the individualized family service plan (IFSP), (2) the individualized education plan (IEP), and (3) the individualized transition plan (ITP). A thorough understanding of the federal law governing services to students with disabilities and an individual state's interpretation of that law is important to successfully navigate school-based services. How this law is written and subdivided directly impacts the types of service plans developed by educational teams at various times in a student's life.

The IFSP is the service plan for students from birth through their third birthday, and the "F" stands for "family," conveying the focus of this education plan. This is a dynamic planning tool that is reviewed every 6 months or more frequently as needed (Colorado Department of Education, n.d.). Services provided for the student are developed by considering the unique aspects of the family system, including cultural background, structure, and available resources. Necessary services identified are typically delivered in the student's home. Each state designates a lead agency that is to be responsible for implementation of Part C. The designated agency does not have to be the state department of education (Mandlawitz, 2006). Further, unlike Part B services, services under Part C are not necessarily free, and community agencies are allowed to charge for educational intervention services on a sliding fee scale (Learning Disabilities Association of America, n.d.). (See Chapter 8 for more information regarding service availability and resources.)

Assurance that there is no gap in the delivery of services as the student turns 3 years of age is the key to a smooth transition from an IFSP to an IEP (Colorado Department of Education, n.d.). The IEP is the primary education plan used for students ages 3 through 21. For all students with disabilities, regardless of their age and grade level, the educational team must strike a balance between the student's need for participation in the general education classroom and the need for more specialized and individualized intervention. Instruction during the elementary and early middle school years typically focuses on academic skill acquisition. Ideally, the inclusive classroom and segregated, or "pull-out," services should be organized in a way that provides optimum development of the student's skills in all areas identified by the IEP. As the student enters the teen years (grades 7–12), inclusion in general education must be balanced with the student's need for special education services to address functional life skills and vocational training. The 1990 reauthorization of the IDEA mandated "transition services" for students in special education who were 16 years of age and older, implying that transition should address all domains of a person's life (Lehman,

Clark, Bullis, Rinkin, & Castellanos, 2002). Thus, beginning in the middle school years, the IEP team should initiate a plan for the student to move from the secondary school setting into a postsecondary employment setting, and the educational focus should begin to incorporate more functional, vocational, and life skills training. Successful transition planning at this stage requires the collaboration of the student's family, school personnel, and relevant community agencies (Lehman et al., 2002). Because independent functioning is generally emphasized for students at this age, a cooperative relationship between home and school may be necessary to ensure that both settings provide consistent learning environments to promote skill generalization in students with autism. The need for communication among key stakeholders during the transition process cannot be overstated (Stormont et al., 2005).

When the individual with autism transitions out of educational services and into adult living, the ITP is used to coordinate ongoing treatment and services as a type of life plan. The ITP outlines what individuals will do during their adult years in terms of continuing education, finding and maintaining employment, and pursuing leisure activities and independent living, whenever possible. Wehmeyer and Palmer (2003) found that high school graduates with mental retardation were more likely to earn more money and live more independently if they were involved in their transition planning and goal setting. According to Arick and colleagues (2005), students with autism are better able to participate in the transition process if visual, organizational, and social supports are provided. Unfortunately, ITPs are too often limited to the services students are already receiving, with most plans being influenced by what is available in the community, rather than providing services students actually need to succeed in the community (Wehman, 1992). The most successful educational transition programs are those that integrate students into the workplace with thoughtful and systematic planning beginning in the middle school years (Lehman et al., 2002). Such programs also provide the students with on-the-job training, place the students in paid employment by the time they reach graduation, and provide social training for students with nondisabled peers (White & Weiner, 2004).

Coordination of Care Differences

There remain significant barriers to adopting the practices that may best support the successful educational transition of youth, including the lack of coordinated efforts across systems (Lehman et al., 2002). Coordination may be achieved through increased communication between local community agencies along with inclusion of the family and the student with autism whenever possible (Lehman et al., 2002; Stormont et al., 2005; Wehman, 1992).

School districts, challenged to address the academic, social, behavioral, and other disparate needs of students with autism through educational programming, frequently work with outside professionals or agencies that can provide expertise in the development of specialized interventions and ongoing consultation to support program effectiveness. Although school districts or families may suggest the use of a community consultant to assist teachers with educational program development, the addition of this third party into the school and family collaboration can be contentious if communication among all parties involved is poor. (Refer to Chapter 12 for more information on school consultation models.)

Johnson and colleagues (2002) emphasize the need for communication about the student as well as tracking and sharing student outcome data in order to improve programs for students with more severe disabilities. They note that it is important for programs supporting transition services to examine student training requirements that are necessary for adult living as well as to engage in systemic planning with the agency that will eventually assume responsibility for the individual after completion of secondary schooling.

SUPPORTING SUCCESSFUL EDUCATIONAL TRANSITIONS

Working as a Team

While many of the factors affecting school-based service provision are outside of the control of any one individual, one person *can* make a difference and cause positive change within the educational team setting. It is also possible for one educational team to have a positive impact across a school community. Some of the keys to facilitating successful navigation through school-based service transitions by the student with autism are for educational team members to be aware of the importance of:

- Knowing the federal law and the state's interpretation of that law.
- Knowing parent rights and how to support those rights.
- Knowing the school district's legal responsibilities.
- Making decisions supported by good assessment data.
- Utilizing educational interventions that are supported by research.
- Making decisions as a team and maintaining good communication skills.

- Maintaining a positive attitude.
- Being creative with intervention development based on available research.
- Getting everyone committed to continuing education of the student.

A thorough understanding of the federal law governing special education services is the best foundation for navigating school-based services and cannot be overemphasized. IDEA 2004 provides the foundation for the role and function of the educational team and its individual members. Those team members not directly educated about special education procedures (e.g., caregivers and general education teachers) may have the most difficult time fully grasping the process and the importance of their role. All members need to understand the rights given to parents through IDEA 2004 as their input is highly valued and protected within the context of the law. Likewise, it is equally important for all team members to understand the responsibilities of the school district as mandated by IDEA 2004. Finally, it is important for team members to realize that the federal law is interpreted differently by each state; thus, professional roles and services provided to students can vary significantly by state.

Because IDEA 2004 encourages teamwork, communication among team members is crucial. During team interactions, active listening and attending are key communication components that will facilitate even the most difficult or contentious meeting process. Ivey and Ivey (2003) have identified four major components of attending behavior, including maintaining appropriate eye contact, listening to voice quality, staying with the topic of conversation, and being aware of one's body language and the body language of others. Through team members' efforts to "hear" one another, all viewpoints are granted validation and areas of compromise can be more easily identified.

Several problems can cause the IEP process to become bogged down, lengthy, and unproductive. In an effort to proactively address potential team communication difficulties, it is very important for a senior administrator to be designated as the IEP meeting facilitator and identified at the beginning of the meeting. He or she should enter with a written agenda outlining the process (not the content) and clarify who is presenting or when it is appropriate to enter into more open dialogue. Additionally, this person should take the responsibility for creating a safe environment while fostering collaboration between the team members. The facilitator should be protective of all participants and actively limit or help to reframe emotional or overtly aggressive forms of communication or behavior in the meeting. The individual facilitating the IEP team meeting should play an active role in making sure procedural guidelines are appropriately followed and discontinue the meeting if necessary to maintain a safe and productive environment. Evaluations and observations that help define a student's needs should precede discussion of specific goals. Goals and benchmarks should precede methodological approaches for achieving those goals and benchmarks. Finally, there should be decisions involving the details of specific classrooms, teachers, schools, placements, and purchased services and equipment (such as transportation). It is important to allow the IEP meeting process to unfold in a manner that will lead to logical outcomes based on the needs, goals, and methodologies identified. If there appears to be a pre-existing agenda for placement, specialized services, or equipment for example, then such an agenda should be identified by the meeting facilitator in a noncritical, nonconfrontational manner that explains the IEP process more thoroughly and indicates where on the procedural agenda such a discussion would take place.

When all educational team members fully understand their role and the role of others in supporting student development, most conflicts can be adequately avoided. Philosophical differences can be bridged, differences in educational plans can be accommodated, and the coordination of care for students becomes easier. It is imperative that school districts support educational team development both fiscally and philosophically. Most importantly, educational teams are part of a larger educational community and when that community emphasizes quality and best educational practices, educational transitions can become negotiable challenges rather than roadblocking problems.

Identifying Successful School Program Components

Although the field of education is placing increasing importance on employing intervention components that have solid research support for their use, such components are not always used. To add to this inconsistency, there is no single intervention or set of interventions that works for every student (Lehman & Klaw, 2003), yet teams composed of individuals who are well versed in research findings may be able to pull examples from the research to modify programs to suit the student's individual and immediate needs.

The heterogeneity of autism diagnostic symptoms requires that interventions be individualized (Freeman, 1997; Schreibman, 2000); however, the guidelines for meeting individual needs across settings and

development are not clear. Extensive research exists regarding the efficacy of various interventions for young students with autism (e.g.,
Odom et al., 2003; Rogers, 2000); however, there is significantly less
research about best educational practices for students with autism in elementary, middle, and high school settings. During a review of recent
research (see section on using peer interventions to increase social skill
development), we discovered that much of the current research for the
later age groups focuses on interventions delivered in inclusive programs, as opposed to segregated classrooms, and the development of
social skills within a school setting is studied primarily for students with
high-functioning autism and Asperger disorder. Very little research exists
regarding academic instruction for individuals with autism, especially
for students with more limited abilities.

Evidence-Based Components

Schools and families may apply interventions regardless of empirical
support for their use. However, educational programs that use applied
behavior analysis (ABA) have the most empirical support for use with
students with autism (Harchik, 2006). Recent research (Eikeseth, Smith,
Jahr, & Eldevik, 2002) that compared eclectic intervention programs to
ABA-based programs yielded clear indications that the students in the
ABA-based programs made more progress. Some propose that educators
of students with autism receive certification in and emphasize the use of
ABA-based techniques as the basis for instruction of students with autism
(Arick et al., 2005; Jacobson, 2000). Regardless of the theoretical under-
pinning of intervention services, as schools design educational programs
for students with autism, they must keep student improvement across
all IEP goals in mind as the primary aim. The New Jersey Department
of Education (2004) describes five components of an effective educational
program for students with autism and these include the following:

1. Provide an educational program that parallels the academic year
   of nondisabled students.
2. Provide a very low student–teacher ratio for all instruction.
3. Provide instruction across all settings, including home, school,
   and community.
4. Provide developmentally appropriate IEP objectives and educational strategies.
5. Provide program and student progress monitoring through adequate and appropriate data collection.

Model Educational Programs

Students with autism are typically served within their school districts; however, sometimes they are enrolled in programs run by outside entities. This seems to be particularly true for those students who are most severely impacted by autism and demonstrate the most severe behavioral symptoms. Several schools created specifically for students with autism exist within the United States. Table 10.1 provides an overview of such schools from across the country, including the Eden Family of Services (Eden Institute, n.d.) in New Jersey; the May Institute (May Institute, 2005) in Massachusetts; the Douglass School at Rutgers (Douglass Developmental Disabilities Center, 2005) in New Jersey; the Princeton Student Development Institute (Princeton Student Development Institute, 2003) in New Jersey; and the Monarch School (Emory Autism Center, n.d.) located in Georgia. These programs typically use empirically validated interventions to teach students at all developmental levels. School attendance is often funded by the students' school districts, with program personnel often working in conjunction with school districts to provide consultation or support. These programs provide a model for education of students with autism, particularly those with more significant needs.

General Classroom Modifications

Public schools have a primary goal of meeting the needs of special education students within the "least restrictive" setting. The definition of "least restrictive" varies from student to student; however, for many students the least restrictive setting is achieved through at least partial inclusion in a general education classroom. Inclusion within the general education setting from an early age may be beneficial to students as they transition through educational programs. McDonnell, Thorson, and McQuivey (1998) reviewed the literature regarding inclusion programs in elementary schools and discovered support regarding the benefits for students with severe disabilities as well as for their nondisabled peers.

Students with autism often have difficulty learning in the typical classroom structure even if they have normal intelligence. "Many of these students are lost in the shuffle of special education, or lost in a regular education setting that focuses heavily on learning methods that are difficult for them" (Daily, 2005, p. 2). Individuals with autism often have difficulty processing large amounts of verbal information, differentiating important from unimportant information, and using effective

TABLE 10.1. Overview: Specialty Programs for Students with Autism

Program	Interventions used
Eden Institute	Discrete-trial training; Picture Exchange Communication System (PECS); low teacher-to-student ratio; parent training and support groups
May Institute	Interventions based in ABA theory; PECS; Social Stories; parent training and home visits
Douglass School	ABA interventions; social skills training; transition services; parent involvement
Princeton Institute	ABA intervention strategies; social and language skill development; transition program coordinated with community agencies; parent involvement
Monarch School	Supports inclusive placements in private and public schools; research-based interventions

executive-functioning strategies for organization and planning, skills typically crucial for school success. Arick et al. (2005) remark on the importance of being aware of anxiety issues in students with autism. Students with autism require a high level of structure in the classroom in order to decrease anxiety and increase academic gains (Olley, 2005). Thus, the inclusive curriculum should have a clear structure in order to address the specific needs that students with autism have for predictability, visual support, organization, and supported transitions. Finally, inclusion programs are not going to be successful unless school staff receive specific training in strategies that provide effective levels of support and instruction to the individual (Kabot, Masi, & Segal, 2003; Strain, Wolery, & Izeman, 1999).

Arick et al. (2005) provide a review of the current research on best instructional practices for students with autism and appropriate curriculum content that lead to best outcomes. Daily (2005) also discusses supports that are necessary for successful inclusion in the classroom. These supports are relevant for students with varying levels of ability and need, although some strategies are more applicable for some students than others. Table 10.2 highlights potentially useful curricular modifications suggested by Arick et al. (2005) and Daily (2005) for the inclusive classroom of a less able school-age student with autism.

Many of the same strategies that are useful for younger students with autism will continue to be helpful as the child grows up, although they may need to be modified for a more age-appropriate presentation. Modifications can include the use of a picture schedule, written schedule, or day planner with assignments, breaks, and rewards clearly indicated. Materials can be organized into different-colored folders that are indicated with the matching color next to the assignment on the schedule. Students should be allowed to put completed work in a "finished" bin or folder. Assignments should be modified to allow the student to practice and prove mastery of work without unnecessary repetition. For students with language and motor difficulties, adaptations can be made to allow them to complete work using file folder activities where they match questions to answers or through the use of educational software. Students should be allowed extra time to process information and complete work. Often, students respond positively to seeing a model of the completed work so they are aware of the teachers' expectations. Another modification involves allowing students to choose a certain number of problems on a worksheet that they will complete. Creativity in curricular modifications and presentations allows students to use their strengths and achieve notable gains.

Roles of Service Providers

Because of the changing and comprehensive needs of the student with autism, there are often many professionals involved in the student's edu-

---

TABLE 10.2. Recommended Curricular Modifications

1. Structure the classroom, home, and work environments with visual schedules and cues.
2. Use strategies that encourage language, communication, and socialization throughout the day.
3. Teach the student how to participate in group discussions.
4. Use scheduling, priming, and other strategies to help reduce disruptive and maladaptive behaviors.
5. Use priming to expose the student to a lesson or activity before it will be taught in the general education classroom.
6. Maintain adequate support from trained paraprofessionals to achieve a low student-to-teacher ratio.
7. Ensure all staff have sufficient training and that regular educators have the ability to provide the type of structured learning environment needed by students.

Note. Adapted from Arick, Krug, Fullerton, Loos, and Falco (2005) and Daily (2005).

cation. Collaboration among service providers is necessary to positively impact educational programming and school transition for the student with autism. In order to develop a more successful educational team, efforts must be made to communicate and to integrate varying skills and philosophies with the overriding goal of meeting the student's needs (Wood, 1998).

Jennett, Harris, and Mesibov (2003) describe "teacher efficacy" as the feeling a teacher has about adequately meeting the needs of the student through knowledge of specialized educational techniques. Underlying the process of inclusion of all students is the assumption that general classroom teachers have a certain amount of knowledge about special education students, teaching techniques, and curriculum strategies (Dow & Mehring, 2001). In order to be effective, educators of students with autism should have comprehensive training to understand autistic-specific impairments. Additional training should include empirically supported instruction and modification strategies, communication and socialization behavior management approaches, IEP development, and data collection (Lord & McGee, 2001; New Jersey Department of Education, 2004). Teachers are ultimately responsible for addressing IEP goals and can most effectively do so if they have a thorough understanding of autism-specific instructional strategies.

Paraprofessionals often play a major role in teaching students with autism both in special education and inclusive settings. Giangreco and Broer (2005) surveyed 737 school employees, including teachers, paraprofessionals, school administrators, and parents of students in special education classrooms, about school practices including the roles of paraprofessionals in the classroom. Their findings indicate that students with disabilities had significant amounts of instructional contact time with paraprofessionals and that these paraprofessionals received very little supervision and training (equivalent to less than 2% of the special education teacher's time) (Giangreco & Broer, 2005). Given these findings, paraprofessionals should receive ongoing training, support, and supervision regarding their performance with the student. This will help ensure that they are able to competently implement specialized instructional strategies and behavior intervention plans, and maintain accurate records to track progress. Because paraprofessionals do not have the educational preparation to work independently with students, they cannot be licensed as an educator by the state department of education. This lack of a license mandates their need to receive monitoring as well as direction of their daily work with students. Many times it is the paraprofessionals who have the most in-depth knowledge of the student, as they spend the most time with the student. For this reason, para-professionals should play a key role on the educational team regarding the student's needs, progress monitoring, and decision making at key educational transition times.

School psychologists are expected to play a significant role in the education of students with autism (Williams, Johnson, & Sukhodolsky, 2005). They are often called on to provide assessments, develop behavior intervention plans, consult with inclusive educational programs, and provide education to school staff about the diagnosis of autism. School psychologists are also often required to interface with the myriad of other professionals involved in the students' educational program. These professionals include those from the school district as well as outside agencies. Additionally, the school psychologist maintains contact and communication with students' families. Because of this, they are key personnel during educational transition times.

Including Caregivers in the Education Process

Families provide the primary source of knowledge about the student and play a pivotal role in the educational process. Caregivers often collaborate with numerous professionals who work with their child across settings, and many caregivers participate in their child's interventions, ultimately developing an expertise in implementing these interventions. It is this involvement that enables the caregiver to inform the educational team about both the student's history and long-term goals during educational transitions. Johnson et al. (2002) discuss the critical role caregivers play in supporting their child's success and encourage schools to "actively engage them in discussions and decisions" and to make sure to meet the multicultural and other needs of caregivers (Johnson et al., 2002, p. 526). Coffey and Obringer (2004) suggest that one way teachers can consider caregivers' perspectives is through home visits and frequent conferences to discuss academic and social issues.

Because of the pervasive needs of students with autism and the intensity of supports required for repetition of learning and skill generalizations across settings, caregivers and teachers must work together to identify goals during IEP meetings and collaborate as the student progresses (Kasari, Freeman, Bauminger, & Alkin, 1999). This collaboration is important in order for the student to make the best possible progress in school, and "parents and school districts together must make a serious and genuine effort to understand the student's real needs and to address them in an appropriate manner" (Mandlawitz, 2002, p. 503).

Using Peer Intervention to Increase Social Skill Development

Educational programming and transitions can be enhanced through emphasis on socialization and the use of peer interventions. Social skills learned by students with autism can assist them as they transition through their educational years. These skills will remain important throughout adulthood. Typically developing peers have been used as part of a broader educational intervention program for a number of years, and research emphasizing empirical support of various types of peer interventions is on the rise. A literature search revealed five journal articles published between 2000 and 2003 that provide reviews of peer-based socialization interventions dating as far back as the early 1980s. Rogers (2000) reviewed interventions that sought to increase peer inter-actions, dividing them into preschool, school-age, and adolescent age groups. Early interventions at the preschool level were reported to have the largest body of published work. Strain and Schwartz (2001) reviewed instructional strategies derived from applied behavior analysis (ABA) and emphasized the need to evaluate social validity (the overall life importance of the skills being learned) and sustainability (the likeli-hood the student will be able to continue demonstrating the skills once learned) of behavior change. Peer-initiated strategies, self-monitoring, and group-oriented contingencies were all underscored as instructional strategies that have demonstrated effectiveness in producing positive social behavior changes in the student with autism. Taylor (2001) found that although studies designed to teach peer social skills to students with autism differed along a number of dimensions (e.g., target of the inter-vention, intervention used), several general conclusions could be drawn from the literature and these include:

1. Some form of teaching or training is necessary, directed either to the peer, the student with autism, or to both.
2. Typical students benefit from learning specific skills for interact-ing with students with autism.
3. Specific reinforcement procedures are required to encourage interaction.
4. Additional strategies may be needed to generalize or maintain interactions.

5. Specific procedures are required to reduce and eliminate adult prompts.
6. Interactions between typical peers and students with autism are more likely to occur when both are taught the necessary skills.
7. It is difficult to ascertain which students with autism will benefit from what types of instructional techniques (e.g., peer-mediated vs. adult-mediated).

A review of peer-mediated interventions conducted by DiSalvo and Oswald (2002) set goals for future research. These goals included improved generalizability (the ability of the student to demonstrate newly learned skills in multiple environments) and social validity of intervention outcomes as well as the inclusion of more comparative studies to facilitate the determination of which interventions are most effective for which outcomes. The most recent review (Odom et al., 2003) examined contributions from single-subject design research for evidence-based practices for preschoolers with autism. Based on their review, intervention practices were categorized into three groups: (1) those with well-established evidence of effectiveness (i.e., adult-directed teaching and differential reinforcement), (2) emerging and effective practices (i.e., peer-mediated interventions, visual supports, self-monitoring, and family member involvement in the intervention), and (3) those practices that were probably efficacious (i.e., positive behavioral support, videotaped models, and incorporating students' choices or preferences into learning tasks). The authors encouraged future researchers to continue to strengthen the available database by including measurements of treatment fidelity (completing the intervention as it was designed), maintenance (supporting the student's continued adequate performance of skills once they are learned), generalization, and social validity.

A review of recent studies that specifically targeted students who were beyond the early intervention years revealed only six studies that investigated intervention efficacy for older students with autism within a segregated classroom setting since the year 2000. Table 10.3 provides a summary of these studies, including the types of intervention used and research design methods. The trend of more research being conducted at the preschool and elementary school levels continues to be supported, as there were numerous studies examining preschool-level interventions not included within this restricted review. Further, only one study specifically targeted students who exhibited severe impairments resulting from an autism diagnosis as opposed to high-functioning autism, Asperger disor-

TABLE 10.3. Characteristics of Interventions for Older Students Included in Reviewed Articles

Study	No. of participants	Education level	Setting	Intervention type	Design type	Design features
Barry & Burlew (2004)	2	Elementary	Segregated	Social stories	Multiple baseline	—
Bauminger (2002)	15	Middle/high	Integrated and segregated	Social–emotional	Pre–post measures	—
Delano & Snell (2006)	3	Elementary	Segregated	Social stories	Multiple baseline	G, SV, M, TF
Kamps et al. (2002)	5	Elementary	Segregated	Social skills/coop learning	Control group	G
Loncola & Craig-Unkefer (2005)	6	Elementary	Segregated	Adult-directed	Multiple baseline	TF
Morrison et al. (2001)	4	Middle	Segregated	Peer/self-monitoring	Multiple baseline	G

Note. G, generalization; M, maintenance; SV, social validation; TF, treatment fidelity; and PE, peer expectancies.

der, or an undifferentiated pervasive developmental disorder without co-occurring mental retardation. Barry and Burlew (2004) are to be commended for their application of the use of social stories to influence choice-making and appropriate play skills. All researchers in this review reported using some experimental design that could allow demonstration of a functional relationship between the intervention and the resulting behavioral change. The most common design feature reported was generalization of behavior (50%). Of the six studies reviewed, four (66%) address at least one treatment design feature highlighted as important for further consideration.

Students with autism moving into secondary education continue to need social, educational, and vocational intervention support. Educational best practices follow from research, and there is currently a *severe* lack of empirical support for academic as well as social interventions, with or without the use of peers, at the secondary level. It is possible for educators to glean information from studies conducted with younger students and adapt these intervention programs to be more age and grade appropriate. When selecting model research projects on which to base interventions, educators should try to find a study that focused on the same skill set and used a research design. Before beginning, it is important to evaluate the students' ongoing need for the selected social skill(s) as they transition to vocational training and adult living settings. Data collection is necessary to help determine if the interventions are making a difference and how skill improvements can be maintained over time and transferred to other settings.

CONCLUSIONS

Transitioning a student with severe autism through a lifetime of educational services can be a daunting and exhausting process for caregivers. Educators and other service providers can assist in building a foundation for successful educational transitions and educational placements. By identifying possible causes of confusion and potential areas of disagreement, educational teams can proactively work together to meet the challenge of educating students with highly specialized needs. Students with autism will also benefit from educational programs that are developed based on the most recent evidence-based practices and include a focus on developing skills that have functional utility in a variety of settings throughout their lives. Further, the adequate development of educational programs can also smooth educational transition difficulties. Unfortunately, there is a dearth of research on academic, behavioral, and especially social interventions for less able students with autism beyond the elementary school years. As additional research addressing these areas of need is made available, it is hoped that the impact on educational programming in meeting the needs of these students will be enhanced.

REFERENCES

American Psychiatric Association. (2000). *Diagnostic and statistical manual of mental disorders* (4th ed., text rev.). Washington, DC: Author.

Arick, J. A., Krug, D. A., Fullerton, A., Loos, L., & Falco, R. (2005). School-based programs. In F. R. Volkmar, R. Paul, A. Klin, & D. Cohen (Eds.), *Handbook of autism and pervasive developmental disorders* (Vol. 2, pp. 1003–1028). Trenton, NJ: Wiley.

Barry, L. M., & Burlew, S. B. (2004). Using social stories to teach choice and play skills to students with autism. *Focus on Autism and Other Developmental Disabilities, 19*(1), 45–51.

Bauminger, N. (2002). The facilitation of social-emotional understanding and social interaction in high-functioning students with autism: Intervention outcomes. *Journal of Autism and Developmental Disorders, 32*(4), 283–298.

Coffey, K. M., & Obringer, S. J. (2004). A case study on autism: School accommodations and inclusive settings. *Education, 124*(4), 632–639.

Colorado Department of Education. (n.d.). *Early childhood connections for infants, toddlers, and families.* Retrieved March 25, 2006, from *www.ryfc.org/ifsp.htm.*

Daily, M. (2005). Inclusion of students with autism spectrum disorders. *New Horizons for Learning.* Retrieved February 15, 2006, from *www.newhorizons.org/spneeds/autism/daily.htm.*

Delano, M., & Snell, M. E. (2006). The effects of social stories on the social engagement of students with autism. *Journal of Positive Behavior Interventions, 8*(1), 29–42.

DiSalvo, C. A., & Oswald, D. P. (2002). Peer-mediated interventions to increase the social interaction of students with autism: Consideration of peer expectancies. *Focus on Autism and Other Developmental Disabilities, 17*(4), 198–207.

Douglass Developmental Disabilities Center. (2005). *Douglass School.* Retrieved March 18, 2006, from *gsappweb.rutgers.edu/DDDC/.*

Dow, M. J., & Mehring, T. A. (2001). Inservice training for educators of individuals with autism. In T. Wahlberg, F. Obiakor, S. Burkhardt, & A. F. Rotatori (Eds.), *Autistic spectrum disorders: Educational and clinical interventions* (pp. 89–107). Oxford, UK: Elsevier Science.

Eden Institute. (n.d.). *The Eden family of services* [Brochure]. Princeton, NJ: Author.

Eikeseth, S., Smith, T., Jahr, E., & Eldevik, S. (2002). Intensive behavioral treatment at school for 4- to 7-year-old students with autism: A 1-year comparison controlled study. *Behavior Modification, 26,* 49–68.

Emory Autism Center. (n.d.). *Monarch School Age Program*. Retrieved March 18, 2006, from *www.psychiatry.emory.edu/PROGRAMS/autism/Monarch. html*.

Freeman, B. J. (1997). Guidelines for evaluating intervention programs for students with autism. *Journal of Autism and Developmental Disorders, 27,* 641–651.

Giangreco, M. F., & Broer, S. M. (2005). Questionable utilization of paraprofessionals in inclusive schools: Are we addressing symptoms or causes? *Focus on Autism and Other Developmental Disabilities, 20,* 10–26.

Harchik, A. (2006, February 8). Eclectic treatments for students with autism have drawbacks. Retrieved March 18, 2006, from *www.masslive.com/metroeastplus/ republican/index.ssf?/base/news-1/1139302850183400.xml&coll=1*.

Ivey, A. E., & Ivey, M. B. (2003). *Intentional interviewing and counseling: Facilitating client development in a multicultural society*. Pacific Grove, CA: Brooks/Cole.

Jacobson, J. W. (2000). Early intensive behavioral intervention: Emergence of a consumer-driven service model. *Behavior Analyst, 23*(2), 149–171.

Jennett, H. K., Harris, S. L., & Mesibov, G. B. (2003). Commitment to philosophy, teacher efficacy, and burnout among teachers of students with autism. *Journal of Autism and Developmental Disorders, 33,* 583–593.

Johnson, D. R., Stodden, R. A., Luecking, R., & Mack, M. (2002). Current challenges facing secondary education and transition services: What research tells us. *Exceptional Students, 68,* 519–531.

Kabot, S., Masi, W., & Segal, M. (2003). Advances in the diagnosis and treatment of autism spectrum disorders. *Professional Psychology: Research and Practice, 34,* 26–33.

Kamps, D., Royer, J., Dugan, E., Kravits, T., Gonzalez-Lopez, A., Garcia, J., et al. (2002). Peer training to facilitate social interaction for elementary school students with autism and their peers. *Exceptional Students, 68*(2), 173–187.

Kasari, C., Freeman, S. F., Bauminger, N., & Alkin, M. C. (1999). Parental perspectives on inclusion: Effects of autism and Down syndrome. *Journal of Autism and Developmental Disorders, 29,* 297–305.

Learning Disabilities Association of America. (n.d.). *Guidelines for the individualized family service plan (IFSP) under Part C of IDEA*. Retrieved March 25, 2006, from *www.ldamerica.org/aboutld/professionals/guidelines.asp*.

Lehman, C. M., Clark, H. B., Bullis, M., Rinkin, J., & Castellanos, L. A. (2002). Transition from school to adult life: Empowering youth through community ownership and accountability. *Journal of Student and Family Studies, 11*(1), 127–141.

Lehman, J. F., & Klaw, R. (2003). *From goals to data and back again: Adding backbone to developmental intervention for students with autism*. New York: Jessica Kingsley.

Loncola, J. A., & Craig-Unkefer, L. (2005). Teaching social communication skills to young urban students with autism. *Education and Training in Developmental Disabilities, 40*(3), 243–263.

Lord, C., & McGee, J. P. (Eds.). (2001). *Educating children with autism*. Washington, DC: National Academy Press.

Mandlawitz, M. R. (2002). The impact of the legal system on educational programming for young students with autism spectrum disorder. *Journal of
Autism and Developmental Disorders, 32,* 495–508.

Mandlawitz, M. (2006). *What every teacher should know about IDEA 2004.*
Boston: Pearson Education.

May Institute. (2005). *May Institute.* Retrieved March 7, 2006, from *www.
mayinstitute.org.*

McDonnell, J., Thorson, N., & McQuivey, C. (1998). The instructional characteristics of inclusive classes for elementary students with severe disabilities:
An exploratory study. *Journal of Behavioral Education, 8,* 415–437.

Morrison, L., Kamps, D., Garcia, J., & Parker, D. (2001). Peer mediation and
monitoring strategies to improve initiation and social skills for students
with autism. *Journal of Positive Behavior Interventions, 3*(4), 237–250.

New Jersey Department of Education. (2004). *Autism quality indicators.* Retrieved
March 6, 2006, from *www.state.nj.us/njded/specialed/info/autism.pdf.*

Odom, S. L., Brown, W. H., Frey, T., Karasu, N., Smith-Canter, L. L., & Strain,
P. S. (2003). Evidence-based practices for young students with autism: Con-
tributions for single-subject design research. *Focus on Autism and Other
Developmental Disabilities, 18*(3), 166–175.

Olley, J. G. (2005). Curriculum and classroom structure. In F. R. Volkmar, R.
Paul, A. Klin, & D. Cohen (Eds.), *Handbook of autism and pervasive
developmental disorders* (Vol. 2, pp. 1003–1028). Trenton, NJ: Wiley.

Princeton Student Development Institute. (2003). *Programs.* Retrieved March
18, 2006, from *www.pcdi.org/programs/school.asp.*

Rogers, S. (2000). Interventions that facilitate socialization in students with
autism. *Journal of Autism and Developmental Disorders, 30*(5), 399–409.

Schreibman, L. (2000). Intensive behavioral/psychoeducational treatments for
autism: Research needs and future directions. *Journal of Autism and Developmental Disorders, 30,* 373–378.

Schulting, A. B., Malone, P. S., & Dodge, K. A. (2005). The effect of school-
based kindergarten transition policies and practices on student academic
outcomes. *Developmental Psychology, 41*(6), 860–871.

Stormont, M., Beckner, R., Mitchell, B., & Richter, M. (2005). Supporting successful transition to kindergarten: General challenges and specific implications for students with problem behavior. *Psychology in the Schools, 42*(8),
765–778.

Strain, P. S., & Schwartz, I. (2001). ABA and the development of meaningful
social relations for young students with autism. *Focus on Autism and
Other Developmental Disabilities, 16*(2), 120–128.

Strain, P., Wolery, M., & Izeman, S. (1998). Consideration for administrators in
the design of service options for young students with autism and their families. *Young Exceptional Students, 1,* 8–16.

Taylor, B. A. (2001). Teaching peer social skills to students with autism. In C.
Maurice, G. Green, & R. M. Foxx (Eds.), *Making a difference: Behavioral
intervention for autism* (pp. 83–93). Austin, TX: PRO-ED.

Wehman, P. (1992). *Life beyond the classroom: Transition strategies for young
people with disabilities.* Baltimore: Brookes.

Wehmeyer, M. L., & Palmer, S. (2003). Adult outcomes for students with cognitive disabilities three years after high school: The impact of self-determination. *Education and Training in Developmental Disabilities, 38*(2), 131–144.

Wells, T., Sandefur, G. D., & Hogan, D. P. (2003). What happens after the high school years among young persons with disabilities? *Social Forces, 82*(2), 803–832.

White, J., & Weiner, J. J. (2004). Influence of least restrictive environment and community based training on integrated employment outcomes for transitioning students with severe disabilities. *Journal of Vocational Rehabilitation, 21,* 149–156.

Williams, S. K., Johnson, C., & Sukhodolsky, D. G. (2005). The role of the school psychologist in the inclusive education of school-age students with autism spectrum disorders. *Journal of School Psychology, 43,* 117–136.

Wood, M. (1998). Whose job is it anyway? Educational roles in inclusion. *Exceptional Students, 64,* 181–195.

▬ ▪ 11 ▪ ▫

Translating Early Intervention into Positive Outcomes

Laurie Sperry
Gary Mesibov

When considering the population of children with autism who have more severe cognitive and language impairments, it is important to recognize it is likely they will continue to need significant amounts of support not only throughout their school years, but throughout their lives. Autism early intervention research reveals that treating children with autism prior to age 5 can have positive long-term benefits (Guralnick, 1997; Dawson & Osterling, 1997). However, outcome studies have reported that while some individuals with autism may achieve near to "typical" maturity, others continue to struggle with impairments throughout their lives (Seltzer et al., 2003). When compared to children with mental retardation (MR), children with autism are more impaired in the areas of socialization, communication skills, and verbal reasoning (Carpentieri & Morgan, 1994). Autism outcome research indicates that early childhood prognostic indicators of successful future functioning includes higher cognitive ability (IQ > 50) and language attainment by age 6 years (Lord & Bailey, 2002). Although these two factors are an important consideration, there is great variability in outcomes for individuals with autism regardless of the type and intensity of intervention provided, suggesting that there are other factors that may contribute to treatment effectiveness (e.g., Gabriels, Hill, Pierce, Rogers, & Wehner, 2001; Luiselli, Cannon, Ellis, & Sisson, 2000). Thus, it is imperative that autism interventionists, educators, and other professionals who work with school-age children and adolescents with autism build upon early intervention efforts in the areas of communication, social skills, behaviors, and adaptive functioning in order to maximize independent functioning and the possibility of attaining a full, rich, and meaningful life.

This chapter examines characteristics of autism that may continue to be problematic for lower-functioning school-age and adolescent individuals with autism. In addition, it provides suggestions and strategies to foster continued development following early intervention, of important life skills that are necessary for more successful transitions by children with autism as they grow up.

PROBLEMATIC AUTISM SYMPTOMS DURING SCHOOL AGE AND ADOLESCENCE

As individuals with autism mature, the expectations of society change and with that, the level of independence expected of them also changes. Individuals with more impaired cognitive and communication abilities are at risk for having poor outcomes by continuing to demonstrate significant impairments in communication, social interaction, and behaviors (Stein et al., 2001). Ineffective communication abilities, improper social skills, and interfering or dangerous behaviors, along with inadequate adaptive living skills, can impair an individual's ability to learn and limit his or her engagement in the activities of daily life such as work, socializing, and leisure activities. These are among the ongoing concerns caregivers have regarding their adolescent and adult children with autism (Fong, Wilgosh, & Sobsey, 1993).

Communication Abilities

Teaching people with autism how to communicate has a considerable impact on them, their families, and other care providers or people in their lives. Outcome research suggests that as a whole, children with autism may make limited progress in the areas of language attainment over time, although some individuals make significant progress in certain areas of language development. Sigman and Ruskin (1999) examined children with autism at two different points in time (Time 1 mean age = 3 years, 11 months; Time 2 mean age = 12 years, 10 months). The mean language age of the group was 18 months when measured at Time 1, and it had only increased to 46 months when the group was measured again 8–9 years later. In a study of 14 men ages 18–39 years with an early diagnosis of autism, impairments in communication, speech prosody, and, especially, the social use of communication, were found to continue to be problematic into adulthood. Communication differences also included self-talk, idiosyncratic use of language, topic perseveration, and repetitive questioning, along with a paucity of spontaneous speech (Rumsey, Rapoport, & Screery, 1985). While there are relatively few longitudinal studies, 146 children with autism who have been followed into adolescence and adulthood have shown differences in self-care, cognitive functioning, and communicative ability with the most remarkable improvements being measured in children who were the youngest at the time the study began (Beadle-Brown et al., 2000). Overall differences in communication did not reach levels of significance between the measurement at Time 1 (1970s) and measurement at Time 2 (1980s); however, specific communication skills did improve significantly. These skills included general comprehension of language, development of grammar, ability to ask questions, articulation, and understanding and use of gestures.

While early interventionists may teach augmentative or alternative communication systems to the child, efforts to continually encourage the child to use these communication skills and systems may be neglected for various reasons as the child enters school age or adolescence. For example, care providers can anticipate the child's needs; therefore, they may not insist that the child use the communication system. The unfortunate, and not uncommon, assumption in this case is that the care provider will always be a part of the child's life throughout adulthood. Another barrier to consistent implementation is the fact that communication systems require a great deal of effort on the part of care providers and teachers to keep them updated and relevant to the communicator. It is imperative that interventionists and careproviders recognize that there are multiple opportunities for the child to practice communication skills throughout the day.

Social Skills

Impaired social skills have pervasive and long-term effects on the ability of people with autism to have quality interactions with their peers, and this further impairs their ability to gain additional social information from their environments (Howlin, 2003). Early portrayals of autism by Kanner (1943) consistently described social interaction impairments among the children in his case studies. Eisenberg's (1956) follow-up study of adolescents and adults, which included 10 of the 11 individuals originally diagnosed by Kanner, suggested that even those individuals who were, for the most part, independent still had significant social impairments. Specifically, these impairments included lack of tact in dealing with others and low levels of social engagement and social responsiveness.

Orsmond, Krauss, and Seltzer (2004) examined the personal and environmental factors most closely related to having friendships, including how often the individuals were involved in social and recreational pursuits, and the types and frequency of peer relationships common among adolescents and adults with autism. Environmental factors most related to the child with autism having friendships included the mother's degree of social engagement, the number of provider agencies involved with the family, and whether the student was in a self-contained versus inclusive educational environment.

What remains unclear is the extent to which a lack of friendships is impacted by a lack of desire or ability to be socially engaged with others. This question may be informed, in part, by the work of Sperry and Mesibov (2005), who examined the perceptions of social challenges experienced by adults with autism within the context of the TEACCH (Treatment and Education of Autistic and related Communication-handicapped CHildren) adult social skills group. Members of the group had specific questions about how to join conversations, assess personal space (i.e., determine how far they should stand away from another person while speaking), and extend conversations. The number of questions they generated related to interpersonal and intimate relationships suggested an interest in the pursuit of such relationships, but might also be suggestive of the differences they encounter in such pursuits.

Behavior Problems

Problem behaviors can include tantrums, destruction of property, and aggression toward self and others (Horner, Carr, Strain, Todd, & Reed, 2000). These behaviors present substantial obstacles to participation in home, school, and community activities by individuals with significant intellectual disabilities and/or autism (Murphy et al., 2005). Problem behaviors can be a source of significant stress for families, care providers, and educators in their efforts to provide appropriate programming and this stress escalates as the child becomes older, larger, and stronger

(Bristol, Gallegher, & Holt, 1993). Problem behaviors are more likely to result in out-of-home placement than any other impairment associated with the person's disability (Black, Molaison, & Smull, 1990). It is essential to consider the levels of care, constant supervision, and management of problem behaviors that families face and the impact on their ability to continue to care for their family members with autism. In a study by Turnbull and Ruef (1996) of children between the ages of 2 and 36 years, parents identified problem behaviors that were of particular concern to them including property destruction, aggression toward self or others, pica, and stigmatizing behaviors including noises and stereotypies. Parents also identified the importance of continued attention to the amelioration of these behaviors as the child with autism enters school age and adolescence to improve their child's functioning in preparation for adulthood. Of particular concern for families was how to provide support for their family member with autism. They requested support in the areas of:

- Teaching their children how to engage in social relationships outside of the family.
- Teaching the family how to structure their home environment.
- Teaching their children how to manage their own stress.
- Helping the family understand *why* a problem behavior occurs.
- Teaching their children how to use meaningful communication systems and make choices.

Adaptive Living Skills

Studies have demonstrated that individuals with autism, compared with matched controls, have inconsistent and lower levels of adaptive behaviors (Burack & Volkmar, 1992; Gillham, Carter, Volkmar, & Sparrow, 2000; Lord et al., 1989). In addition, there is evidence to suggest that specific to individuals with autism, adaptive abilities appear to decline or to not progress as they age, regardless of cognitive ability levels (Liss et al., 2001; Siperstein & Volkmar, 2004). This lack of progress is sometimes exacerbated by assigning a one-to-one assistant to the child with autism whose job it becomes to complete the activities of daily living for the child. Therefore, it is essential that staff view themselves as supports who can help to maximize independence rather than fostering dependence. Dependence on staff may seem less problematic when children with severe disabilities are very young, but as the children get older it becomes more pronounced and discrepant and may become part of a learned routine of helplessness.

Case Example

John is a young adult with autism who works in the kitchen at a large university. He works 40 hours a week and lives in a group home with other adults with autism and mental retardation. John was not taught the social skill of how to get a friend's attention appropriately. To gain the attention of his coworkers he gets very close to them and begins to speak in a very loud voice. When he gets too close, his coworkers take a step backward, which results in John taking a step forward and increasing his volume. When his coworkers continue to move backward, he may grab their arm. This has caused significant alarm on the part of his coworkers and concern on the part of his employer that John may grab a customer. While John means no harm, it has caused his coworkers to avoid him.

As outlined in the LEAP (Learning Experiences: An Alternative Program for Preschoolers and Parents) program (Strain & Cordisco, 1994), very young children can begin to be taught basic social skills, the first of which is to how get a friend's attention appropriately. This becomes the springboard for teaching about social communication, sharing, accepting new ideas, and giving compliments to others. While these do not represent the full spectrum of skills necessary to navigate the social world they are designed to provide entrée into social exchanges, maintain and extend social exchanges, and increase the person's social cachet.

Social impairments are a significant obstacle to the successful inclusion of students with autism. The environmental modifications and emphasis on teaching specific social and communication skills present in early childhood settings may become less prevalent as the child enters adolescence. Therefore it is important to continue to build on the work of early interventionists. Social skill deficits can be mitigated through intensive intervention that incorporates ongoing and deliberate interactions with peers who are typically developing and includes multiple opportunities to practice social skills across multiple exemplars (Strain, 1987).

TREATMENT ELEMENTS TO ADDRESS ENDURING IMPAIRMENTS

As previously described, the communication, social, behavioral, and adaptive living impairments in autism continue into adolescence, impacting every facet of an individual's existence such as being able to communicate basic wants and needs, enjoying friendships, living independently, and being employed. Over the years there has been a dichotomy of exclusively teaching people with disabilities either self-help skills *or* academic skills. More recently, there has been a shift away from teaching functional skills to students with severe disabilities in favor of an emphasis on social skills and membership. Billingsley and Albertson (1999) remind us that functional skills and social membership are not mutually exclusive, rather they are interdependent. A paucity of self-help skills on the part of the person with disabilities can result in diminishing status with typical peers (Evans, Salisbury, Palombaro, Berryman, & Hollowood, 1992). On the other hand, strict adherence to a functional skill model can lack the individualization necessary to make it successful in meeting the unique needs of the person with disabilities.

Teaching Meaningful Communication Systems

Teaching individuals with autism communication systems so that they can make choices has the power to increase their engagement and productivity and to decrease problem behavior. One way to keep communication at the forefront in children's lives as they age is to constantly consider communication challenges and build the use of communication skills into daily routines and activities (i.e., arrival and departure routines, getting attention appropriately from an adult or peer, making choices, using an augmentative or alternative communication system to make a request or initiate an interaction). Communication can be encouraged by developing a functional, universally understandable system that reflects things the student would want to communicate about, a means of doing so (objects, pictures), and multiple opportunities to communicate those messages across settings and people (Layton & Watson, 1995). Augmentative and alternative forms of communication can include sign language, an object communication box, picture symbols, the written word, or choice boards. They can also include assistive technology devices, especially those with natural-sounding voice output capability and a range of messages, or even a simple paper and pencil. Young children may want to communicate about basic wants and needs, and favorite objects, activities, or people. Adolescents may want to communicate about snacks, music, TV or video games. The point is, the device should provide students a way to communicate about what is important to them.

Individuals with autism, even those who are significantly impaired, are capable of showing preferences and making choices. Teaching a student how to make choices can provide a worthwhile, meaningful, and lifelong skill that can be generalized to multiple environments. Individuals with autism can be taught to make choices by presenting choices within work tasks. For example, telling the student with autism, "It's time to work" is not presented as a choice. Rather, a choice can be embedded into work tasks by stating, "Here are six tasks [based on student's IEP]. Pick three." This can be done by creating a work system that uses nonordered specific tokens to indicate that three tasks must be completed, but having six tasks available so students create their own matching system. They take a token off their work system and match it to the task of their choice. If a student picks the same task over and over and the concern is that the other tasks are not being chosen, efforts could be made to limit the number of choices or to rotate the tasks out to maintenance. Also, one could require that certain tasks be completed and the choice would be the order in which they were performed.

Choices can be incorporated in leisure time: "It's time for recess, what do you want to play, and who are you going to pick for your buddy?" Choices could also be incorporated into behavioral self-management. A child hands over the break card (see Figure 11.1) and is directed to a menu of choices containing pictures that display the following: I need a break, I can go sit in the calm-down area and count; take a walk; swing in the swinging chair for 5 minutes; scratch my back with my back scratcher. In particular, this obviates the need for staff to physically direct a child who is displaying problem behavior by giving the

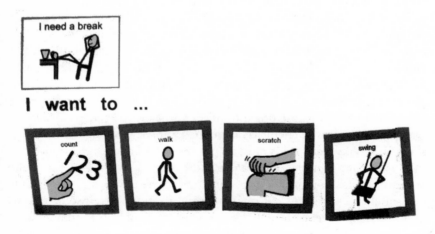

FIGURE 11.1. Students can be taught to request a break using the break card as a replacement skill for using problem behavior to escape or avoid a task, activity, or person. These choices reflect activities the student can choose from during his break to self-calm before returning to work.

child control over his or her environment. Furthermore, attempting to physically direct an adolescent who is engaging in problem behavior becomes a difficult, if not impossible, task for support staff.

Teaching Social Skills

Social skills are often of primary importance for individuals to engage with families and their communities. Providing opportunities for full membership, not just in schools, but in the communities in which families and children reside should be a goal of inclusive programming (Odom et al., 1996). A starting point could be an inclusive preschool that creates a culture of friendship that extends to all of its members. Social skills are explicitly taught, reinforced, and valued. According to parent report, benefits of inclusion for children without disabilities include increased self-esteem, self-confidence, and an appreciation for individual differences (Brown, Odom, Li, & Zercher, 2004). It can be extremely difficult for the student with autism, the school staff, and other students if inclusion is delayed until the student is older. Rather, if inclusion, to the maximum extent possible, is done from the time the student enters school and throughout his or her school years, it will become standard operating procedure for all of the students and staff.

The past few decades have witnessed an evolution in the understanding of and interventions related to improving the social behaviors of students with autism. Originally viewed as enhancing a skill deficit, social skills training began to address and change negative peer attitudes, followed by a movement toward considering the entire social ecology of the student with autism with combined social skills training for both the child and any and all social agents that may be encountered in the child's daily environment (Strain & Hoyson, 2000). While this attitudinal shift has resulted in increasing the generalization of social skills across multiple settings and exemplars, it represents a silo approach to teaching social skills as a separate domain independent of other areas of performance such as motor, cognitive, communication, behavior, and adaptive skills. Teaching social skills must be part of a comprehensive, empirically supported intervention, rather than addressing a particular set of skills in a discrete fashion during a specific time of the day. Social opportunities should be embedded in ongoing daily routines (Strain & Hoyson, 2000). Certain elements are necessary to maximize the number and quality of social opportunities. First, students with autism need access to typically developing peers. The number of their social interactions is greater when they have access to neurotypical peers than when they are placed in self-contained, special education classrooms (Guralnick,

1990). Inclusion also provides numerous opportunities to interact with what Strain, Odom, & McConnell (1984) describe as "relevant social agents." While placement in an inclusive environment is a good first step, it does not guarantee acceptance by the typical peers, nor does it necessarily mean that the child with autism will model the desired behaviors (Guralnick, 1990).

Access to Typical Peers to Teach Social Skills

Access to typical peers, as early as possible, is essential for promoting the development of appropriate social behaviors (Strain et al., 1984) and should be continued throughout the life of the person with autism. A peer buddy approach has been found to be effective during early school years (Laushey & Heflin, 2000). Although less studied in the older school-age and adolescent autism population, this peer buddy approach could be used to increase the generalization of social skills to novel environments. (Refer to Chapter 10 for more information about peer models.) A peer buddy approach for adolescents and adults may include membership in a club that reflects their special interests (e.g., chess, math, computers, photography, trains). It could also include manager or player positions on intramural or varsity teams. To ensure the success of a peer buddy approach, teachers can start with their most socially responsive typical peers. In other words, the students who have demonstrated confidence, social maturity, and patience when working and playing in the classroom make the best initial candidates. An adult facilitator should be available to provide, when appropriate, strategies to help students interact with each other, rather than serving in the role of problem solver. For example, if a student with autism and his peer buddy are struggling over the use of an item, the adult facilitator can encourage them to employ problem-solving strategies they have learned in the classroom. These strategies could include sharing, taking turns, setting a timer, offering a trade, or using something else. These are critical social skills for all children and ultimately provide the foundation for negotiation skills needed by all people in postschool environments.

Another way to embed social interactions is to consider the number of things adults do for children in a classroom setting. Are these activities that students could be doing for each other? Take, for example, passing out materials. The simple act of having a student pass out materials creates an opportunity for several social interactions and even more exchanges: The receiving student's attention is secured ["Brian—"]; the item is offered ["here are your markers"]; a response is given (sign, voice output, or picture symbol) ["Thanks"]; a final response is given

["You're welcome"]. These exchanges create multiple opportunities to practice social skills in a contextualized setting. If this same principle were applied across the day, across the number of students in the classroom, the number of social opportunities would grow exponentially.

Capitalizing on Special Interests to Teach Social Skills

Boyd, Conroy, Mancil, Nakao, and Alter (in press) found that incorporating the restricted interests of children with autism into their social interactions resulted in an increase in social initiations with typical peers compared to when a neutral item was used during the interactions. The behavioral differences of people with autism are often more tolerated by others when the individual has expertise in specific areas (Grandin, 1996; Howlin, 1997). Some people with autism are able to parlay their circumscribed interest into a career focus (Grandin, 1996). Asperger (1944) noted that it was the special interests that often led people with autism to become accomplished in their career fields. Teaching a child with autism who enjoys numbers how to play card games such as Uno would provide an opportunity to capitalize on a special interest as a way of creating a connection with peers and expanding the person's social leisure skills. Consider the special interests of persons with autism and how those can be used to make social interaction more attractive or to serve as an entrée into social circles (hobbies, clubs, teams), or simply to enrich their lives.

Providing Structured Environments to Manage Behaviors and Increase Independence

TEACCH is a statewide system of support for individuals with autism in North Carolina that emphasizes structuring the environment to reduce maladaptive behaviors and promote independent functioning in individuals with autism. There are four types of structure defined by the TEACCH system: physical structure, daily schedules, individual work systems, and visual structure.

Van Bourgendien, Reichle, and Schopler (2003) examined the effectiveness of the Carolina Living and Learning Center (CLLC), a residential treatment center based on the principles of TEACCH and structured teaching, and how placement at the center impacted the functioning of adults with autism and significant disabilities. The CLLC offers a structured learning program designed to modify the environment to increase the understanding of the individual with autism. The goal of its program for severely disabled adults is to increase their ability to function as independently as possible, thereby increasing their ability to access their communities more fully and independently. Visual supports, including object and picture instructions, visual work systems, daily schedules, and color coding, allow the residents to capitalize on their visual strengths and increase their independence, rather than becoming dependent on staff prompts (see Figure 11.2). Furthermore, teaching life skills in a naturalized context in the environments in which they will be used has been shown to be effective in allowing the residents at the CLLC to generalize their skills to the community. This study also showed that using modified communication strategies and positive, proactive behavioral supports and strategies resulted in a reduction of challenging behavior. The investigators in this study found that settings that had lower rates of visual, communication, and positive behavior supports had comparative increases in challenging behavior over the same time period. An important point made by the authors is that these types of specialized supports are comparable to the use of hearing aids

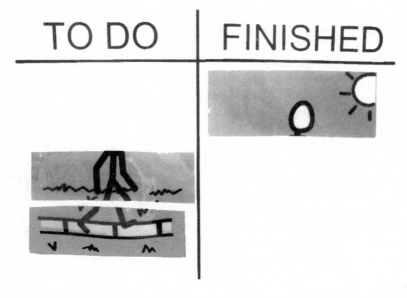

FIGURE 11.2. The walking card can be used to set parameters around the behavior of pacing. The student can be taught to walk the high school track as a calming activity. Each time he or she walks a lap, the student takes part of the picture and transfers it from left to right. When the picture is completed on the right, the student is finished walking.

or prescription glasses. It would be inconceivable to remove those types of assistance if the person had a visual or hearing impairment, yet as is often the case, visual supports are often "faded" over time with the justification that the person with autism "knows his schedule or is too high functioning for that support." The response to that argument might be to compare it with asking people to hand over their eyeglasses, day planner, or PDA and see how independently and efficiently they would be able to function.

Physical Structure

Physically structuring the environment is a way to add meaning and context. It provides the person with autism additional information about what is supposed to happen in that area. It is a way of establishing clear boundaries and minimizing, to the extent possible, visual and auditory distractions. Setting up a structured environment has been shown to reduce self-stimulation and increase on-task behavior (Duker & Rasing, 1989). Bookcases, room dividers and tables can all be utilized to create physical structure within a room, with each area having a clear purpose. Boxes can be labeled with words, pictures, or even objects so that students with autism can help with cleanup. These labeled boxes can then be matched to the visual supports on the bookcases and shelves throughout the room.

Physical structure can be achieved in early childhood by having clearly defined areas that communicate what is going to happen in those areas (play area, one-to-one work, small group, circle, snack area) and minimize auditory and visual distractions. For adolescents the general areas would include work tables, desks, a computer station, a domestic area, and a recreation and leisure area where the students might listen to music, look at books (especially those that reflect their special interests), play board games, look at magazines, play hand-held video games, and listen to their MP3 players. It is particularly important that students have an understanding that certain things happen in certain places, especially as they get older. What begins in early childhood as "I eat in the snack area and play in the play area" can translate into "I get dressed and undressed in the locker room," as illustrated in the case example provided below in the section on work systems.

Schedules

Visual schedules, which should be introduced during the early intervention years and continued through elementary grades and adolescence, can have positive effects on the independence and functioning abilities of adults with autism. A visual schedule identifies which events will occur during the day and their sequence, allowing the person with autism to anticipate what will happen next. Routines can help individuals with autism stay organized and efficient. The activities and routines of daily living should be identified, task analyzed, and then structured using visual supports for people with autism. This strength-based approach capitalizes on their strong visual skills, and they get into the routine of checking their schedule, which increases flexibility as the order of the pictures or the schedules and words themselves can be changed. This approach also capitalizes on the individual's ability to adhere to routines and often, once a routine is learned, it can be used for a lifetime.

Visual schedules can be presented in the form of actual objects, pictures, icons, or written words. For individuals with autism who are significantly impaired, a visual schedule may be a collection of objects that allows them to move from place to place or activity to activity with minimal physical or verbal prompting from others. For example an object schedule for an adolescent's daily activities could be represented as follows: a notebook = math, a stapler = office work; a CD = break; and a lunch ticket = lunch in the cafeteria. Additionally, visual schedules can be used in the home environment to increase independent living skills. A picture schedule for home might include pictures of getting up, eating breakfast, brushing teeth, showering, getting dressed, walking out to the bus stop, and getting on the bus.

Work Systems

A work system allows persons with autism to understand what they have to do, how much they have to do, how much progress they are making, and what is going to happen next. A practical way to increase independence is to conduct an activity analysis to determine what visual supports and skills the individual needs to complete all or part of an activity and what the individual actually does during that activity. The discrepancy between what is expected and what actually occurs can be used as a starting point to determine what skills need to be taught so the person with autism can successfully complete all or part of the activity as independently as possible.

Case Example

Andre is a middle school student who swims with his class at the community pool each week. He uses a visual work system to help him remember to take his clothes off *inside* the locker room and put his swim suit on *before* going out to the pool. The pictures on his work system include the following: Step 1—Take off clothes; Step 2—Put clothes in locker; Step 3—Put swim suit on; Step 4—Take a shower; and Step 5—Swim in pool. This tells Andre how many steps he has to complete (how much work), what steps he has to take (what work), a way of measuring their progress (he turns the pictures over as he finishes each step), and what happens next (swim in pool).

Visual Structure

Visual structure provides clarity by highlighting the relevant information in a task or activity and providing a sequencing mechanism for effectively combining and completing the individual components of a task. The strategies mentioned earlier are effective in decreasing the anxiety and subsequent problem behavior of persons with autism and increasing their ability to work successfully and as independently as possible.

Case Example

Ron is a high school student with autism who works in his school library. His job is to put together routing slips that are used to determine where books go in the school. He has visual instructions that show pictures of the following: Picture 1—a folded piece of paper; Picture 2—a rubber band going around the folded piece of paper; Picture 3—the piece of paper being stapled. Ron also has a detachable sentence strip at the bottom of his instructions that says, "I need more _____." He has been taught to hand this sentence strip, plus the picture of what he needs more of, over to his work supervisor.

CONCLUSION

This chapter began by asking what to teach the population of children with autism who have more severe cognitive and language impairments to best prepare them for positive adult outcomes. Our approach has been to focus on those skills, behaviors, and foundations that can be identified in early childhood and promoted throughout one's educational experiences. By targeting important priorities early and cultivating the development of skills in those areas, the expectation is that we should be able to promote more positive outcomes and more meaningful and productive lives for these students. The framework we have used is to identify potential problems in late adolescence and adulthood that are related to learning patterns and related characteristics in autism and to start emphasizing appropriate remedial strategies in preschool and continue with them throughout a student's educational experiences.

We have proposed that the very early preschool years should be devoted to fundamental issues like making the world meaningful and comprehensible to our students. We should also establish organizational strategies for moving around the classroom, understanding the daily routine, and working on organized tasks and activities. We should cultivate the use of visual strategies and the identification and adherence to visual cues and information. Once these fundamental learning strategies and understandings are established, then the educational program can build on them to develop necessary cognitive, social, and personal skills.

Based on the literature and our discussions in this chapter, the basic skills that are needed for successful and productive adult functioning include self-management, functional communication, appropriate social skills, activities of daily living, and vocational skills. In addition, there is the ability to communicate effectively, exercise reasonable choices, and participate in a variety of social and leisure activities that are meaningful and enjoyable. The best way to achieve these desired ends is to provide early childhood programs that provide the necessary foundations for learning and exploring and then build upon these foundations by emphasizing areas for skill development that have been identified through the literature and clinical practice as being the most important for successful adult outcomes.

REFERENCES

Asperger, H. (1944) Die "autistischen Psychopathen" in Kindesalter. *Archives fur Psychiatrie und Nervenkrankheiten, 117,* 76–136.

Beadle-Brown, J., Murphy, G., Wing, L., Gould, J., Shah, A., & Holmes, N. (2000). Changes in skills for people with intellectual disability: A follow-up of the Camberwell Cohort. *Journal of Intellectual Disability Research, 44*(1), 12–24.

Billingsley, F. F., & Albertson, L. R. (1999). Finding a future for functional skills. *Journal of the Association for Persons with Severe Handicaps, 24*(4), 298–302.

Black, M. M., Molaison, V. A., & Smull, M. W. (1990). Families caring for a young adult with mental retardation: Service needs and urgency of community living requests. *American Journal on Mental Retardation, 95,* 32–39.

Boyd, B. A., Conroy, M. A., Mancil, G. R., Nakao, T., & Alter, P. J. (in press). Effects of circumscribed interests on the social behaviors of children with autism spectrum disorders: Use of structural analysis analogues. *Journal of Autism and Developmental Disorders.*

Bristol, M. M., Gallagher, J. J., & Holt, K. D. (1993). Maternal depressive symptoms in autism: Response to psychoeducational intervention. *Rehabilitation Psychology, 38,* 3–9.

Brown, W. H., Odom, S. L., Li, S., & Zercher, C. (2004). Ecobehavioral assessment in inclusive early childhood programs: A portrait of preschool inclusion. *Journal of Special Education, 33,* 138–153.

Burack, J., & Volkmar, F. (1992). Development of low- and high-functioning autistic children. *Journal of Child Psychology and Psychiatry and Allied Disciplines, 33,* 607–616.

Carpentieri, S., & Morgan, S.B. (1994). Brief report: A comparison of patterns of cognitive functioning in autistic and nonautistic retarded children on the Stanford-Binet-Fourth Edition. *Journal of Autism and Developmental Disorders, 24,* 215–233.

Dawson, G., & Osterling, J. (1997). Early intervention in autism. In M. J. Guralnick (Ed.), *The effectiveness of early intervention* (pp. 307–326). Baltimore: Brookes.

Duker, P. C., & Rasing, E. (1989). Effects of redesigning the physical environment on self-stimulation and on-task behavior in three autistic-type developmentally disabled individuals. *Journal of Autism and Developmental Disorders, 19,* 451–460.

Eisenberg, L. (1956). The autistic child in adolescence. *American Journal of Psychiatry, 1112,* 607–612.

Evans, I. M., Salisbury, C. L., Palombaro, M. M., Berryman, J., & Hollowood, T. M. (1992). Acceptance of elementary-aged children with severe disabilities in an inclusive school. *Journal of the Association for Persons with Severe Handicaps, 17,* 205–212.

Fong, L., Wilgosh, L., & Sobsey, D. (1993). The experience of parenting an adolescent with autism. *International Journal of Disability, Development and Education, 40,* 105–113.

Gabriels, R., Hill, D., Pierce, R., Rogers, S., & Wehner, B. (2001). Predictors of treatment outcome in young children with autism: A retrospective study. *Autism, 5*(4), 407–429.

Gillham, J. E., Carter, A. S., Volkmar, F. R., & Sparrow, S. S. (2000). Toward a developmental operational definition of autism. *Journal of Autism and Developmental Disorders, 30,* 269–278.

Grandin, T. (1996). Making the transition from the world of school into the world of work. Retrieved October 25, 2005, from *www.autism.org/temple/transition.html.*

Guralnick, M. J. (1990). Social competence and early intervention. *Journal of Early Intervention, 14,* 3–14.

Guralnick, M. J. (1997). Second-generation research in the field of early intervention. In M. J. Guralnick (Ed.), *The effectiveness of early intervention,* (pp. 3–20). Baltimore: Brookes.

Horner, R. H., Carr, E. G., Strain, P. S., Todd, A. W., & Reed, H. K. (2000, April 12). *Problem behavior interventions for young children with autism: A research synthesis.* Paper presented at the Second Workshop of the Committee on Educational Interventions for Children with Autism, National Research Council, University of Oregon, Eugene, OR.

Howlin, P. (1997). *Autism: Preparing for adulthood.* London: Routledge.

Howlin, P. (2003). Implications for the differentiation between autism and Asperger syndrome. *Journal of Autism and Developmental Disorders, 33*(1), 3–13.

Kanner, L. (1943). Autistic disturbances of affective contact. *Nervous Child, 2,* 217–250.

Laushey, K. M., & Heflin, L. J. (2000). Enhancing social skills of kindergarten children with autism through the training of multiple peers as tutors. *Journal of Autism and Developmental Disorders, 30*(3), 183–193.

Layton, T. L., & Watson, L. R. (1995). Enhancing communication in nonverbal children with autism. In K. Quill (Ed.), *Teaching children with autism: Strategies to enhance communication and socialization* (pp. 73–103). New York: Delmar.

Liss, M., Harel, B., Fein, D., Allen, D., Dunn, M., Feinstein, C., et al. (2001). Predictors and correlates of adaptive functioning in children with developmental disorders. *Journal of Autism and Developmental Disorders, 31,* 219–230.

Lord, C., & Bailey, A. (2002). Autism spectrum disorders. In M. Rutter & E. Taylor (Eds.), *Child and adolescent psychiatry* (pp. 664–681). Oxford, UK: Blackwell Scientific.

Lord, C., Rutter, M., Goode, S., Heemsbergen, J., Jordan, H., Mawhood, L., et al. (1989). Autism diagnostic observation schedule: A standardized observation of communicative and social behavior. *Journal of Autism and Developmental Disorders, 19,* 185–212.

Luiselli, J., Cannon, B. O., Ellis, J., & Sisson, R. (2000). Home-based behavioral intervention for young children with autism/pervasive developmental disorder: A preliminary evaluation of outcome in relation to child age and intensity of service delivery. *Autism, 4*(4), 426–438.

Murphy, G. H., Beadle-Brown, J., Wing, L., Gould, J., Shah, A., & Holmes, N., (2005). Chronicity of challenging behaviours in people with severe intellectual disabilities and/or autism: A total population sample. *Journal of Autism and Developmental Disorders, 35*(4), 405–418.

Odom, S. L., Peck, C. A., Hanson, M., Beckman, P., Kaiser, A., Leiber, J., et al. (1996). Inclusion at the preschool level: An ecological systems analysis. *SRCD Social Policy Report, 10,* 18–30.

Orsmond, G. I., Krauss, M. W., & Seltzer, M. M. (2004). Peer relationships and social and recreational activities among adolescents and adults with autism. *Journal of Autism and Developmental Disorders, 34*(3), 245–253.

Rumsey, J. M., Rapoport, M. D., & Screery, W. R. (1985). Autistic children as adults: Psychiatric, social and behavioral outcomes. *Journal of the American Academy of Child Psychiatry, 24*(4), 465–473.

Seltzer, M. M., Wyngaarden Kraus, M., Shattuck, P. T., Orsmond, G., Swe, A., et al. (2003). The symptoms of autism spectrum disorders in adolescence and adulthood. *Journal of Autism and Developmental Disorders, 33*(6), 565–581.

Sigman, M., & Ruskin, E. (1999). Continuity and change in the social competence of children with autism, Down syndrome, and developmental delays. *Monographs for the Society for Research in Child Development, 64*(1, Serial No. 256).

Siperstein, R. & Volkmar, F. (2004). Report: Parental reporting of regression in children with pervasive developmental disorders. *Journal of Autism and Developmental Disorders, 34*(6), 731–735.

Sperry, L. A., & Mesibov, G. B. (2005). Perceptions of social challenges of adults with autism spectrum disorder. *Autism: The International Journal of Research and Practice, 9*(4), 363–378.

Stein, D., Ring, A., Shulman, C., Meir, D., Holan, A., Weizman, A., et al. (2001). Brief Report: Children with autism as they grow up: Description of adult inpatients with severe autism. *Journal of Autism and Developmental Disorders 31*(3), 355–360.

Strain, P. S. (1987). Comprehensive evaluation of young autistic children. *Topics in Early Childhood Special Education, 7*, 97–110.

Strain, P. S., & Cordisco. L. (1994). LEAP preschool. In S. L. Harris & J. S. Handleman (Eds.), *Preschool education programs for children with autism* (pp. 225–244). Austin, TX: PRO-ED.

Strain, P. S., & Hoyson, M. (2000). The need for longitudinal, intensive social skill intervention: LEAP follow-up outcomes for children with autism. *Topics in Early Childhood Special Education, 20*(2), 116–122.

Strain, P. S., Odom, S. L., & McConnell, S. (1984). Promoting social reciprocity of exceptional children: Identification, target behavior selection and intervention. *Remedial and Special Education, 5*(1), 21–28.

Turnbull A. P., & Ruef, M. (1996). Family perspectives on problem behavior. *Mental Retardation, 34*(5), 280–293.

Van Bourgondien, M. E., Reichle, N. C., & Schopler, E. (2003). Effects of a model treatment approach on adults with autism. *Journal of Autism and Developmental Disorders, 33*(2), 131–140.

Volkmar, F. (2003). *Healthcare for children on the autism spectrum: A guide to medical, nutritional and behavioral issues.* Bethesda, MD: Woodbine House.

▬ ▬ 12 ▢ ▢

School Consultation and Interventions for Middle School and High School Students with Autism

Brian R. Lopez
Dina E. Hill
Sandy Shaw
Robin L. Gabriels

Individuals with autism who have lower cognitive and communication skills frequently place unique demands on educators and the school system that may require outside consultation with a professional who has expertise in autism. For example, these children and adolescents may exhibit multiple challenging behaviors (e.g., self-injurious behaviors, aggression, masturbation, perseveration on nonfunctional routines, or extreme responses to subtle sensory stimuli), limited functional communication, poor social awareness, and unique cognitive profiles that can affect their ability to learn. Teachers are frequently ill equipped to address these behavioral and cognitive extremes, and few teachers have specialized training in the evidence-based practices for autism that are needed to make lasting change in this population.

Given the legal requirement of the Individuals with Disabilities Education Act (IDEA; Public Law 105-17) and No Child Left Behind, educators are required to demonstrate that they are "highly qualified" in evidence-based practices and strategies (EBPS) in order to meet the needs of their students with autism and to educate those students in the least restrictive environments. This means that educators must be able to effectively implement EBPS, such as applied behavioral analysis, naturalistic learning approaches, incidental teaching, positive behavioral supports, assistive technology, and social skills curricula, and to make adaptations to the environment within least restrictive settings (Lord & McGee, 2001). For many smaller districts and rural communities it is difficult to identify special education teachers or therapists with these particular skills and talents. This problem is frequently confounded by the fact that many educators are unable to access specialized training in evidence-based practices for children with autism due to a lack of support for training and assistance. In fact, on average, it takes 12 years to implement research findings on EBPS into daily educational practices (Ayres, Meyer, Erevelles, & Park-Lee, 1994; Walker, 2004).

There is a current lack of professionals trained to meet the specific needs of these more severely impaired individuals with autism (Scheuerman, Webber, Boutot, & Goodwin, 2003). This has resulted in an increased reliance on autism consultation to assist school districts in meeting the needs of their students with autism. Autism consultants are often called upon to provide a variety of services to multidisciplinary educational teams in an attempt to address a range of educational programming issues. An autism consultant can assist an educational team in improving an individual's adaptive, social, and functional communication skills and in decreasing problematic behaviors, with the desired outcome of increasing the student's ability to access the educational curricula. In addition, consultation with autism experts can provide a means of disseminating training and supporting educators in the use of EBPS for children with autism.

This chapter reviews general school consultation models, the critical components to effective autism consultation, ways a consultant can assist the educational team (e.g., reducing challenging behaviors, improving family involvement, and developing specialized curricula and systematic instruction), and potential barriers to the consultative process. Finally, we demonstrate the potential of autism-specific consultation through three case studies, beginning with an example of consultation with classroom teachers regarding an individual with autism (case-based consultation), then moving to describe consultation with a broader scope to train multiple educators in one school district about how to intervene with problem behaviors (topic-based consultation), and finally moving to an even broader consultation model (systems-based consultation) to improve autism identification and evaluation methods across school districts.

MODELS OF SCHOOL CONSULTATION

Mental health consultation, ecobehavioral consultation, and organizational and systems consultation are the most traditional approaches to consultation (Reynolds & Gutkin, 1998). Caplan's (1963) definition of consultation is one of the most widely used in the school consultation literature:

> The process of interaction between two professional persons—the consultant, who is a specialist, and the consultee, who invokes his help in regard to a current work problem with which the latter is having some difficulty, and which he has decided is within the former's area of specialized competence. The work problem involves the management or treatment of one or more clients of the consultee, or the planning or implementation of a program to cater to such clients. (p. 470)

Historically, school consultation started with mental health approaches that were traditionally psychoanalytic in nature and focused on both prevention and remediation for individuals, consultees, programs, or administrators. Caplan (1970) and Caplan and Caplan (1983), whose writings have largely influenced the conceptualization and implementation of this model, focused primarily on consultee-centered case consultation. Consultee-centered case consultation involves identifying possible impediments educators face when working with children, such as lack of professional knowledge, professional skills, sufficient self-confidence, or sufficient professional objectivity (Gutkin & Curtis, 1998). In the mental health consultation approach, the consultant works with the consultee to resolve the identified impediment and thereby indirectly addresses the child's concerns. Although the mental health consultation approach is one of the most commonly used models of school consultation, the outcome research for this approach has been limited. In the case of children with autism, approaches based in psychoanalytic theory would seem less beneficial than models based more in behavioral theory. However, we found no research on the use of the mental health consultation model with this population.

The ecobehavioral consultation model, as described by Gutkin and Curtis (1998), uses behavioral principles within a systems orientation in order to incorporate environmental variables that impact a child's behavioral functioning. The advantages of this model include the methodological rigor of a behavioral approach and the acknowledgment that a child's school functioning is impacted by not only variables within the school setting, but by variables outside of that setting as well. Ecobehavioral consultants work with consultees "to identify and manipulate relevant person–environment relationships to improve, eliminate, and/or prevent identified problems" (Gutkin & Curtis, 1998, p. 616). With this approach there are four steps in the consultation process:

- Step 1: As with mental health consultation, the problem is identified and defined in measurable terms.
- Step 2: The consultant and consultee develop hypotheses as to why the behaviors are occurring and interventions to address the behaviors.
- Step 3: The treatment interventions are implemented and data are collected to determine effectiveness.
- Step 4: An evaluation of the overall process is completed to ensure that the identified problems were effectively addressed.

The ecobehavioral consultation model has been scrutinized via outcome research and has been found effective for addressing a variety of behavioral issues (Gutkin & Curtis, 1998). However, the model's effectiveness with the autism population is not known at this time. We would suggest that such an approach could be highly effective when working with individuals with autism.

The organizational and systems consultation model focuses not on the individual but rather on the organization or system, ranging from classrooms, schools, and school districts to the state educational system (Gutkin & Curtis, 1998). The rationale for this model is that children and educators work more effectively in functional systems. Important strategies in this model include involving all relevant stakeholders and using a collaborative problem-solving approach. Again, specific studies of organizational and systems consultation involving the autism population are not available. However, the implementation of evidence-based practices for students with autism lags well behind the research (Walker, 2004), suggesting at least some impediments at a systems level, and the need for change at the systems level for services provided to children with autism is apparent. For example, this model could be effective at helping a system implement positive behavior supports across the entire organization to systematically teach new skills and to improve use of skills, thereby reducing challenging behaviors that are frequently observed in lower-functioning individuals with autism.

A Possible Consultation Model for Autism

Although there are no autism-specific models of school consultation, the conjoint behavioral consultation (CBC) model, developed by Sheridan and colleagues (e.g., Sheridan, Kratochwill, & Elliott, 1990; Sheridan & Steck, 1995; Sheridan, Kratochwill, & Bergan, 1996), appears promising for use with this population. Sheridan and Kratochwill (1992) described CBC as an indirect model of service delivery whereby the consultant works with both educators and parents to facilitate home and school collaboration regarding a variety of child-related problems. CBC involves four stages of consultation:

1. *Problem identification stage*: The consultant, parents, and educators identify the problematic behaviors, and baseline data are collected in both the home and school settings.
2. *Problem analysis stage*: A functional analysis of the problem is completed, and a treatment plan is developed.
3. *Treatment implementation stage*: The treatment plan is implemented in both settings, and objective data are collected to help make informed decisions about its effectiveness.
4. *Treatment evaluation stage*: The data are analyzed to determine if the treatment plan has been effective, and if it hasn't been effective then ideas are generated about how it should be changed.

CBC has undergone extensive research in a variety of areas and has been found to be (1) more effective than consultation provided in isolation to either school professionals or in a home setting (Sheridan & Colton, 1994); (2) acceptable to school psychologists as a method of service delivery (Sheridan & Steck, 1995); (3) effective with children with emotional and behavioral difficulties (Wilkinson, 2005); and (4) acceptable to parents and teachers (Sheridan et al., 2004; Wilkinson, 2005). Given the difficulties that individuals with autism face when trying to generalize skills learned in one setting to other settings, CBC appears to be a natural choice for autism consultants.

UNDERPINNINGS OF AUTISM SCHOOL CONSULTATION

There are several components that should be considered when aiming to develop productive and successful relationships between the consultant and the consultee around autism-related issues. The following expectations, or core characteristics, were adapted from the general school consultation research (Erchul & Martens, 2002; Gutkin & Curtis, 1990):

- The central component of this teaming process is that it is mutually respectful, nonhierarchical, cooperative, and voluntary.
- The consultation consists of a triadic relationship between the consultant, the educational team, and the student and parent. Research in the field of autism has demonstrated that the active involvement of parents in the educational process greatly increases the effectiveness of educational strategies (Hurth, Shaw, Izeman, Whaley, & Rogers, 1999; Iovannone, Dunlap, Huber, & Kincaid, 2003; Lord & McGee, 2001; Powers, 1992).
- When working with children with autism, sensitive information is shared between the team and consultant, and this information is always held in confidence by the consultant and consultee.
- The consultee is actively involved in the problem-solving activities and is integrally involved across the life of the consultation with planning the implementation of selected strategies. This is one of the best ways parents and educators learn how to implement the EBPS beyond the consultation period.
- Finally, the educational team retains the right to reject or accept any of the consultant's suggestions or recommendations. This creates a positive feedback loop that allows the consultant and educational team to generate alternative solutions.

While implementing these core characteristics of autism consultation and in congruence with effective educational practices for children with autism (Iovannone et al., 2003), an autism consultant's goal is to directly address the consultee's primary concern and implement EBPS across settings. Regardless of the setting (school, home, or community), the research supports the implementation of a range of evidence-based practices (Rogers, 1998). Therefore, it is important to identify an autism consultant who can implement a variety of interventions as opposed to one who espouses a single approach. Additionally, consultation for a specific aspect of autism (e.g., sensory deficits) does not appear to affect other areas of autistic deficits or overall skill development (Rogers, 1998). Thus, most effective consultations should address the needs of individuals with a diverse range of strategies and approaches.

Autism Consultation Topics

An autism consultant can assist an educational team in increasing the ability of individuals with autism to access the educational curricula by improving academic instruction so that it best matches the individual's needs, abilities, and strengths. The autism consultant can assist the educational team in developing behavioral intervention plans based on providing positive behavioral supports, implementing systematic instruction, developing structured environments, adapting specialized curriculum content, and increasing family involvement in the educational process as reviewed as follows.

Positive Behavioral Supports

Challenging behaviors (e.g., aggression, self-injurious behaviors, masturbation, property damage, or unpredictable emotional outbursts) frequently cause school staff extreme distress and affect their ability to educate students with autism. One of the most effective ways to understand the purpose of challenging behaviors and to develop successful educational plans that promote the learning of new skills and the reduction (and eventual elimination) of challenging behaviors is through the development of positive behavioral supports (PBS) (Fox, Dunlap, & Buschbacher, 2000; Horner, Carr, Strain, Todd, & Reed, 2002). PBS take an ecological approach to reducing challenging behaviors by viewing the individual's systems, settings, and lack of skills as parts of the problem. More specifically, in a PBS approach behavior is viewed as purposeful, and the purpose of the behavior can be determined through a comprehensive functional behavioral analysis (FBA). The functional behavioral analysis then guides the development of a specialized curriculum, structured instruction, and professional development through ongoing training. The FBA will also dictate new skills that need to be taught to help the individual better perform tasks. PBS are used to increase quality of life, decrease problem behaviors, and improve an individual's access to individualized curriculum. Not only are PBS highly effective for individuals with autism, but the IDEA requires the individualized education plan (IEP) team to consider using PBS to address behavior that impedes the child's learning and/or the learning of others [Section 614 (d)(3)(B)].

Specialized Curriculum

Based on the results of an individualized assessment, an autism consultant can assist in the development of a specialized curriculum using positive behavioral supports and systematic instruction to directly address the student's behavioral difficulties, communication skills, social deficits, and recreational activities (Olley, 1999). For example, consultants may need to work with the educational team to develop or expand the functional communication skills of children with limited language. Additionally, given that many individuals with autism have significant motor delays and difficulties regulating their arousal levels across settings and activities (Baranek, 2002), the consultant and educational team may need to develop a plan to systematically address an individual's sensory and motor processing impairments and teach skills that compensate for these neurological deficits. Regardless of the presenting problem, a specialized curriculum needs to be developed that addresses the specific skills and deficits observed in individuals with autism (Dunlap & Robbins, 1991). Curriculum content for older individuals who have autism and intellectual deficits needs to increase those skills that improve the individuals' ability to functionally manipulate their environment in a meaningful way and to improve their quality of life, their adaptive skills, and their current skill level.

For an autism consultant to develop specialized curriculum content for students with autism who also have intellectual disabilities, the consultant will need to take the following steps:

- Gather information from the student's educational record.
- Observe the student in multiple environments (e.g., the school system, the home environment, and community-based activities).
- Interview parents, educators, and other outside treating professionals.
- Based on all of the data, develop a comprehensive behavioral intervention plan that emphasizes positive behavioral supports (see Carr et al., 1999) to manage behaviors, make very specific recommendations to build new skills that will lead to long-term independence and suggest systematic instruction strategies that can help the teacher better implement the curriculum.

Systematic Instruction and Objective Data

The use of positive behavioral supports and behavioral principles will allow the consultant to formulate a plan that uses systematic instruction, which is vital to the success of an educational program. Systematic instruction includes altering the teaching environment, identifying teaching approaches for each IEP goal, ensuring staff have the skills to implement teaching procedures, and adjusting the instruction based on the objective data collected (Hurth et al., 1999; Westling & Fox, 2000).

Objective data allow the consultant and the IEP team to systematically evaluate the individual's progress over a given duration and to determine if the teaching approaches and strategies are having the desired outcomes. Given that autism consultants may rely on applied behavioral principles (see Cooper, Heron, & Heward, 1987, for a complete review of applied behavioral principles), the autism consultant should be expected to assist the IEP team in developing goals and behavioral objectives that are easily observed and measurable. Objective data can assist in directing the need for modifications to the individual's educational plan. In addition, having objective data about a disputed methodology or educational approach at a due process hearing can be a major factor that influences the outcome of these cases (Yell & Drasgow, 2000; Yell, Katsiyannis, Drasgow, & Herbst, 2001).

Children who have autism and intellectual disabilities learn skills at different rates (e.g., some might be nonverbal, but able to complete long division). Therefore, tracking objective data on each of the IEP or treatment goals is vital to showing the efficacy of the chosen educational strategies. An autism consultant can help develop objective data tracking methods and assist in the analysis of the data. Collecting objective data is a major tenet of applied behavior analysis (ABA) and allows the educational team to alter the educational plan during and between IEPs to most effectively meet the child's needs.

Ongoing Training by Consultants

Given that the educational demands of children with autism are very different from those of other children, many districts rely on teams that are specifically trained in evidence-based practices. However, not every district has this luxury. One of the critical functions of an autism consultant is to provide ongoing training and mentoring to the educational team, which should include the family. Over the past 30 years, researchers have investigated how to most effectively train professionals and paraprofessionals to meet the multifaceted needs of individuals with autism (McGee & Morrier, 2005). Based on this research, ongoing training will need to consist of mentoring, active demonstration of how to implement applied behavioral principles and strategies, and training about the development and implementation of positive behavioral supports and structured concepts and strategies. In addition, the training consultant should provide ongoing supervision to ensure the fidelity of the implementation of strategies and to guide the adaptation of the educational plans to ensure the long-term success of the team. For providers and educators in rural districts, receiving this ongoing coaching, mentoring, and supervision is a challenge that technology is starting to bridge (e.g., use of teleconferencing, Web broadcasting, and digital video capture). When seeking consultation for training purposes, securing an autism consultant who can provide this ongoing mentoring and direct feedback is critical to the overall success of others' abilities to implement these principles and strategies. Similarly, involving the family in this training can help improve the overall success of the programs implemented.

Family Participation

Parent involvement is considered one of the most important components of "best practices" when educating children with autism (Hurth et al., 1999; Iovannone et al., 2003; Lord & McGee, 2001). When considering seeking consultation from an autism specialist, it is important to talk directly with family members about their perspective on how an autism consultant can improve their child's educational experience. Families' belief systems and sociocultural characteristics need to be fully integrated into effective educational plans as well (Lynch & Hanson, 1998). Family involvement can be accomplished through collaborative goal setting, parent and sibling support groups, regularly scheduled meetings, classroom observations, in-home consultation, informational resources, and community service referrals.

Incorporating families' preferences into the educational plan, encouraging families to be involved in all autism-related trainings, and having families meet with their child's educational team during regularly scheduled staff meetings can substantially decrease the risk of unwanted litigation and due process hearings. More important, family involvement in all aspects of the educational plan is vital when educating individuals with autism who have significant cognitive and adaptive deficits, as their involvement will allow the educational team to capitalize on the individual's preferences and interests, which can then be used to exponentially increase the effectiveness of the educational plan. Regularly scheduled meetings and parent involvement in autism-related training will increase the consistency of the educational approaches employed across settings (i.e., home, school, and community) and with both parents and educators, thereby improving the efficacy of the educational plan, the child's adaptive skills, and parents' access to the educational curricula. Finally, an autism consultant can be a highly effective negotiator for the child's best interests when the educational team and the family are at odds. This can also help to reduce the possibility of litigation.

Barriers to Progress

In our clinical experience, we have identified several barriers that inhibit an educational team's ability to implement an autism consultant's recommendations. One of the biggest barriers is a lack of commitment by the school administration to allow school personnel opportunity to complete the preparation work needed for program implementation. An example of lack of commitment by school administration is when school districts hire an autism consultant to assist with a highly aggressive, cognitively impaired individual with autism, but they do not reduce the number of students in the teacher's classroom, provide a specific educational assistant for the student, increase the amount of time educators can spend preparing for classroom interventions, or block out specific class periods when the teacher and behavioral aides are available to systematically plan teaching opportunities. Clinical experience suggests that teachers need approximately 15 minutes of educational planning for every hour of intervention. As the school staff and educational assistants become more familiar with the educational plan and specific teaching strategies, the planning time can be reduced by half. The importance of sufficient planning to the overall success of any educational plan cannot be overstated, especially an educational plan for an individual with autism who also has impaired cognitive abilities. Thus, a lack of administration support for educator preparation time can be a significant barrier to success.

Another common barrier to success is the district's strict adherence to a state's standards and benchmarks. States have specific standards and benchmarks for each grade, and it is very difficult for children with autism and significant cognitive impairments to be at grade level even in their best-developed splinter skills (usually visual–spatial skills; see Minshew, Goldstein, & Siegel, 1997), much less in all areas of development. One critical component to developing an effective consultation plan is for the autism consultant to suggest ways of adapting the educational curricula to best fit the needs of the individual and to implement specialized instruction to support the child in maximizing his or her potential. This consultation process usually requires the participation of the special education administrators and the student's special education teacher to ensure that the child's needs are being meet while adhering to components of the state's standards and benchmarks.

SUMMARY

Lower-functioning individuals with autism present many unique challenges to educational teams that frequently require specialized knowledge and skills to remediate. Behavioral consultative models (i.e., the conjoint behavioral consultative model) can be highly effective for addressing a range of autism-related concerns. While supporting the educational team, an autism consultant will employ a host of evidence-based strategies and approaches to bring about measurable changes in an individual's skills and abilities. The following three case studies demonstrate a range of topics autism consultants can address. The first case study focuses on how consultation improved the educational plan for a lower-functioning, medically complex individual with autism. The second demonstrates how autism consultants can address specific issues that repeatedly emerge in a school district. Finally, the last case study focuses on the use of videoconferencing to assist a rural district in making organizational change to screen for autism.

CASE STUDIES

The following sections describe three different examples of consultation moving from the individual to two examples of broader systems-level school consultation. The case-based consultation example that follows presents a hypothetical case derived from a combination of many clinical case consultations.

Case-Based Consultation: Working with a Specific Student

Robert is an adolescent male high school student, diagnosed with autism, mental retardation, a seizure disorder, and mild cerebral palsy. He engages in inappropriate behaviors associated with autism, including self-stimulatory behaviors, physical aggression, and resistance to performing given tasks. Robert has moderate mental retardation and is nonverbal, although he is proficient in using a dynamic communication device to communicate his wants and needs. Robert has seizures when his temperature spikes. Thus, to decrease the chance of his contracting colds and the flu, his hands and educational equipment need to be consistently cleaned and sanitized. Due to mild cerebral palsy, Robert is not able to participate in most fine-motor tasks and he is not able to use writing implements. Although Robert ambulates independently, he regularly loses his center of gravity and balance when walking across campus. Within the past year, he has fallen seven times, resulting in sprained ankles, cuts and bruises, and a broken arm.

Currently, Robert attends school in an autism classroom with seven other students and a staff-to-student ratio of 5:8. Robert generally requires the assistance of the teacher or an aide for the majority of the school day, as he is often unable to perform the given tasks due to motor skill deficits or refuses to complete them. Robert also requires assistance throughout the day to clean and sanitize himself and his equipment, to help him ambulate safely across campus, and to assist him in using and carrying the communication device. This level of support directs attention away from the other students in the classroom, contributing to an increase in their rate of inappropriate behaviors. In addition to Robert's actual need for staff assistance, the classroom staff feels that Robert is accustomed to receiving a high level of attention from staff so that when they attempt to work with the other students in the class, he engages in negative attention-seeking behaviors (e.g., throwing objects and yelling). Robert's IEP team, including his teacher, school principal, school psychologist, and district administrator, agreed to seek outside consultation and assistance to address these issues.

The consultant met with the IEP team to discuss Robert's educational and behavioral needs as well as the overall needs of students in his current classroom. The consultant conducted a functional behavior analysis, gathering data on his inappropriate behaviors (e.g., self-stimulatory behaviors, physical aggression, and resistance to performing given tasks) and observed the effects of Robert's behavior on other students in the classroom. The results of the school observation and functional analysis were consistent with the impressions of the classroom staff. Robert required constant supervision and assistance throughout the school day due to health, medical, motor, and behavioral issues.

Robert's need for a high level of teacher support had begun to compromise the staff's ability to work with other students in the classroom. By pulling a staff member away from the class to work directly with Robert, the other students in the class did not receive the attention they needed, resulting in increased inappropriate behaviors from them as well. When Robert was pulled out of the classroom for speech therapy or occupational therapy, the other students were much calmer and more compliant. Additionally, school staff were observably more capable of meeting the needs of the other students in the class without Robert's presence. The consultant reviewed the findings with the IEP team. Robert's classroom placement was considered appropriate for his current educational and behavioral needs. However, he required full-day assistance due to his high level of individual need. Recommendations were made to the school district regarding a full-day school aide for Robert.

Additionally, recommendations were made for ongoing training and mentoring of school staff. The consultant worked directly with Robert's teacher to implement positive behavioral supports by creating and modifying class activities and individual work activities to meet his motor deficits. The classroom environment was organized to further assist with Robert's independent functioning. Robert received an assistive technology assessment and, as a result, was granted access to adaptive learning devices (an adaptive word-processing device to take the place of writing and a computer touch screen that employs specific learning software) to further accommodate his motor deficits. Robert's school staff and family members were trained in all components of the behavior intervention plan, including the implementation of positive behavioral supports (preventative interventions such as the one-to-one aide and adaptive learning devices) and reactive behavior plans (i.e., addressing behaviors when they occur).

With regard to treatment implementation, the consultant initially worked with Robert while his teacher and newly assigned full-day aide observed and charted data. This provided them with the opportunity to observe the consultant implementing the behavior intervention plans, creating a clear visual structure within the classroom environment (e.g., creating a visual schedule system with pictures, developing physical barriers by using bookshelves and brightly colored tape to demarcate specific locations for activities, and using a digital timer to signal the end of activities and remind Robert to check his schedule); modifying class activities (e.g., simplified tasks and reduced task demands to build up Robert's willingness to participate in educational activities by alternating between preferred activities and less preferred, academic activities); and incorporating the assistive technology devices into his curriculum. Gradually, within the first week, his teacher, his assigned aide, and the consultant alternated working with Robert. The consultant provided suggestions and support during this process. As Robert's teacher and assigned aide developed competence implementing the behavior intervention plans and the modified curriculum, the consultant continued to observe and provide feedback. This transition took place over a period of 3 weeks.

Thereafter, the school district requested that the consultant remain on Robert's case to consistently monitor his program and behavior intervention plans, as well as to assist the teacher in modifying Robert's curriculum. The consultant met with the teacher and the assigned aide once a month to review his progress and program needs. The consultant also observed and assisted Robert's classroom staff for up to 6 hours per month over the next 3 months. By the fourth month, the consultant decreased consultation and observation time to only once per month and assisted in the classroom only when the teacher deemed it necessary.

The results from the changes in Robert's program, including changes in staffing, creating and modifying curriculum to better meet his learning needs, and implementing behavior intervention plans, resulted in a significant decrease in his inappropriate behaviors and an increase in compliance in performing given tasks. Robert learned to use the assistive technology equipment and enjoyed learning through computer programs. He also benefited greatly from the increased and consistent assistance from the assigned aide. Over time, the assigned aide was able to gradually fade the level of assistance provided to further increase Robert's independent functioning. Within 9 months, Robert was proficient in utilizing the adaptive devices and the computer programs so that he functioned independently with learned tasks. At that time, the assigned aide was faded out to part-day assistance, where the aide was assigned to small group activities to help modify those activities and to assist when Robert ambulated across the campus. Robert continued to demonstrate the need for part-day, one-on-one assistance throughout high school due to continued health issues, motor skill deficits, and the need for modified educational tasks. However, Robert's behavioral problems decreased and his level of independence increased, allowing classroom staff to work with the other students in his class.

Topic-Based Consultation

Challenging or aggressive behaviors, such as throwing or destroying objects along with hitting, kicking, or biting self or others, are commonly observed in young children with autism (Horner, Carr, Strain, Todd, & Reed, 2002). When the child with autism physically matures, entering middle and high school settings where there are more expectations for sitting and attending in desk-filled classrooms, these behaviors can present a serious safety risk to teachers and other students. Examples from clinical experience demonstrate that school districts often respond to challenging behaviors of individuals with autism by either repeatedly calling parents to pick up their children from school or by suspending these individuals from school for a period of time. In more extreme cases, schools have called law enforcement officers to physically restrain these individuals and take them to the nearest emergency room. Without a proactive plan to prepare teachers and aides to address the potential challenging behaviors of individuals with autism, school districts are simply setting up school staff to struggle with each case as the need arises. This process can be time consuming and ultimately more costly for the school district. A topic-based consultation approach can provide school districts with a plan to proactively train school staff to understand the various functions of an individual's challenging behaviors and implement strategies that not only address but also prevent challenging behaviors.

Once school districts have identified personnel from a variety of school settings who have or will have children with autism assigned to their classrooms, the first step for the consultant is to conduct a series of intensive (all-day) training workshops that involve a combination of didactic and hands-on instruction. This training should involve the following components.

• *Teach an understanding of the core and associated features of autism.* School personnel need to have a working knowledge of how the core features of autism present unique challenges when teaching this population. This will involve the consultant explaining in detail what is known about the unique learning styles and different coexisting issues (e.g., speech and language delays, sensory sensitivities, or medical issues) present in this population. Following this, there should be a review of how this knowledge base of the "nature of the autism" translates into an understanding the function of these individuals' behavior problems and identification of effective intervention approaches. Cox and Schopler (1993) use the metaphor of an iceberg to explain the importance of not only addressing the obvious behaviors (visible tip of the iceberg), but also considering the underlying core impairments of autism and other reasons for the behavior (what lies beneath the obvious tip of the iceberg) in order to more effectively address or change the behavior presentations of the individual with autism. Finally, it may be helpful to enlist the support of other disciplines (e.g., speech–language pathologists and occupational therapists) to give presentations on their area of expertise and explain how they can support classroom teachers in better understanding and addressing the behavior problems in this population. (See Chapters 1–6 for more information about understanding behaviors and associated problems in the individual with autism.)

• *Teach functional behavior assessment strategies.* Although the process of collecting data to understand the function of presenting behavior problems in individuals with autism may at first glance appear too time-consuming for teachers and aides, a consultant's clear explanation of the necessary components of a functional assessment may help to reinforce the idea that behaviors can be understandable and manageable. Explaining that the general function of most behaviors is to either gain access to something or to avoid something may also provide a framework for teachers and aides to begin categorizing otherwise misunderstood behaviors. The initial components of a functional behavioral assessment involve collecting information (through observation and interview) about the nature of the behavior problem, the contexts in which the behavior occurs or does not occur, the antecedents and consequences related to the behavior, and the communication ability of the individual with autism (Foster-Johnson & Dunlap, 1993). Following this process, hypotheses are developed about the purposes and maintaining factors of the behaviors, and then with this information an intervention plan can be developed. One of the most effective ways to train individuals in the use of functional behavioral assessments is through cases that the trainees are currently experiencing, through hands-on examples, and through ongoing coaching and mentoring.

• *Teach cognitive and behavioral intervention techniques.* Appendix 12.1 provides a list of strategies derived from behavioral learning theory and principles of ABA that have been proven effective with individuals with autism (e.g., Matson, Benavidez, Compton, Paclawskyj, & Baglio, 1996; Rogers, 1998), along with the use of visual cues and structure (e.g., Hume, Loftin, & Odom, 2005; MacDuff, Krantz, & McClannahan, 1993). These strategies are not included as a comprehensive list, but are a general overview to provide a frame of reference for positive and proactive behavior intervention and management options (i.e., positive behavioral supports). It is also important for the consultant to incorporate peer models for enhancing the social interactions of the individual with autism. (See Chapter 10 for a discussion of the use of peer models with individuals with autism.) It is suggested that the consultant provide a combination of video clips of case examples and hands-on demonstration, as well as opportunities to practice these behavior intervention and management strategies in order to reinforce the concepts with trainees. It may also be necessary to allow time for trainees to present case examples from their classroom settings and to problem-solve how to address behavior problems specific to certain cases.

• *Review and demonstrate strategies to modify the classroom environment.* Studies of children with autism in their natural environment have demonstrated that the introduction of external structure (e.g., visual cues and physical organization) and individualized, predictable routines can help increase a child's engagement in on-task behaviors and decrease behavior problems (Hume, 2005; MacDuff et al., 1993; Mesibov, Browder, & Kirkland, 2002). There is also evidence to support alternating activity schedules between preferred (activities not associated with challenging behaviors) and less preferred activities (those that evoke challenging behaviors) in order to decrease the likelihood of behavior problems occurring throughout the individual's day (O'Reilly, Sigafoos, Lancioni, Edrisinha, & Andrews, 2005). The structured teaching methods of Division TEACCH (Treatment and Education of Autistic and related Communication-handicapped CHildren)

include strategies for modifying the physical environment to minimize visual distractions and enhance comprehension of expectations
(Schopler, Mesibov, & Hearsey, 1995). (Also see Chapter 11 for more
information on developing structured environments to manage behaviors.) In addition to providing trainees with both a didactic overview
and hands-on practice of these strategies, it may also be necessary for
the consultant to visit each classroom setting to help teachers make
appropriate modifications to their classroom environments specific to
the needs of the individuals in their classrooms, while taking individual
building space limitations into account.

• *Provide ongoing topic-based training or individual classroom
consultation.* Finally, it is important for the consultant to be available
on an ongoing basis to classroom teachers and aides to continue to reinforce and monitor the implementation of the concepts and strategies
taught during the workshops. This will help to ensure not only that
there is follow-through of the skills taught, but also that techniques
taught are appropriately modified and applied to meet the individual
needs of the student with autism.

Systems-Based Consultation

Through the Southwest Autism Network (SWAN) and the Rural Early
Access to Child Healthcare (REACH) Network, we frequently provide
autism consultative services to rural communities across New Mexico.
REACH is a telehealth program whose goal is to increase access to specialty services for children with disabilities who live in rural communities. We recently used REACH's videoconferencing technology to help a
rural district make substantial systems change in its evaluation practices.

Like many system-based consultations, this particular relationship
started with a case-based consultation and was quickly expanded to
include a system-based consultation paradigm. During an initial meeting
the consultation team and school administrators set a goal of improving
the district's evaluation procedures for children with autism. Our primary goal with the rural district was to develop an efficient and effective
system to determine if a child met the educational exceptionality criteria
for autism.

Based on the model developed by Noland and Gabriels (2004), our
first step was to identify two teams of professionals that would serve as
the district's autism specialists. Each team had a school psychologist,
speech therapist, occupational therapist, and special education teacher.
These two teams were then assigned to work with either children
between 3 and 8 years old or with children older than 9 years. As part of

the consultative agreement, the director of special education for the district was also to participate in the training. We saw this as essential to ensure sustainability and implementation of systems change.

After identifying the two evaluation teams, we then developed a screening and referral process for each of the age groups. For example, for the older group, a referral was made by a teacher or parent, a set of questionnaires was sent to the family, and then classroom and community observations were scheduled. If any of the parent/teacher questionnaires were positive, the individual was then scheduled for a complete psychoeducational evaluation.

We also scheduled a series of training sessions on the essentials of identifying children and adolescents with autism and on autism-related instruments, questionnaires, and tests. The consultants first demonstrated test administration via videotaped examples, which were shown to the rural teams during weekly videoconference case discussions. The teams started to conduct assessments while digitally videotaping the evaluations. These digital videotapes were then sent to SWAN for review and critique. Each team member received specific feedback during the regularly scheduled videoconferences. During these conferences, the SWAN team discussed specific behaviors that were consistent with a diagnosis of autism and those behaviors that were not. We were also able to co-score several Autism Diagnostic Observation Schedules (ADOS) while the test was administered by using IP-based videoconferencing technology (i.e., live Internet-based interactions). For each student, SWAN participated in a case discussion to review all of the testing and to assist the team in arriving at an appropriate assessment of educational exceptionality. We are continuing to use these case-based discussions to hone team members' understanding of the diagnostic profile of children with autism and their clinical judgment in identifying individuals with autism.

After the system-based consultation goals were achieved, the rural district and SWAN explored ways to continue the consultative relationship and to provide training in family participation, development of specialized curricula, data collection of IEP goals, and implementation of systematic instruction approaches. Currently, as we complete the autism evaluations, we are observing the children in their educational settings via digital videotaping. These videos are then reviewed during the regularly scheduled, case-based videoconferences and serve as a means to train the team on multiple approaches to teaching children with autism. We are now seeing that the teams feel more effective in identifying children with autism and in developing educational plans, and they are starting to provide direct consultations to other educators.

REFERENCES

Ayres, B. J., Meyer, L. H., Erevelles, N., & Park-Lee, S. (1994). Easy for you to say: Teacher perspectives on implementing most promising practices. *Journal of American Speech and Hearing, 19,* 84–93.

Baranek, G. T. (2002). Efficacy of sensory and motor interventions for children with autism. *Journal of Autism and Developmental Disorders, 32,* 397–422.

Caplan, G. (1963). Types of mental health consultation. *American Journal of Orthopsychiatry, 33,* 470–481.

Caplan, G. (1970). *The theory and practice of mental health consultation.* New York: Basic Books.

Caplan, G., & Caplan, R. B. (1983). *Mental health consultation and collaboration.* San Francisco: Jossey-Bass.

Carr, E. G., Horner, R. H., Turnbull, A. P., Marquis, J., Magito-Mclaughlin, D., McAtee, M. L., et al. (1999). *Positive behavior support for people with developmental disabilities: A research synthesis.* Washington, DC: American Association on Mental Retardation.

Cooper, J. O., Heron, T., & Heward, W. L. (1987). *Applied behavior analysis.* Upper Saddle River, NJ: Prentice Hall.

Cox, R. D., & Schopler, E. (1993). Aggression and self-injurious behaviors in persons with autism: The TEACCH approach. *Acta Paedopsychiatrica, 56,* 85–90.

Dunlap, G., & Robbins, F. R. (1991). Current perspectives in service delivery for young children with autism. *Comprehensive Mental Health Care, 1,* 177–219.

Erchul, W. P., & Martens, B. K. (2002). *School consultation: Conceptual and empirical bases of practice.* New York: Kluwer Academic Publishers.

Foster-Johnson, L., & Dunlap, G. (1993). Using functional assessment to develop effective, individualized interventions. *Teaching Exceptional Children, 25,* 44–50.

Fox, L., Dunlap, G., & Buschbacher, P. (2000). Understanding and intervening with children's challenging behavior: A comprehensive approach. In A. M. Wetherby & B. M. Prizant (Eds.), *Autism spectrum disorders: A transactional developmental perspective* (Vol. 9, pp. 307–331). Baltimore: Brookes.

Gutkin, T. B., & Curtis, M. J. (1990). School-based consultation: Theory, techniques, and research. In T. B. Gutkin & C. R. Reynolds (Eds.), *The handbook of school psychology* (2nd ed., pp. 577–611). New York: Wiley.

Gutkin, T. B., & Curtis, M. J. (1998). School consultation theory and practice: The art and science of indirect service delivery. In T. G. C. Reynolds (Ed.), *Handbook of school psychology.* New York: Wiley.

Horner, R., Carr, E. G., Strain, P. S., Todd, A. W., & Reed, H. K. (2002). Problem behavior interventions for young child with autism: A research synthesis. *Journal of Autism and Developmental Disorders, 32,* 423–446.

Hume, K., Loftin, R., & Odom, S. (2005, May). *Effects of an individual work system on the independent academic work skills in children with autism.* Paper presented at the 4th International Meeting for Autism Research (IMFAR), Boston, MA.

Hurth, J., Shaw, E., Izeman, S. G., Whaley, K., & Rogers, S. J. (1999). Areas of agreement about effective practices among programs serving young children with autism spectrum disorder. *Infants and Young Children, 12,* 17–26.

Iovannone, R., Dunlap, G., Huber, H., & Kincaid, D. (2003). Effective education practices for students with autism spectrum disorder. *Focus on Autism and Other Developmental Disabilities, 18,* 150–165.

Lord, C., & McGee, J. P. (Eds.). (2001). *Educating children with autism.* Washington, DC: National Academy Press.

Lynch, E. W., & Hanson, M. J. (1998). *Developing cultural competence: A guide for working with children and their families* (2nd ed.). Baltimore: Brookes.

MacDuff, G. S., Krantz, P. J., & McClannahan, L. E. (1993). Teaching children with autism to use photographic activity schedules: Maintenance and generalization of complex response chains. *Journal of Applied Behavior Analysis, 26*(1), 89–97.

Matson, J. L., Benavidez, D. A., Compton, L. S., Paclawskyj, T., & Baglio, C. (1996). Behavioral treatment of autistic persons: A review of research from 1980 to the present. *Research in Developmental Disabilities, 17,* 433–465.

McGee, G. G., & Morrier, M. J. (2005). Preparation of autism specialists. In F. R. Volkmar, P. P. Rhea, K. Ami, & D. C. Cohen (Eds.), *Handbook of autism and pervasive developmental disorders: Assessment, interventions and policy* (Vol. 2, pp. 1123–1160). Hoboken, NJ: Wiley.

Mesibov, G., Browder, D., & Kirkland, C. (2002). Using individualized schedules as a component of positive behavioral support for students with developmental disabilities. *Journal of Positive Behavioral Support, 4,* 73–79.

Minshew, N. J., Goldstein, G., Siegel, D. J. (1997). Neuropsychological functioning in autism: Profile of a complex information processing disorder. *Journal of the International Neuropsychological Society, 3,* 303–316.

Noland, R. M., & Gabriels, R. L. (2004). Screening and identifying children with autism spectrum disorder in the public school system: The development of a model process. *Journal of Autism and Developmental Disorders, 34,* 265–277.

Olley, J. G. (1999). Curriculum for students with autism. *School Psychology Review, 28,* 595–606

O'Reilly, M., Sigafoos, J., Lancioni, G., Edrisinha, C., & Andrews, A. (2005). An examination of the effects of a classroom activity schedule on levels of self-injury and engagement for a child with severe autism. *Journal of Autism and Developmental Disorders, 35*(3), 305–311.

Powers, M. D. (1992). Early intervention for children with autism. In D. E. Berkell (Ed.), *Autism: Identification, education and treatment* (pp. 225–252). Hillsdale, NJ: Erlbaum.

Reynolds, C. R., & Gutkin, T. B. (1998). *The handbook of school psychology* (Vol. 3). New York: Wiley.

Rogers, S. J. (1998). Empirically supported comprehensive treatments for young children with autism. *Journal of Clinical Child Psychology, 27,* 168–179.

Scheuerman, B., Webber, J., Boutot, E. A., & Goodwin, M. (2003). Problems with personnel preparation in autism spectrum disorders. *Focus on Autism and Other Developmental Disabilities, 18,* 197–206.

Schopler, E., Mesibov, G. B., & Hearsey, K. (1995). Structured teaching in the

TEACCH system. In E. Schopler & G. B. Mesibov (Eds.), *Learning and cognition in autism* (pp. 243–268). New York: Plenum Press.

Sheridan, S. M., Erchul, W. P., Brown, M. S., Dowd, S. E., Warnes, E. D., Martin, D. C., et al. (2004). Perceptions of helpfulness in conjoint behavioral consultation: Congruence and agreement between teachers and parents. *School Psychology Quarterly, 19,* 121–140.

Sheridan, S. M., & Kratochwill, T. R. (1992). Behavioral parent–teacher consultation: Conceptual and research considerations. *Journal of School Psychology, 30,* 117–139.

Sheridan, S. M., Kratochwill, T. R., & Bergan, J. R. (1996). *Conjoint behavioral consultation: A procedural manual.* New York: Plenum Press.

Sheridan, S., Kratochwill, T., & Elliott, S. (1990). Behavioral consultation with parents and teachers: Delivering treatment for socially withdrawn children at home and school. *School Psychology Review, 19,* 33–52.

Sheridan, S. M., & Steck, M. C. (1995). Acceptability of conjoint behavioral consultation: A national survey of school psychologists. *School Psychology Review, 24,* 633–647.

Walker, H. M. (2004). Commentary: Use of evidence-based interventions in schools: Where we've been, where we are, and where we need to go. *School Psychology Review, 33*(3), 398–407.

Westling, D. L., & Fox, L. (2000). *Teaching students with severe disabilities* (2nd ed.). Englewood Cliffs, NJ: Prentice Hall.

Wilkinson, L. A. (2005). Bridging the research-to-practice gap in school-based consultation: An example of using case studies. *Journal of Educational and Psychological Consultation, 16,* 175–200.

Yell, M. L., & Drasgow, E. (2000). Litigating a free appropriate public education: The Lovaas hearings and cases. *Journal of Special Education, 33,* 205–214.

Yell, M. L., Katsiyannis, A., Drasgow, E., & Herbst, M. (2001). Developing legally correct and educationally appropriate programs for students with autism spectrum disorder. *Focus on Autism and Other Developmental Disabilities, 18,* 182–191.

Appendix 12.1

Positive Behavior Intervention and Management Strategies

1. Use **"First do this, then get that" directives** with the "first" item being something more difficult for the individual with autism and the "then" item being something more enjoyable. If the individual has limited understanding or requires visual reminders to stay on task, this direction can be communicated with the aid of pictures such as a two-picture schedule.

   - *Example:* "[Individual's name], first clean up [difficult activity], then play on the computer [preferred activity]."
   - *Example:* "First clean dishes [independent work activity], and then we will have a thumb war [individual identifies an activity as a reward]."

2. **Provide visual structure.**

   - Create an object, picture, or word schedule for the individual with autism that alternates between preferred and less preferred activities.
   - Use a *digital timer* to indicate how much time an activity takes and when it will be finished.
   - Provide a mini-schedule or list of step-by-step expectations for group, classroom work, or chore activities.

3. **Lower expectations during difficult times.** Lower expectations for individuals with autism so that they can complete adult-directed tasks *quickly and successfully,* and are able to move on to more enjoyable/preferred activities.

4. **Have the individual go to a quiet or relaxation area** on a regular basis to practice having independent fun and quiet time. This area should be a place away from potential distractions (e.g., reduced number of people, fewer visual distractions, less auditory distraction). Individuals can then go to this location when they appropriately request a break or can go on a regular basis as part of their daily schedule, not just when they are upset and need to calm down. The goal is to have individuals begin to associate feeling positive with this area so they can more quickly calm down when they need to. A time limit should be set for this area, such as 10 or 15 minutes, so that the individual does not use this area to isolate indefinitely. This area might have a comfortable place to sit (e.g., beanbag chair, blanket, mat) and a *few* interesting objects with which to fiddle (e.g., squishy balls, glitter wands, light spinners/chasers). See Groden, Baron, & Groden (2006) for more information about ways to teach individuals with autism how to cope with stress and use relaxation strategies.

(continued)

5. **Use a calm, low voice and as few words as possible** when addressing an agitated individual with autism, and consider videotaping for review of responses. When parents and educators observe the videos at a later time, they frequently find that they have inadvertently exacerbated the situation by giving the individual too many commands or by using too many words.

6. **Use positive language,** for example, avoid saying "Don't do that" and rather redirect the individual with autism by saying, "How about this" or "Try this." Provide a visual example or demonstration, or an alternative idea/ solution.

7. **Provide choices that are equally reinforcing.** Give individuals with autism choices between two behaviors or activities to help them feel like they have some control in the situation.

   - *Example:* "[Individual's name], you can choose to either listen to music or read a book during this time."

8. **Ignore mild upset behaviors** so that they don't develop into more out-of-control problem behaviors. Avoid engaging individuals with autism in verbal arguments. Tell them briefly and calmly, "When you use inside voices, you can do [preferred activity]."

9. **Provide individuals with time to complete requested tasks.** Try counting to 5 or 10 before repeating a direction or use a timer to signal when activities need to be completed. Many individuals with autism require additional time to process directions and, with every repetition of the direction, the individual with autism must process the direction from the beginning. It is also important to check in with individuals to make sure they comprehended the statement by asking them, "What are you to do?" Individuals will frequently process information without looking directly at the adult who is talking to them, so it should not be assumed that they did not hear the instructions. Before repeating the instructions, check the individual's comprehension of the expectation.

10. **Provide fidget materials** to help the individual with autism remain focused during less preferred activities such as large groups.

11. **Use natural consequences** when the individual's actions cause a problem.

    - *Example:* "You can have computer time starting at 3:00 P.M. for 15 minutes. So the faster you finish [activity] or get calm, the more time you'll have on the computer."
    - *Example:* If the child gets angry and spits or throws things, the natural consequence is to have him or her clean up the mess after calming down, but before moving on to the next preferred activity.

12. **Increase positive time together.** Teach classroom peers how to have fun with the individual who has autism. The more they can have fun together on a routine basis, the more the individual with autism can learn how to engage with others in positive versus negative ways.

13. **Acknowledge positive behaviors.** Catch the individual being good and provide positive attention. The goal is to provide motivation for individuals to engage in positive behaviors. The general rule is to catch them five times doing a positive behavior for every one time they are corrected. It is important to specifically state to the child what he or she is doing well.

   * *Example:* While giving the individual a high five say, "[Individual's name], I like the way you raised your hand when you wanted to speak."
   * *Example:* "[Individual's name], you did a good job listening."

14. **Build on strengths.** Use the individual's strengths to help shape positive behavior.

   * *Example:* Have individuals with autism share their special interest with the group or be a teacher's assistant.

15. **Teach emotional regulation skills.** Teach individuals to request a break (e.g., verbally or by signing, picture exchange, or object exchange) or to indicate when they are done with a task. When teaching emotional regulation, it is important to read individuals' subtle behavioral cues that indicate when they are becoming frustrated and have them request to stop the activity. Immediately respect the request and, over time, extend the duration or number of items to be completed before stopping the activity.

13

Criminal Justice Issues and Autistic Disorder

Alicia V. Hall
Michele Godwin
Harry H. Wright
Ruth K. Abramson

The literature indicates that individuals with disabilities are more likely to become involved in the criminal justice system than persons without disabilities (Lord & McGee, 2001). The likelihood of a person with any developmental disability becoming a victim of crime is four to ten times higher than that of the general population of nondisabled individuals (Sobsey & Doe, 1991). Individuals with a disability are vulnerable to being victims of a variety of crimes including economic crimes, child abuse and neglect, and sexual assault. Moreover, studies have shown that there is a high probability of frequent and repeated victimization because the perpetrators tend to be caregivers or family members, and an individual with a disability can be unable to verbally report an attack or to fight off the attacker (Sobsey & Doe, 1991). Research also indicates that individuals with autism will have up to seven times more contacts with law enforcement during their lifetimes than the general population (Curry, Posluszny, & Kraska, 1993).

Although individuals with a disability are generally more likely to be victims of a crime, they can also be the perpetrators of a crime. This is of particular concern for individuals with autism because of the social, communication, and behavioral impairments specific to the diagnosis, which can increase their vulnerability to a variety of forensic issues. For example, the social impairments that are a defining diagnostic feature of autism (American Psychiatric Association, 2000) can impair the way individuals with autism understand social rules and values. These social deficits can also impair their ability to understand how their behaviors affect others and, in turn, affect how individuals with autism are understood by personnel in the criminal justice system. The only known study to address the prevalence of forensic issues in autism documented that as many as 15% of the juveniles evaluated in a Swedish forensic setting were diagnosed with autism (Siponmaa, Kristiansson, Jonson, Nyden, & Gillberg, 2001).

This chapter will highlight how the core diagnostic features of autism and resulting behaviors can make this population vulnerable to involvement with law enforcement, either as victims or perpetrators of a crime. The goal is to promote discussions between personnel in the law enforcement and criminal justice system and the community of autism-specific professionals and caregivers to develop a better understanding of how to intervene in cases involving individuals with autism.

NONCRIMINAL ISSUES AND SAFETY MEASURES

Noncriminal Issues

Law enforcement may be called to intervene in a situation involving an individual with autism for a variety of noncriminal reasons. For example, persons unfamiliar with children who have autism might misinterpret their behaviors, such as head banging while loudly repeating a specific phrase in an agitated manner, as bizarre or disruptive. In addition, these behaviors in an older child or adolescent with autism can be interpreted as quite odd, even threatening, by laypersons, thus prompting them to call the police. In these cases, the police may be told to respond to a report of a "mentally ill" person or to someone suspected of using drugs. Demonstrating inappropriate social boundaries, such as standing in close proximity to or touching strangers, has also resulted in individuals with autism being involved with the police. For example, there is a documented case of a boy with autism whose special interest was tickling women, even those whom he did not know, under their arms. This resulted in legal involvement because the boy's motivation for this behavior was misinterpreted as sexual when, more likely, it was his way to initiate social interaction (Davis & Schunick, 2002). Another example of possible police involvement might be a well-meaning stranger reporting suspected child abuse after observing a parent restraining an out-of-control child with autism in public. The amount of force necessary to hold a child with autism may look suspicious to a layperson.

Finally, a common reason the police might be called to intervene is elopement. Elopement is a situation in which individuals with autism escape from home or school, or from parents and caregivers in public (Debbaudt, 2002). One difficulty with elopement is that persons with autism may not realize they are missing or lost. Adults and children with autism can wander off with the thought of going to a favorite place or to see something that interests them. They may not be able to communicate to someone that they want to leave or, if they have communication skills, they may not understand why it is important to do so. Police involvement can occur either when the parent discovers the person is missing or when the person is found in an environment where his or her presence causes problems or is perceived as inappropriate.

Two examples illustrate the impact of elopement on the parent, the individual with autism, and the community. The first example involves children with autism who elope when out in the community with their parents or caregivers, and the second example illustrates more serious consequences of elopement. Ben, a preschooler, loved the sound of falling water. One day, while at the mall with his parents, he ran off. With the help of mall security personnel, Ben was found standing at a fountain in the middle of the mall. Ben was so engrossed in this special interest that he did not respond to either of his parents. Because there was no other way to confirm that these were in fact the parents of this child, the security personnel were very reluctant to release Ben to his parents (Githens, 1998). In the second case, Tobias, a preschool-age child, eloped from the house in the middle of the night. Tobias's father awoke at 4:00 A.M. to prepare to go to work. He noticed a light on and the front door standing wide open. The father immediately checked Tobias's room to find him gone. As his parents were searching the neighborhood for Tobias, a police officer stopped them. They informed the officer of the situation and the officer followed them home. Once the parents were home, the officer informed them that Tobias was involved in a hit and run accident. Tobias was pronounced dead at the local hospital on arrival ("Autistic Boy Killed," 2006). As police officers began to investigate the incident, they questioned the parents in a way that suggested that they felt that the parents had been neglectful. This added to the stress of the situation for the parents.

Safety Measures

There are several safety measures caregivers can take to decrease the likelihood of children leaving the home without notice.

Alarm Systems

If the child or adult with autism tends to elope, families may need an alarm system. Along with setting up an alarm system, it can be helpful for parents to get to know their neighbors and to educate them about their child's special needs. Neighbors can then be on the alert and notify parents if they see something unusual.

The alarm systems available have a wide cost range. There are simple systems from drugstores or discount chains that set off chimes or an alarm each time a door or window is opened. There are more expensive security systems and services provided by companies such as Brinks or ADT. There are also perimeter alert systems that are set off if anyone or anything crosses into or out of the property. In some states the cost of an alarm system may be reimbursable. Such is the case in Pennsylvania, where children with autism who are also mentally retarded can receive assistance under the Family Driven Support Services program (*www.dpw.state.pa.us/Disable/AutismAffairs*; see autism taskforce).

Transmitter receiver alarm systems are available for use outside of the home and are extremely reliable and easy to use. These systems allow parents to attach the receiver, which comes in a variety of shapes (e.g., animals or balls), to their child's shoe or belt. If the child wanders off, the parents can press the transmitter on their key chain and the receiver chirps, alerting the parents to their child's location. There are other transmitter receiver systems that allow parents to set a distance, anywhere from 6 to 30 feet. When the child goes beyond the set distance, the parents' transmitter will beep, letting them know that their child has wandered off. A more expensive option is a handheld GPS system. This system allows parents to pinpoint the exact location of a missing child. However, these systems are limited in that they rely on cell towers or satellites to locate the child. Therefore, a GPS signal could be interrupted by cloud cover, lack of a cell tower, or a building's roof, preventing a child from being found immediately.

Identification Cards

Children who will tolerate wearing a medical alert bracelet should have one. There are types of ID bracelets that have pictures on one side and personal information on the other. These bracelets look more like jewelry and this may increase the child's willingness to wear one. For children who will not tolerate wearing a medical alert or ID bracelet on their wrist, parents can consider threading it through a shoelace, attaching it to a belt, or using it as a zipper pull on a jacket. (See Chapter 9 for specific information about medical alert bracelets.)

Parents can also make a preprinted card with a brief description of autism and some of their child's personal information on one side of the card. On the other side of the card, parents can attach a family picture. Both the parents and the child should carry a copy of the card in a wallet or pocket, as this will help provide proof to officials that this is their child. This could prevent a long wait in a security office or police station. Parents should also make similar cards for their child's teachers with a picture of the teacher and child in the classroom. This will be helpful if a child elopes from school or during field trips.

Another identification strategy is to make a temporary tattoo using specialized paper available from office supply or craft stores. On the tattoo, parents can put the child's first name, their first names, and an emergency cell phone number. The tattoo can be placed somewhere on the child (e.g., upper shoulder or high on the back) so that an officer will find it when looking for identification. The tattoo should not be put anywhere that is easily seen by the public, as this can present a safety risk. Another alternative is putting identification information on the inside of clothing.

FORENSIC PSYCHOLOGY

Although noncriminal and safety issues are the most common ways children and adults with autism encounter law enforcement, there is a subpopulation of individuals with autism that will come into contact with the criminal justice system as victims of or defendants in crimes. This often presents a problem for parents and professionals who are unfamiliar with the criminal justice system. The following section provides an overview of the issues that will affect persons with autism in the criminal justice system.

The court will evaluate any person with a developmental disability who is charged with a crime. A mental health professional, such as a forensic psychologist or psychiatrist, will perform this evaluation. Forensic psychology is the branch of psychology that combines psychological and legal concepts, and experts in that field are called to provide testimony regarding criminal and/or civil matters. The practice of forensic psychology addresses a number of areas. The most common area of practice is assessing individuals' competency or understanding of the court process at various stages (i.e., trial, sentencing, medical decisions) or their mental state at the time of the offense (capacity). To aid in understanding both of these concepts, a brief review is provided next.

Competency to Stand Trial

An individual charged with a crime must first be competent to proceed with all aspects of the legal process for that process to be considered fair. Issues regarding a defendant's competency to stand trial have been particularly significant in the area of forensic psychology. There are three rationales for why individuals being tried should be competent. First, defendants must be able to assist their attorney with collecting information about their case to aid in their defense (Stafford, 2003). Second, defendants must be able to choose an appropriate attorney for their case, participate in the court by confronting their accusers, and, if elected to do so, possess an ability to provide meaningful testimony. Individuals who do not fully understand the court proceedings during their trial are being denied their Sixth Amendment rights to *due process* (Melton, Petrila, Poythress, & Slobogin, 1997). The third rationale addresses the notion that if defendants do not understand the reasons why they are being punished, the objective of that phase of the proceedings does not carry the same meaning (Stafford, 2003). Therefore, defendants should be able to understand the entire criminal court process and have the ability to stand trial, to be sentenced, to participate in probation revocation proceedings, and to revoke the use of the insanity defense.

Legal Standard for Competency to Stand Trial

In most states there are two prongs to the competency evaluation. The first prong is that the individual must possess a factual and rational understanding of the court proceedings. An individual who is factually competent or has a basic understanding of the court proceedings would be likely to:

- Have an awareness of the charges being brought against him or her.
- Understand and follow the court proceedings (e.g., know the purpose of a trial).
- Know the roles of various courtroom officials including the

judge, jury, prosecuting attorney, defense attorney, and possible witnesses.

- Have an awareness of the police report and the circumstances surrounding his or her arrest.
- Have knowledgeable awareness of the plea options available and the consequences associated with each plea (e.g., pleading guilty would likely lead to sentencing and punishment).

The second prong addresses defendants' capacity to cooperate with their attorney to aid in their defense. For example, if defendants believe that their attorney is biased in some way or is on the side of the prosecutor, their competency would be considered questionable, given that they would view their attorney as functioning in an adversarial role rather than as one who provides assistance to them. If defendants have sufficient rational understanding of court process and capacity to cooperate with their attorney, then they are able to proceed with their court case and are found competent to stand trial (Stafford, 2003).

A mere diagnosis of a mental impairment, such as autism, does not automatically render a person incompetent to stand trial (*Feguer v. United States,* 1962; *Swisher v. United States,* 1965). However, the core symptoms of autism may, in fact, render a defendant with autism incompetent to stand trial. For example, impairments in communication may impede an individual's ability to consult with and assist counsel. Likewise, a defendant with autism may have severe cognitive deficits that prevent him or her from comprehending simple legal concepts such as "guilt" or "innocence." In the cases reviewed, as a general rule, defendants with more severe impairments were held to be incompetent while those defendants with less severe impairments proceeded to trial. For example, Raymond Frye, who was charged with transporting a stolen vehicle in interstate commerce, was found incompetent to stand trial after a psychiatrist stated that Frye had several mental impairments, including "autistic and unrealistic thinking," which resulted in, among other things, "markedly impaired judgment and insight" (*Frye v. Settle,* 1958, p. 12). The psychiatrist concluded, and the court agreed, that Frye was incompetent to stand trial (*Wieter v. Settle,* 1961).

Competency to Stand Trial: Evaluations for Special Populations

The majority of the people who are referred for a competency evaluation also have a major mental illness classified by the DSM-IV-TR (American Psychiatric Association, 2000). The bulk of the research on trial evaluations for special populations has centered on addressing competency issues for individuals with such mental illnesses as schizophrenia and mood disorders. However in recent years, the question of how to assess and make determinations of competency has shifted to include the importance of competency issues for persons with mental retardation. According to Everington and Luckasson (1992), defendants who have been diagnosed with mentally retardation are in jeopardy of passing through the entire legal process without being able to fully understand or participate in the process because of their cognitive limitations. This issue is especially important to the autism community since an estimated 70% of individuals with autism are also mentally retarded (Happe & Frith, 1996). Given the sometimes subjective nature of determining competency for individuals diagnosed with mental retardation and the potential for evaluator error, a specific instrument, the *Competence Assessment for Standing Trial for Defendants with Mental Retardation* (CAST-MR), was developed by Everington and Luckasson in 1992. This measure contains 50 questions, including 40 multiple choice, that cover three areas: basic legal concepts, skills to assist defense, and understanding case events. The goal of asking questions in a multiple-choice format is to ensure that accurate results will be obtained. This format has been cited as being appropriate for individuals with mental retardation (Everington & Luckasson, 1992). However, there is limited research on evaluating the competency status of individuals with autistic disorder.

Capacity

As noted in the previous section, once individuals are deemed competent to stand trial, they may proceed with all aspects of their criminal case. Most often when individuals are labeled competent to stand trial, they are then able to enter a plea by working with their attorney to make an informed choice based on the evidence and facts of the case. To be held accountable for almost all crimes, the law specifies that the mental state of the accused at the time the offense was committed be classified as "intentional," "knowing," "purposeful," "malicious," "reckless," or "negligent" (American Law Institute, 1980–1985; Estrich, 1998; Warboys, Burrell, Peters, & Ramiu, 1994). Melton and colleagues (1997) described the insanity defense as being the most controversial issue in criminal law. Due to the nature of the disorder, many people with autism are unaware that their behavior is inappropriate or may not be able to control their behavior, especially behaviors that are driven by repetitive or restrictive interests.

FEATURES OF AUTISM AND VICTIMS OF CRIMES

This section reviews the characteristics specific to the population of individuals diagnosed with autism that can affect their capacity to make valid decisions, and thus their level of accountability for offenses.

Children with autism are at increased risk of physical and sexual abuse, due in part to their tendency to be socially isolated and have poor communication skills (Howlin & Clements, 1995). Individuals with autism who are at particular risk of sexual abuse include those with long-term dependency on caregivers, a tendency toward unquestioning compliance, and poor communication skills, along with a lack of knowledge about sex, sexuality, and sexual abuse (Ammerman, Hersen, & Lubetsky, 1988; Howlin & Clements, 1995). Although individuals with autism may be incapable of accurately reporting abuse due to their cognitive and communication deficits, parents and clinicians need to be aware of behavioral warning signs that may be indicative of physical and sexual abuse. Howlin and Clements (1995) assert that children with autism display significant changes in their behavior as a result of abuse. These children tend to have significant increases in aggressive and self-injurious behaviors, as well as increases in mood swings, hyperactivity, and sleep disturbances. Engaging in sexual acting-out behaviors can also be indicative of physical and sexual abuse in children with autism (Mandell, Walrath, Manteuffel, Sgro, & Pinto-Martin, 2005). Additionally, children may have a sudden onset of aversion or fearful responses to people or places with which they were previously comfortable. Other studies of adults with developmental disabilities have found that behaviors associated with sexual abuse are similar to those of typically developing individuals, including suicidal, delinquent, and sexualized behaviors (Sequeira & Hollins, 2003; Sequeira, Howlin, & Hollins, 2003). It is essential that parents, clinicians, and police do not attribute these behavioral changes to the fact that the child has autism, but rather investigate them as indications of possible abuse.

FEATURES OF AUTISM AND CRIMINAL OFFENDERS

There are several areas in which a person with autism is more likely to get into trouble with the law as an offender. The first area is violating social norms through such actions as trespassing and stealing. The second area is aggressive behavior, often as a result of disruption of routine. The third area includes instances of inappropriate social boundaries due to social naiveté, such as approaching or touching strangers, stalking, sexual harassment, or other sexual offenses. The final area is property damage, such as starting fires or throwing objects. The concept of whether persons with autism are victims or perpetrators of crimes may be a complicated decision tempered by the specific circumstances of the act that brought the individual into the criminal justice system.

This section provides examples from documented cases to illustrate and support various points. The majority of the cases cited involve adults with autism and higher cognitive abilities who were living with parents or in an assisted living facility when the offenses occurred. There are few adolescent cases cited in the literature because juvenile records are sealed and the public does not have access to them under the Freedom of Information Act unless the child is charged as an adult.

When individuals with autism are detained by police or otherwise confronted by the criminal justice system, it is often because they have violated a social norm through such activities as trespassing or stealing. For example, David, an adolescent, had interests similar to those of children much younger than him. His favorite play activities were similar to those of the young girls on his block. He liked to jump rope, ride bicycles, and run with them when they were playing tag. One day, David could not find his friends so he began looking in the windows of his neighbors' homes trying to find them. A neighbor saw David peeking into the bedroom window of one of his little girlfriends and called the police. David was arrested as a Peeping Tom and potential sexual predator (Holmes, 1998).

Obsessions and compulsions combined with impulsivity can lead to behaviors in stores that may look like vandalism or shoplifting (Davis & Schunick, 2002). Arranging objects in a particular order or pattern is often a tendency in individuals with autism. For example, when in a store, a child with autism might be compelled to rearrange store merchandise according to color, size, or in any number of other ways. Persons with autism who exhibit this behavior may be trying to bring order to an environment that they may perceive as chaotic. The store clerk may have no understanding of the person's intent and thus interpret this behavior as vandalism and try to stop it. The disruption of this behavior might cause great distress for the child with autism, possibly leading the child to hit the clerk or to have a tantrum, causing the clerk to call the police.

Aggressive behavior by an older child or adolescent, such as hitting or biting children or teachers, has led to police involvement (Davis & Schunick, 2002). For individuals with autism, aggression may result when their routine is disrupted or if they are overstimulated. Many times, the intent behind the behavior is not to cause bodily harm to another person, but rather to escape an unfavorable situation. Aggressive or violent behavior can also be a form of retaliation for intense teasing and bullying by peers at school or in the community. For example, in a case in South Carolina, a 35-year-old male with Asperger disorder was charged with and found guilty of murder because he killed his neighbor. The neighbor had come over to his house and demanded repayment of a loan. The neighbor and the adult with Asperger disorder got into an argument and began a fistfight. During this fight, the adult with Asperger disorder went to his bedroom, got his gun, and shot his attacker several times with a .38 caliber revolver. Next, he got another gun and fired a single shot into the neighbor's head. When asked why he shot the victim so many times, the adult with Asperger disorder stated he wanted to be sure the victim did not get up and kill him like he had seen the "bad guys" do in the movies (Schwartz-Watts, 2005).

Violent behavior may also result from an individual with autism being overwhelmed by particular sensory issues or because his or her anxiety increased to feelings of panic. Schwartz-Watts (2005) reported another case in which the oversensitivity to touch of a 22-year-old individual with Asperger disorder led to the death of an 8-year-old boy. While sitting outside, a young boy on a bike struck up a brief conversation with the defendant. As the boy turned to leave, he ran over the defendant's foot. The defendant pulled out a concealed gun and shot the boy. He was charged with capital murder and sentenced to life in prison.

In each of the previous cases, the defendants' reactions were far greater than the original assault warranted. These reactions demonstrate the tendency of this population to form literal interpretations of social situations and to sometimes act accordingly. Individuals with autism tend to miss information that is inferred or implied. This tendency is demonstrated by the case of a woman with Asperger disorder who was arrested for shoplifting because she took a purse that she knew her mother wanted. She intended to pay for the purse next year because she had seen a sign on the shop window that said, "Take home what you want today with no payments until January of next year!" (Doyle & Iland, 2004). She interpreted the words on the sign literally and completely missed its inference of credit.

Individuals with autism are often naive. Their social naiveté can be exacerbated by a limited comprehension of sophisticated emotions such as love, which can lead to mistaking social attraction or friendship for romantic love (Berney, 2004). Therefore, persons with autism can find themselves charged with such crimes as stalking, sexual harassment, or other sexual offenses. A young man with an autism spectrum disorder liked a young woman in his small town. He often waited for her in places where she was likely to be and talked about his favorite topics. She tried to "brush him off." He thought that maybe someday she would be his girlfriend. The young woman felt stalked and harassed and filed a restraining order. This upset the young man, and he decided to write a note of apology and put it on her desk at the office where she worked while she was out to lunch. This violated the restraining order and he was arrested (Doyle & Iland, 2004). This young man mistook the young woman's kindness as a sign of romantic interest.

Social naiveté can also lead individuals with autism to misinterpret other relationships and leave them open to exploitation (Berney, 2004; Debbaudt, 2002). Two examples illustrate this well. A 27-year-old male with autism spectrum disorder often took women from his neighborhood shopping for lingerie, thinking this could be a prelude to sexual contact. However, the women would leave after he made the purchase. He also allowed these women to use his telephone to set up drug deals, believing that this would result in sexual favors, although they never actually discussed such an arrangement (Murrie, Warren, Kristiansson, & Dietz, 2002). Police have reported that persons with autism can become unwitting accomplices in other peoples' criminal schemes. One such case involved counterfeiting United States money. An individual with excellent computer skills and access to sophisticated printing equipment was encouraged by his "friends" to make counterfeit money (Debbaudt, 2002). In these two examples, the individuals' social naiveté led them to seek out social relationships in very ill-advised ways.

The final area where individuals with autism can encounter law enforcement is property damage. Property damage offenses such as arson may result from overriding obsessions and preoccupations or ruminative thinking. There are two cases that exemplify this point. Barry-Walsh and Mullen (2004) report a case in which a young man with Asperger disorder was charged with arson. KA, a 24-year-old, had overriding preoccupations with listening to a particular radio station. A local religious radio station set up a new broadcast on a frequency close to his favored station. This interfered with his listening between the hours of 7:00 and 10:00 P.M. He wrote a number of letters to the radio station asking them to stop interfering with his favored broadcasts. Following a further unsuccessful communication, he walked to the radio station and burned it down. Second, there is the case of a 31-year-old male with Asperger disorder who was charged with 11 counts of arson. For 2 months, he broke into summer homes in his neighborhood and set them on fire. During his evaluation, he disclosed that over the year he had become increasingly preoccupied with those who had wronged him in the past and increasingly convinced that he needed to avenge himself.

When apprehended by police, he immediately confessed to the crimes and explained that they were a means of revenge against people who had harassed him during his youth. There was no relationship between the summer homes and his schoolmates. However, this individual described details of the houses that had reminded him of the houses of the peers who had bullied him. He reported feeling satisfied after the fires (Murrie et al., 2002).

These cases illustrate that persons with autism have difficulty predicting how their behavior will influence the outcome of a situation. This results in their embarking on actions without understanding the consequences; setting fires may result in a building's destruction or an assault may end in death. Clearly, these men had no appreciation for the serious nature of their actions or the fact that someone could have been seriously injured or killed.

KEEPING THE PERSON WITH AUTISM OUT OF THE CRIMINAL JUSTICE SYSTEM

The diagnostic features of autism, including the lack of social understanding, poor social-communication skills, and restricted, repetitive, stereotyped behaviors and interests, can also present problems when persons with autism have to interact with professionals (e.g., evaluators and investigators) within the criminal justice system. This section provides (1) suggestions for enhancing the social interaction abilities of the individual with autism to avoid criminal involvement, (2) strategies for addressing issues that may arise during the course of involvement with the legal system, and (3) suggestions for training professionals in the criminal justice system about the unique needs and problems of individuals diagnosed with autism.

Enhancing Social Interaction Abilities

Parents may ask professionals: "How can we prevent our child from being charged with a criminal offense?" One way is to help the child develop as many prosocial skills as possible. Parents should be reminded that any unusual behavior that may be perceived as endearing in a young child with autism may be interpreted as odd or threatening when their child becomes older and larger in stature. It is therefore important that parents teach children with autism clear rules about appropriate social behavior from a young age, particularly regarding obsessional interests.

Howlin (1997) suggests that with an autistic child, it is generally better to establish strict rules during childhood that can be relaxed in adulthood rather than to implement stricter rules in adulthood, which may then be resented.

Given the tendency for individuals with autism to adhere rigidly to rules, their responses can appear inappropriate in social situations. For example, it is appropriate to hug and kiss a family member in greeting, but this is generally an inappropriate greeting for a complete stranger. To keep this from happening, parents should teach appropriate social behavior and understanding of social rules in a concrete, demonstrative manner using such methods as social stories (Gray, 1993, 2002), and role play. Social stories present information about social situations. They have been very useful in teaching children with autism prosocial behaviors. Social stories help children with autism understand why certain behaviors are appropriate. Providing a justification for the appropriate behavior can increase the likelihood that the individual will engage in the behavior. Social stories also help children with autism understand social cues and others' expectations during social situations.

Legal System Involvement: Issues and Strategies

Interviewing the Accused

Due to deficits in communication and social functioning, individuals with autism who are accused as perpetrators of an offense may exhibit behaviors that are misinterpreted as being hostile and uncooperative. Evaluators or police investigators unfamiliar with the diagnostic features of this population may interpret behavior by persons with autism in the following ways:

1. The inability to quickly process and respond to requests, commands, and questions as a result of cognitive and communication deficits may be misinterpreted as stalling or being uncooperative. For individuals with autism, as stress increases their ability to communicate often decreases (Debbaudt, 2002).
2. Inattention, staring off into space, or constant fidgeting with objects may be seen as avoidance behavior or nervousness due to guilt.
3. Difficulty with abstract thinking and perspective taking may hinder the ability to make inferences about other people's thoughts and feelings.

4. Poorly modulated eye contact, such as avoiding eye gaze or staring, may be mistaken for a sign of a guilty conscience or perceived as hostile or insincere.
5. Odd or bizarre body movements (rocking, hand flapping, or mimicking the body language and mannerisms of the investigator), strange verbal behaviors (shrieking, repeating sounds), or the presence of echolalia may be perceived as attempts to feign mental illness.

Another potential problem when evaluating this population is that in formal interviews individuals with autism may misjudge the friendliness or politeness of the evaluator or investigator as a sign of friendship and confess to an offense they did not commit to make their new "friend" happy (Debbaudt, 2002).

It is important for parents to work with professionals within the criminal justice system to make them aware of the particular impairments that characterize individuals with autism. This will help these professionals to at least consider consultation with experts in the field of autism in order to identify more effective criminal evaluation methods with this population.

The Individual with Autism and Sentencing

If an individual with autism is found guilty of an offense, there are some behavioral issues that must be addressed with the judge and/or jury during the sentencing phase. One common behavioral feature of individuals with autism who commit crimes is a deficit in empathy (Murrie et al., 2002; Wing, 1981). During a trial, this behavior can be viewed as coldhearted or unfeeling, thus increasing the likelihood that the decision makers in the case will not be lenient with the defendant. There was a case in Florida involving a group of teenagers who had committed arson. One of the boys had Asperger disorder. During the hearing, the typically developing adolescents showed and expressed remorse, but the adolescent with Asperger disorder did not. He was sentenced to a correctional facility, while his "friends" got probation (Debbaudt, 2002). The shoplifting case mentioned earlier provides another good example. The young woman's behavior in court, including lack of eye contact with the judge and lawyers, a fixed grin on her face, and the repetitive behavior of continuously lining up pencils, was interpreted as rude and increased her sentence. The judge gave her the maximum penalty possible, stating that her grin was an insult to the court, along with the fact that she did not appear to pay attention to the proceedings or show remorse (Doyle

& Iland, 2004). It is the responsibility of the professional (the forensic evaluator or autism expert) during the sentencing phase to make sure the judge understands that the deficit in empathy is a feature of autism because it may be used as a mitigating factor that explains the perpetrator's lack of insight to police, prosecutors, or jurors and may lead them to be more compassionate toward the person with autism.

Postadjudication

For individuals with autism who have been convicted of an offense, the question of disposition arises. Depending on the nature of the offense, the outcome could be probation or incarceration. There are issues that need to be addressed in both situations that will increase the likelihood of successfully completing the sentence.

The Arc of New Jersey provides wrap-around services for individuals with developmental disabilities who get into trouble with the law. The most groundbreaking service the Arc provides is the Personalized Justice Plan (PJP). The PJP is presented to the court system as an alternative to incarceration. It emphasizes the use of least restrictive, community-based alternatives to incarceration as early as possible in the criminal justice process, while holding individuals accountable for their behavior. When presented as a special condition of probation or parole, the PJP can help stabilize the individual in the community due to how supports are identified, coordinated, and monitored. Once clients are placed on probation or parole, the program monitors the PJP until the clients complete their sentences. Monitoring can be weekly, biweekly, monthly, or annually, depending on the needs of the individual. The goal of PJP in every case is to help clients successfully complete their probation or parole. This program has been very successful, and 93.5% of the individuals who complete the program have not reoffended (D. Goobic, personal communication, April 26, 2006).

Nightingale (2003) asserts that individuals with autism can be successful in diversion or probation programs that incorporate language that is simplistic so that the individuals will understand what is being asked of them. Novel situations can be especially upsetting for individuals with autism; even those individuals with adequate receptive language may have difficulty understanding what is expected of them until they are acclimated to their new environment. Prior to the initial meeting of the staff in the diversion or probation program, it may be beneficial to create a picture story using photographs of the persons with whom the individual with autism will work and the venues where they will meet in order to ease any anxiety about novel situations or people. Visual cues are commonly used to help individuals with autism anticipate events (Schopler, Lansing, & Waters, 1983). These visual cues can also be used to teach the program rules. In programs that have a token economy it is important to discover what is valuable to the individual with autism. Taking the special needs of the autism population into account can increase the likelihood that the person with autism will invest in the diversion program and be successful.

Incarceration is very difficult for persons with autism because there is a risk of these individuals becoming victims of violence and bullying. Other inmates may read their direct manner and odd behaviors and characteristics as an invitation to exploit and control the individual with autism. Untrained correctional workers, those in law enforcement, and those who work in the medical field (i.e., physicians and nurses) may view an individual with autism as someone who is rude and difficult (Debbaudt, 2004; D. Swartz-Watts, personal communication, November 16, 2005). This perception makes it less likely that they will be supportive of or even come to the defense of the individual with autism if necessary. Autism-specific social deficits may make it more difficult for these individuals to get along with prison staff, and, as a result, the individual with autism may frequently spend time in seclusion, making good behavior privileges, like work opportunities, difficult to earn. As "good behavior privileges" are one criterion for parole, this situation may make sentences longer (Debbaudt, 2004). Thus, training correctional facility staff about the issues pertaining to individuals with autism is crucial.

Training Criminal Justice Professionals

One of the most important issues surrounding autism and the criminal justice system is the training of first responders (police, fire, paramedics) regarding autism. Because of the lack of basic knowledge about developmental disabilities in the criminal justice system, many autism advocacy groups and autism societies provide generic and specialized training sessions for any number of target audiences including defense and prosecuting attorneys, court officials, judges, police officers, parole officers, and community service agencies. Training curricula are designed to meet the diverse needs and interests of the target audience. For example, the South Carolina Autism Society uses the Autism and Informed Response (AIR) program. The AIR program is an awareness training program for police, firefighters, and EMS personnel that was developed by the South Carolina Autism Society and is used across the United States (www. scautism.org). The training consists of videotapes and handouts that describe situations and behaviors that may bring individuals with autism to the attention of first responders. The trainers in the AIR program are parents of children with autism who are also first responders. Parent trainers have found that emergency personnel tend to listen when they describe actual incidents or potential emergencies involving their child. Parent trainers have great credibility and add an important "personal touch" to information about autism (C. Niederhauser, personal communication, June 19, 2006). The New Jersey Chapter of the Arc *(www. arcnj.org)* is another organization that provides services to the criminal justice system, through the Developmental Disability (DD) Offenders Program. The DD Offenders Program helps the criminal justice system overcome the lack of understanding of developmental disabilities by providing technical assistance to attorneys who represent these individuals, case management assistance, and education and training to the community.

Debbaudt and Brown (2006) suggest implementing an Autism Response Team (ART) that would consist of first responders (FR) and criminal justice agencies (CJA). The goal of the ART would be "to ensure positive, informed responses, and just resolutions . . . when an individual on the spectrum comes into contact with first responders in an emergency or CJA situation" (p. 7). The duties and responsibilities of the ART may include the following:

1. Develop state-certified law enforcement and first responder training courses.
2. Assist and consult with FR and CJA personnel from first contact to the closing of a case.
3. Develop and disseminate information to the autism community that can be used to avoid or prepare families for an emergency or criminal justice contact.
4. Promote partnerships between the autism community, law enforcement, and the community at large.
5. Assist in creating a 911 database that would alert the FR that an individual with special needs is on the scene.

The ART could be a valuable resource for the criminal justice system and the autism community.

CONCLUSIONS

Individuals with autism are at risk for having more contacts with law enforcement than members of the general population as either a victim or a perpetrator of crime. This population is susceptible to economic crimes, child abuse and neglect, and sexual assault, with a high probability of repeat victimization. Additionally, a subgroup of individuals with autism may be more likely to encounter problems with the law as perpetrators. Not only is it critical to educate individuals with autism about issues of safety and appropriate social behaviors throughout their lives, but it is equally important to educate professionals in the criminal justice system about the unique behavioral, social, and communication features of the autism diagnosis to improve the likelihood that these individuals will be better understood by and treated more appropriately in the criminal justice system.

REFERENCES

American Law Institute. (1980–1985). *Model penal code and commentaries.* Philadelphia: Author.

American Psychiatric Association. (1994). *Diagnostic and statistical manual of mental disorders* (4th ed.). Washington, DC: Author.

Ammerman, R., Hersen, M., & Lubetsky, M. (1988). Assessment and treatment of abuse and neglect in multi-handicapped children and adolescents. *International Journal of Rehabilitation Research, 11*(3), 313–314.

Autistic boy killed in a hit-in-run collision. (2006, July 24). Available online at: *http://www.autismconnect.org/news.asp?section=00010001&itemtype=news&id =5830*

Barry-Walsh, J. B., & Mullen, P. E. (2004). Forensic aspects of Asperger's syndrome. *Journal of Forensic Psychiatry and Psychology, 15*(1), 96–107.

Berney, T. (2004). Asperger syndrome from childhood into adulthood. *Advances in Psychiatric Treatment, 10,* 341–351.

Curry, K., Posluszny, M., & Kraska, S. (1993). *Training criminal justice personnel to recognize offenders with disabilities.* Washington, DC: Office of Special Education and Rehabilitative Services News.

Davis, B., & Schunick, W. G. (2002). *Dangerous encounters: Avoiding perilous situations with autism.* London: Jessica Kingsley.

Debbaudt, D. (2002). *Autism, advocates and law enforcement professionals.* London: Jessica Kingsley.

Debbaudt, D. (2004). Beyond guilt or innocence. *Leadership Perspectives in Developmental Disability, 4*(1).

Debbaudt, D., & Brown, M. (2006, Spring). The Autism Response Team: A concept whose time has come. *Autism Spectrum Quarterly,* 7–10.

Doyle, B. T., & Iland, E. D. (2004). And justice for all—Unless you have autism: What the legal system needs to know about people with autism spectrum disorders. Retrieved July 3, 2006, from *asdatoz.com.*

Estrich, S. (1998). *Getting away with murder: How politics is destroying the criminal justice system.* Cambridge, MA: Harvard University Press.

Everington, C. T., & Luckasson, R. (1992). *The competence assessment for standing trial for defendants with mental retardation (CAST-MR) manual.* Worthington, OH: IDS Publishing.

Feguer v. United States, 302 F.2d 214 (8th Cir. 1962).

Frye v. Settle, 168 F. Supp. 7 (W.D. Mo. 1958).

Gillberg, C. (1998). Asperger syndrome and high-functioning autism. *British Journal of Psychiatry, 172,* 200–209.

Githens, P. B. (1998). Law enforcement and autism: A chapter perspective. *The Advocate, 31*(3), 3–10.

Gray, C. (1993). Social Stories: Improving responses of students with autism with accurate social information. *Focus on Autistic Behavior, 8,* 1–10.

Gray, C. (2002). *My Social Stories book.* London: Jessica Kingsley.

Happe, F., & Frith, U. (1996). The neuropsychology of autism. *Brain, 119*(4), 1377–1400.

Holmes, D. L. (1998). *Autism through the lifespan: The Eden model.* Bethesda, MD: Woodbine House.

Howlin, P. (1997). *Autism: Preparing for adulthood.* New York: Routledge.

Howlin, P., & Clements, J. (1995). Is it possible to assess the impact of abuse on children with pervasive developmental disorders? *Journal of Autism and Developmental Disorders, 25*(4), 337–354.

Lord, C., & McGee, J. P. (Eds.). (2001). *Educating children with autism.* Washington, DC: National Academy Press.

Mandell, D. S., Walrath, C. M., Manteuffel, B., Sgro, G., & Pinto-Martin, J. A. (2005). The prevalence and correlates of abuse among children with autism served in comprehensive community-based mental health setting. *Child Abuse and Neglect, 29,* 1359–1372.

Melton, G. B., Petrila, J., Poythress, N. G., & Slobogin, C. (1997). *Psychological evaluations for the courts: A handbook for mental health professionals and lawyers* (2nd ed.). New York: Guilford Press.

Murrie, D., Warren, J., Kristiansson, M., & Dietz, P. E. (2002). Asperger's syndrome in forensic settings. *International Journal of Forensic Mental Health, 1,* 59–70.

Schopler, E., Lansing, M., & Waters, L. (1983). *Teaching activities for autistic children: Individualized assessment and treatment for autistic and developmentally disabled children.* Austin, TX: PRO-ED.

Schwartz-Watts, D. M. (2005). Asperger's disorder and murder. *Journal of the American Academy of Psychiatry and the Law, 33,* 390–393.

Sequeira, H., & Hollins, S. (2003). Clinical effects of sexual abuse on people with learning disability: Critical literature review. *British Journal of Psychiatry, 182,* 13–19.

Sequeira, H., Howlin, P., & Hollins, S. (2003). Psychological disturbance associated with sexual abuse in people with learning disabilities—case-control study. *British Journal of Psychiatry, 183,* 451–456.

Siponmaa, L., Kristiansson, M., Jonson, C., Nyden, A., & Gillberg, C. (2001). Juvenile and young adult mentally disordered offenders: The role of child neuropsychiatric disorders. *Journal of the American Academy of Psychiatry and the Law, 29,* 420–426.

Sobsey, D., & Doe, T. (1991). Patterns of sexual abuse and assault. *Sexuality and Disability, 9,* 243–259.

Stafford, K. P. (2003). Assessment of competence to stand trial. In A. M. Goldstein (Vol. Ed.) & I. B. Weiner (Series Ed.), *Handbook of psychology: Vol. 11. Forensic psychology* (pp. 359–380). Hoboken, NJ: Wiley.

Swisher v. United States, 237 F. Supp. 921 (W.D. Mo. 1965).

Warboys, L., Burrell, S., Peters, C., & Ramiu, M. (1994). *California juvenile justice special education manual*. San Francisco: Youth Law Center.

Wieter v. Settle, 193 F. Supp. 318 (W.D. Mo. 1961).

Wing, L. (1981). Asperger's syndrome: A clinical account. *Psychological Medicine, 11*, 115–129.

Index

"f" following a page number indicates a figure; "t" following a page number indicates a table.